# Guidebook on Preclinical Conservative Dentistry Q & A



*Edited by*

**K.S. Karthikeyan**

CBS

**CBS Publishers & Distributors Pvt. Ltd.**

NEW DELHI • BANGALORE • PUNE • COCHIN • CHENNAI (INDIA)

ISBN : 81-239-0707-9

First Edition : 1999
Reprint : 2000, 2001, 2002, 2005,
2006, 2009, 2010, 2011



Published by Satish Kumar Jain and produced by V.K. Jain for
CBS Publishers & Distributors Pvt. Ltd.,
CBS Plaza, 4819/XI Prahlad Street, 24 Ansari Road, Daryaganj,
New Delhi - 110002, India. • Website: www.cbspd.com
e-mail: delhi@cbspd.com, cbspubs@vsnl.com, cbspubs@airtelmail.in
Ph.: 23289259, 23266861, 23266867 • Fax: 011-23243014

*Branches:*

- ***Bengaluru:*** Seema House, 2975, 17th Cross, K.R. Road, Bansankari 2nd Stage, Bangalore - 560070 Ph.: 26771678/79 Fax: 080-26771680 • e-mail: bangalore@cbspd.com
- ***Pune:*** Bhuruk Prestige, Sr. No. 52/12/2+1+3/2, Narhe, Haveli (Near Katraj-Dehu Road by Pass), Pune-411051 Ph.: +91-20-32404169 • Fax: 020-24464059 e-mail: pune@cbspd.com
- ***Kochi:*** 36/14, Kalluvilakam, Lissie Hospital Road, Cochin - 682018, Kerala • e-mail: cochin@cbspd.com Ph.: 0484-4059061-65 • Fax: 0484-4059065
- ***Chennai:*** 20, West Park Road, Shenoy Nagar, Chennai - 600030 e-mail: chennai@cbspd.com Ph.: 044-26260666-26202620 Fax: 044-45530020

*Printed at* :
J.S. Offset Printers, Delhi

**DEDICATED TO**

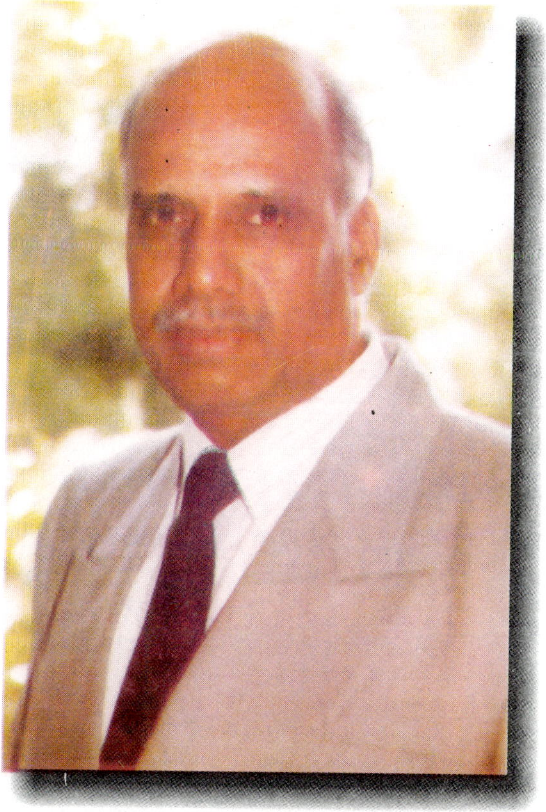

**Dr. A. PARAMESWARAN** B.Sc., MDS
***My mentor, a noble person***

# FOREWORD

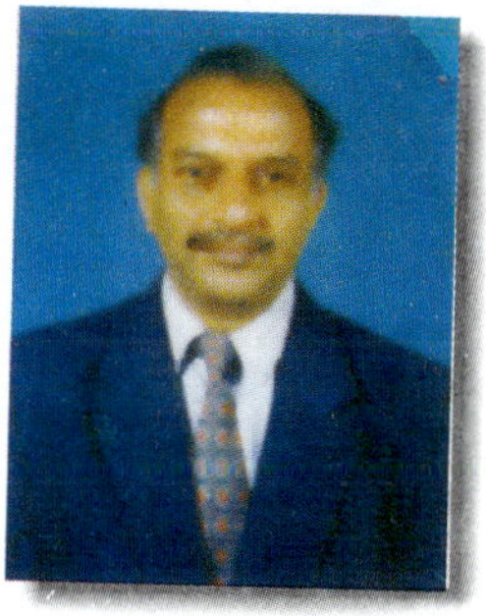

*Principal*
*Meenakshi Ammal Dental College*

*Dr. K.S. Karthikeyan qualified as dental surgeon in 1971 and completed his post graduation in Conservative Dentistry and Endodontics in 1985.*

*He was awarded gold medal in Anatomy, Medicine, Prosthodontic and the best outgoing student medal for the year 1970.*

*Earlier he served in Tamilnadu Government Medical Services under various capacities in rural areas until he completed his post graduation. He joined as a teacher in Madras Dental College and took keen interest in disseminating the knowledge of the science of dentistry to the students.*

*He has co-edited two books namely "Recent Advances in Operative Dentistry" & "Multiple ways for Dental Hygiene" in regional language. He strives hard to communicate with the public through his periodic publications. He takes lot of interest in research and has also presented many scientific papers in various conferences, nation wide.*

*A dedicated teacher and a dynamic clinician he shares his knowledge with the budding dentists by simple easy to follow presentation.*

*He has published "Guide Book on Preclinical Conservative Dentistry" for students in a Question and Answer format which is dedicated to his own teacher.*

*I am sure this book will be useful to the students during preparation of Viva-voce -*

CHENNAI
JANUARY 1999

**Dr. E. MUNIRATHNAM NAIDU**

# PREFACE

*My dear friend,*

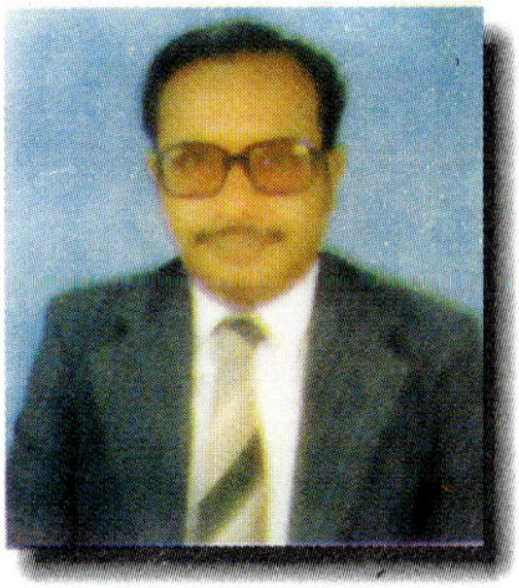

*You have bought this book as a second year student, with a hope that this will be of some help to you in passing the preclinical O.D.S. exams. Frankly, I would have felt the same, had I bought the book when I was a student. Though our teachers insist that accumulation of knowledge, is more important than acquiring a degree, our aim is inclined towards the latter.*

*I don't pretend that anything contained in this book is original and mine. It is knowledge distilled from great books and wonderful teachers I have come across. If this book is of some use to you, a preclinical student, my purpose is served. If you feel like thanking someone after reading this book, please thank*

*1)* **Mr. RADHAKRISHNAN**, *the managing trustee of Meenakshiammal Dental College and numerous other educational institutions for his financial support,*

*2)* **Dr. E. MUNIRATHNAM NAIDU**, *Principal, Meenakshiammal Dental College, who strives for excellence in education and gave unconditional freedom in bringing this book,*

*3)* **Dr. A. PARAMESWARAN**, *my inspiration.*

*4) My loving family of* **my wife and two wonderful daughters**, *whose affection supported me*

*5)* ***Dr. V. Mahesh Kumar*** *and* ***Dr. Joseph Maxim****, for the excellent get up, format and finish of this book.*

*6) The team of dental surgeons of Meenakshiammal Dental College especially* ***Dr. Suseela, Dr. Vasanthi Santhanam, Dr. J. Selvakumar, Dr. Chitra Sarvotham, Dr. Priya Dr. Mamta Harilal Nichani, and Dr. Bhuvan Shome*** *who gave invaluable suggestions and assistance during the formative stages of the book.*

*I thank them sincerely and I hope you will join with me.*

*With best wishes*

Affectionately yours,

CHENNAI
JANUARY 1999

Sd/-
**Dr. K.S. KARTHIKEYAN MDS.**

# CONTENTS

# CHAPTER : I

# INTRODUCTION

**1. WHAT IS OPERATIVE DENTISTRY?**

**A :** Operative Dentistry is a branch of Dentistry that deals with diagnosis, treatment and prevention of diseases of the calcified parts of teeth, pulp and periapical region. As the treatment mainly consists of replacing the lost portion of tooth to normal function and appearance, it is also known as **restorative dentistry.** As the emphasis given in this speciality is conservation and preservation of healthy natural tooth substance, it is also called **conservative dentistry.**

**2. WHAT ARE THE RESTORATIONS COMMONLY DONE IN OPERATIVE DENTISTRY?**

**A :** Fillings, Crowns, inlays , veneers, core buildups and onlays are some of the common restorations done in operative dentistry.

**3. WHAT ARE FILLINGS?**

**A :** Filling is a term commonly used to denote a restoration prepared intraorally to fill up a cavity in the tooth.

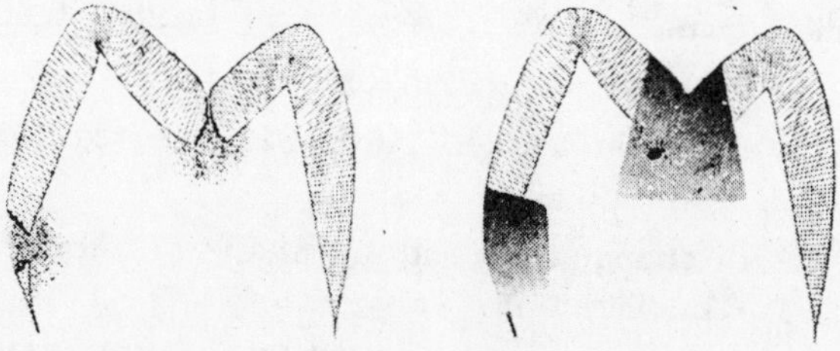

*Fig. 1.1. Filling (carious tooth & Filled tooth)*

**4. WHAT MATERIALS ARE COMMONLY USED AS FILLINGS?**

**A :** Silver amalgam, Glass ionomer, composite resin filling materials, reinforced Zinc Oxide are commonly used filling materials. Gold foil and silicate cement are rarely used direct filling materials.

5. **WHAT ARE CROWNS?**

**A :** Crowns are restorations prepared to cover all or most of surfaces of the tooth. It may be a full crown (when all the surfaces of the tooth are covered) or Three fourth or Four fifth crown (when all surfaces except labial or buccal surface are covered)

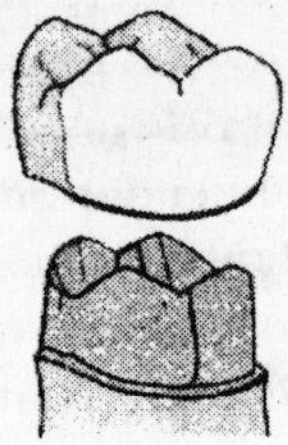

*Fig. 1.2. Full Crown*

6. **WHEN ARE CROWNS PREPARED?**

**A :** i. In diseased or damaged teeth, when the destruction is shallow but wide, involving many surfaces (eg., hypoplasia) a crown is prepared.

ii. In grossly damaged teeth, a crown is prepared as a reinforcing (strengthening) restoration to hold the remaining weakened parts of the tooth. (eg., fractured or deep carious tooth).

iii. Crowns are also prepared in healthy teeth

a. to mask defective formation (eg., peg laterals)

b. to retain a fixed partial denture (eg., Major retainer of a bridge)

c. to change the contour - shape of a tooth (for occlusal rehabilitation)

7. **WHAT MATERIALS ARE USED FOR PREPARING CROWNS?**

**A :** Cast gold, containing varying percentages of gold, Non-gold noble alloy (silver palladium or palladium Silver alloys) Nickel-Chromium, Chrome cobalt alloys (Base metal alloys) are examples of custom made metallic crowns. Feldspathic porcelain crowns, Reinforced (aluminous) Porcelain crowns, porcelain fused to Metal crowns, cerestore crowns (cast porcelain crown by injection moulding) Dicor crowns (Castable ceramic crowns) are examples of custom made non-metallic (tooth coloured) crowns. Acrylic resin crowns are custom made non metallic temporary crowns. Poly carbonate crowns are commercially available (ready made) temporary anterior tooth coloured crowns. Stainless steel and Aluminium crowns are commercially available (ready made) metallic temporary crowns for posterior teeth.

**8. WHICH ARE BETTER, CUSTOM MADE OR COMMERCIALLY AVAILABLE CROWNS?**

**A :** Custom made crowns are superior because they are made for individual prepared teeth. Their marginal fit, adaptation and contour (shape) are always superior. Ready made commercially available crowns do not have accurate fit and adaptation. Though they are available in different sizes, careful selection and suitable adjustments are mandatory to have a reasonable fit and they are best used as temporary crowns. The only superiority of commercially available crowns over custom made crowns is the absence of crown fabrication time.

**9. WHAT ARE INLAYS AND ONLAYS?**

**A :** Inlay is an intracoronal restoration fabricated extra orally and cemented (luted) into the prepared tooth. An inlay may cover one or more cusps (to protect a weakened cusp) but not all the cusps of the occlusal surface. An onlay is an intracoronal restoration covering all the cusps, fabricated extra orally and cemented into place.

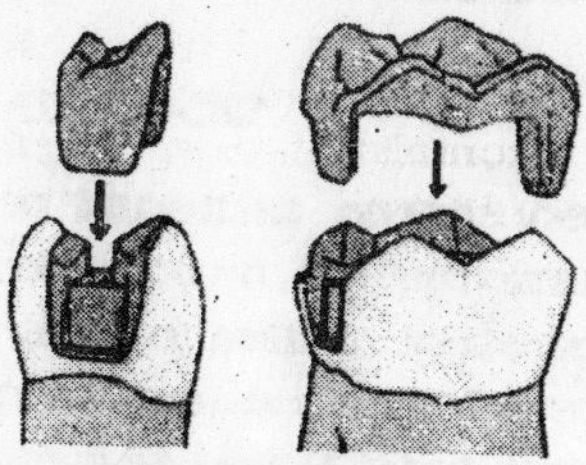

*Fig. 1.3. Inlay & Onlay*

**10. FROM WHAT MATERIALS ARE INLAYS AND ONLAYS MADE?**

**A :** Conventional gold alloys, low gold alloys, non-gold alloys, base metal alloys are alloys used to fabricate inlays and onlays. Porcelain fused to metal, reinforced porcelain, castable glasses, cerestore porcelain, laboratory processed composites. These are examples of tooth coloured inlays. Machined porcelain (CAD CAM PORCELAIN) is the latest chair side fabrication technique in inlay fabrication, wherein the inlay is machined from a preformed porcelain block of superior quality. Acrylic resins are used for making temporary inlays.

**11. WHAT ARE VENEERS?**

**A :** Veneers are thin restorations made on the labial surface of a hypoplastic or discoloured tooth to mask a defect and have better aesthetic result. Veneers can also be part of a crown. Veneers may cover one or more metallic surfaces of the crown.

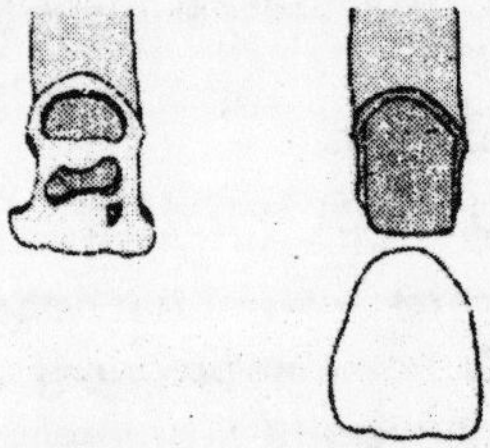

*Fig. 1.4. Veneers*

**12. HOW ARE VENEERS MADE?**

Though veneers could be made directly over a tooth, for better aesthetic results, veneers are made indirectly in the laboratory over dies or models and later luted into position.

**13. WHAT MATERIALS ARE USED FOR PREPARING A VENEER?**

**A :** Porcelain veneers and laboratory processed composite veneers are superior. An acrylic resin veneer could be used as a temporary veneer.

## 14. WHAT ARE CORE BUILD UPS?

**A :** Whenever crowns are made, good foundation is necessary. In teeth with wide and shallow destruction, natural tooth substance will be the foundation (core) around which a crown can be built up. In grossly mutilated carious or fractured teeth, enough natural tooth material might not be available to serve as a core. To provide adequate grip (retention) and strength (resistance) for the crown, the lost tooth substance is built up over the damaged tooth and then the crown is prepared over the built up core.

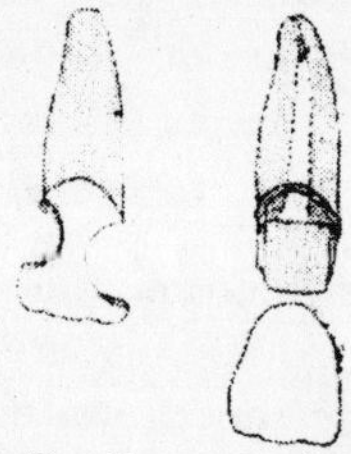

*Fig. 1.5. Core build up*

## 15. WHAT MATERIALS ARE USED FOR CORE BUILD UP?

**A :** Silver amalgam, composite resin, glass ionomer, compomer, metal modified glass ionomer are some materials used for direct core build ups. Pins in vital teeth and posts in non-vital teeth are sometimes used for better tie up of the core with the remaining tooth substance. In some non-vital teeth, a cast post and core are made as a single casting over which a crown could be made.

## 16. HOW ARE RESTORATIVE MATERIALS CLASSIFIED?

**A :** i) **Depending upon durability:**

(a) Temporary (b) permanent

ii) **Depending upon area of usage:**

(a) Anterior (b) Posterior

iii) **Depending upon its chemical nature:**

| (a) Metallic | (b) Non-Metallic |
|---|---|
| 1. SILVER AMALGAM | (1) CERAMIC : Porcelain & its improved versions |
| 2. DIRECT FILLING GOLD | (2) DENTAL CEMENTS : Silicate, Glass Ionomer, Zinc Oxide Eugenol |
| 3. CAST GOLD ALLOYS | (3) COMPOSITE RESINS |
| 4. BASE METAL ALLOYS | |

iv) **Depending upon the fabrication technique :**

(a) Intra orally made incrementally added non-adhesive restoration : These materials are placed directly in the tooth in a plastic (softened) state and allowed to harden. Placement of these restorations need only a single appointment with the dentist. Examples are (1) Silver Amalgam (2) Direct Filling Gold (3) Silicate Cement (4) Zinc Oxide Eugenol Cement.

(b) Extra orally made cemented restorations :

Due to technical difficulties during fabrication (like necessity of high temperature, pressure etc.,) certain materials can not be directly prepared in the mouth of the patient. They are best prepared in a laboratory and the finished and polished restoration is later cemented on to the tooth. Examples are (1) Porcelain (2) Cast Gold Alloys (3) Base Metal Alloys (4) Laboratory Processed Composite.

(c) Acid etched bonded restorations :

Enamel is etched to create micropores into which enamel bonding agents are applied, allowed to harden and help retain the restorations.

Presently dentine bonding agents are also used over conditioned dentine to help bond the restoration. Example is composite resin.

(d) Adhesive restorations :

The restorative material chemically bonds with enamel and dentine. Example is glass ionomer cement.

(V) **Depending upon its appearance :**

(a) Tooth coloured restorations (i) Composite resins (ii) Acrylic resins (iii) Silicate cements (iv) Glass ionomer (v) Resin modified glass ionomer (vi) Porcelain (vii) Cerestore procelain (viii) Dicor (ix) CAD CAM porcelain (x) Hiceram

(b) Non tooth coloured restorations (I) Silver amalgam (ii) cast gold (iii) Direct filling gold (iv) Zinc Oxide Eugenol cement (v) Metal modified glass ionomer (vi) Base metal alloy restorations.

**17. WHAT IS CAVITY PREPARATION?**

**A :** Cavity preparation is a series of procedures done by a dentist, on the tooth to be restored, to make the tooth fit to receive the restorative material.

**18. WHY IS CAVITY PREPARATION NECESSARY BEFORE RESTORING A TOOTH?**

**A :** (1) The diseased portion of the tooth should be completely removed to avoid further progression of the disease or its recurrence (eg., Dental caries)

(2) The disease might have progressed in an irregular shape. The cavity should be given an appropriate shape to obtain best mechanical properties of the restorative material (better strength, grip etc.,)

**19. HOW IS CAVITY PREPARATION DONE?**

**A :** Cutting tools called burs and diamond points are used in a hand held device called handpiece. These rotary instruments are operated either by electricity or compressed air. The burs revolve at a very high speed and cut the tooth structure easily. After gross cutting of the cavity with rotary instruments, finer adjustments are done with hand held instruments or special burs used in slow speed handpieces.

**20. IS CUTTING OF A TOOTH ABSOLUTELY NECESSARY BEFORE ANY RESTORATION?**

**A :** Cavity cutting may not be necessary before giving an adhesive or acid etched restoration, provided the tooth to be restored is free from Dental caries. But even if cavity cutting is not done in such teeth, "tooth preparation" should be done.

**21. WHAT IS MEANT BY "TOOTH PREPARATION"?**

**A :** Before giving an adhesive or acid etched restoration, the surface of the tooth should be thoroughly cleaned to remove surface contaminants, plaque, pellicles & materia alba. The enamel and dentine should be conditioned and primed to receive the restorative materials. These steps are called "tooth preparation".

**22. WHAT IS PRECLINICAL OPERATIVE DENTISTRY?**

**A :** Preclinical operative Dentistry is a Branch of Operative Dental Surgery wherein practical training is given in cavity preparation and restoration of teeth with various materials in dummy models in simulated oral environment.

**23. WHY IS THE SUBJECT PRECLINICAL OPERATIVE DENTISTRY IMPORTANT?**

**A :** Oral cavity is a small area. There exist the confining atmosphere of lips, cheek and palate with the constantly mobile tongue. To prepare a cavity in such a restricted area, greater skill is needed. Repeated cavity preparations in extracted natural teeth hones the skill and efficiency of the student. By doing the cavities of correct width & depth in the dummy models, a student is able to juxtapose his acquired skill in the clinical patient easily. Preclinical training increases the psychomotor skills and student gains confidence to handle live tissues later.

# CHAPTER : 2

# CAUSES OF LOSS OF TOOTH STRUCTURE

**1. WHAT ARE THE CAUSES OF LOSS OF TOOTH STRUCTURE?**

**A :** The commonest cause of loss of tooth structure is dental caries. Other causes are trauma (resulting in fracture of tooth), attrition, abrasion, erosion, resorption, hypoplasia, malformations and iatrogenic (dentist induced).

**2. WHAT IS DENTAL CARIES?**

**A :** Dental caries is a bacterial disease affecting the hard tissues of the teeth (i.e., enamel, dentine and cementum) When caries extends to pulp, it causes pulpal inflammation & most of the time, pulpal death.

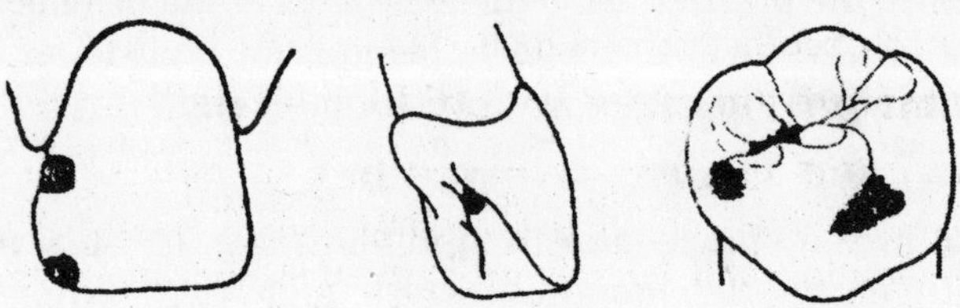

*Fig. 2.1. Dental caries*

**3. WHICH BACTERIA CAUSE DENTAL CARIES?**

**A :** It has not been possible to pinpoint a single micro-organism as the causative factor, though streptococcus mutans and Lactobacillus acidophilus have been associated with carious lesions. The causative organisms are acidogenic (acid producing) and aciduric (capable of living in an acid medium).

**4. IF ACIDOGENIC AND ACIDURIC BACTERIA ARE PRESENT IN THE MOUTH, WILL CARIES START IN A TOOTH?**

**A :** Normally, human mouth harbours plenty of bacteria. They do not always cause disease. Mere presence of streptoco ccus mutans or Lactobacillus acidophilus around the tooth can not initiate caries. Only when fermentable carbohydrates stagnate around teeth and bacteria utilize the food particles for energy by breaking down the carbohydrate molecules, acid byproducts are formed which can demineralize the hard portions of the teeth. The role of dental plaque at this stage is important in caries formation.

**5. WHAT IS DENTAL PLAQUE? WHAT IS ITS ROLE IN CARIES FORMATION?**

**A :** Dental plaque is a tenacious membrane formed around teeth and it consists mainly of salivary mucin and microoganisms. If the organisms in the plaque are predominantly streptococcus mutans, the acids produced as byproducts of bacterial metabolism reduce the plaque pH and the minerals in enamel are dissolved by the acids, thereby initiating the caries. However, caries is not a continuous disease. If the bacterial metabolic activity ceases, the pH rises and remineralisation of the demineralised area can occur. A cariogenic plaque can provide an acidic atmosphere for caries activity to progress.

**6. HOW ARE PLAQUE ELIMINATED?**

**A :** Oral hygiene procedures like toothbrushing, flossing, rinsing with antiseptic mouth washes and oral prophylaxis (mechanical cleaning and polishing in the Dental clinic) can eliminate plaque from the mouth for a brief period. However plaque can form again within a few hours.

**7. DOES IT MEAN CARIES IS INEVITABLE?**

**A :** If the plaque formed is non cariogenic (having a low proportion of acidogenic organisms) demineralization of tooth does not occur. The present emphasis in caries prevention is not complete plaque elimination but plaque control.

**8. WHICH PORTIONS OF THE TEETH ARE AFFECTED BY CARIES?**

Caries usually affects the crown of the tooth and starts in enamel. After spreading through enamel, it affects dentine. Sometimes, when gingival recession is present, caries attacks the cementum and dentine and is known as root caries. In deep cavities, after penetrating dentine, uncontrolled caries affects the pulp and through the apical foramen, the periodontium.

**9. WHAT ARE THE SIGNS & SYMPTOMS OF CARIES?**

**A :** Caries in enamel initially is seen as a white spot, when the tooth is dry. It can not be seen on a wet tooth. When the lesion takes up pigments, it appears brown or black. On probing, it yields to pressure. Later when caries spreads to dentine, patient starts feeling hypersensitivity to thermal changes and sweet and sour substances. The loss of tooth structure leads to cavity formation and resultant food impaction. When caries is limited to dentine, patient usually has only discomfort and not pain. But when caries reaches pulp, usually severe pain occurs.

**10. WHAT IS THE DIFFERENCE BETWEEN PAIN AND HYPER-SENSITIVITY?**

**A :** Hypersensitivity is usually milder than pain. It usually vanishes with cessation of the stimulus that started it. Hypersensitivity occurs only after a stimulation (provocation) and stops when the stimulus is removed. Pain may be a consequence of a stimulus or may be spontaneous. Pain is usually continuous while hypersensitivity is transient. Hypersensitivity can never be spontaneous.

**11. HOW DOES DENTIST MANAGE CARIES?**

**A :** Dentist advises the patient about preventing caries. He also removes the part of the tooth affected by caries and restores the tooth.

**12. IS IT ALWAYS POSSIBLE TO RESTORE A CARIOUS TOOTH?**

**A :** Most of the time, it is possible to restore a carious tooth. The type of restoration and the duration of treatment might vary depending upon the severity, extent of damage and the tissue involved. Restoring and retaining a natural tooth is more beneficial (more comfortable & less expensive) to the patient rather than extraction & providing artificial tooth. Small cavities in enamel & dentine are cleaned and simple fillings are made. When caries has affected the pulp, suitable endodontic treatment is given followed by stronger restorations.

**13. HOW ARE CARIES CLASSIFIED?**

**i) Depending on the rapidity of progress:**

(a) ACUTE CARIES (b) CHRONIC CARIES (rampant caries)

**ii) Depending on the location :**

(a) PIT & FISSURE CARIES

(b) SMOOTH SURFACE CARIES

**iii) Depending on the tissue involved :**

(a) ENAMEL CARIES (b) DENTINE CARIES

(c) CEMENTAL CARIES (root caries)

**iv) Depending on the patient's age :**

(a) NURSING BOTTLE CARIES (b) SENILE CARIES

**v) Depending on the origin:**

(a) PRIMARY CARIES (b) SECONDARY CARIES

(c) RESIDUAL CARIES

**vi) Depending on extent of lesion :**

(a) INCIPIENT (reversible) CARIES

(b) CAVITATED CARIES

**14. WHAT IS ACUTE CARIES?**

**A :** Rapidly progressing caries is known as acute caries. Many teeth are affected and lesions are soft to touch and are light in colour. Progress of caries is in months. Periods of demineralization are more and continuous than remineralization.

**15. WHAT IS CHRONIC CARIES?**

**A :** Slowly progressing caries is known as chronic caries. The lesions affect fewer teeth & lesion is dark and hard. Periods of remineralization after demineralization reflect changes in oral environment. The slow rate of caries allows time for extrinsic pigmentation.

**16. WHAT ARE PIT AND FISSURE CARIES?**

**A :** Caries occuring in the pits & fissures of the occlusal, buccal or lingual surfaces (which serve as stagnation area for food debris) are called pit & fissure caries. In pit & fissure caries of enamel, the lesion is triangular in shape with the apex of the triangle near the pit & base near the Dentino enamel junction. At the Dentino enamel junction, there is lateral spread of decay, undermining the overlying enamel (backward decay). In dentine, carious lesion spreads towards pulp in a triangular fashion, again with the base near Dentino enamel junction.

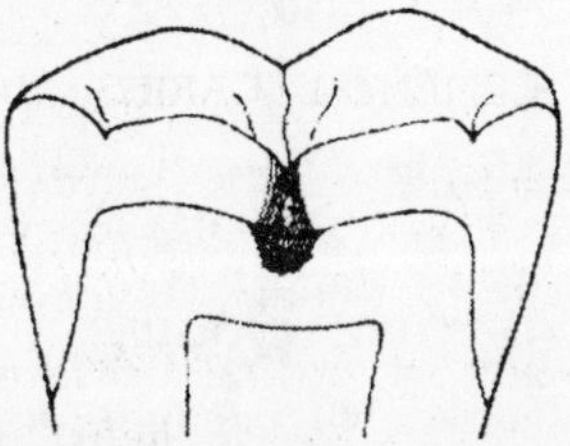

*Fig. 2.2. Pit and fissure caries*

**17. WHAT ARE SMOOTH SURFACE CARIES?**

**A :** Caries occuring on the smooth surface of enamel that is habitually unclean and usually covered by cariogenic plaque. The progress of lesion in enamel is triangular in cross section with its base on outer enamel surface and apex towards the Dentino enamel junction. At the Dentino enamel junction, there is lateral spread of decay (backward decay) undermining the enamel. In dentine, the carious lesion spreads towards the pulp in a triangular fashion, again with the base near the dentino enamel junction.

## 18. WHAT IS ENAMEL CARIES?

**A :** The initial carious lesion in enamel could be an incipient lesion or a cavitated one. In incipient carious lesion, there is no structural loss but subsurface enamel demineralization is present. It looks white & opaque when the tooth is dry. As such there is no hole in the tooth. In cavitated caries the caries has progressed further with collapse of the intact surface layer & loss of surface integrity. During the normal course, an incipient carious lesion is capable of being remineralized by salivary calcium and phosphate and might not need any restoration. A cavitated lesion usually needs a restoration. Be it an incipient caries or cavitated caries, the patient does not have any hypersensitivity as long as the carious lesion is in enamel only.

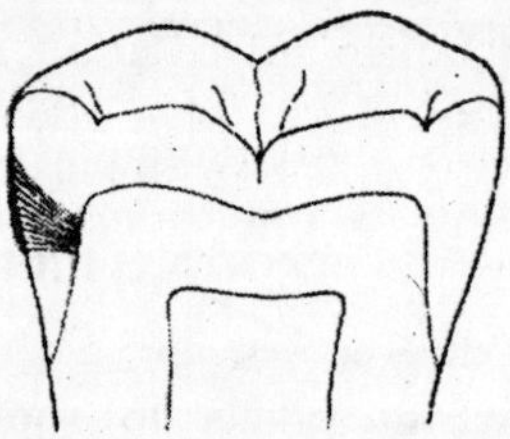

*Fig. 2.3. Enamel caries*

## 19. WHAT IS DENTINE CARIES?

**A :** A cavitated caries, after penetrating through enamel, spreads laterally, along the dentino enamel junction to undermine overlying intact enamel. It also demineralizes the under-

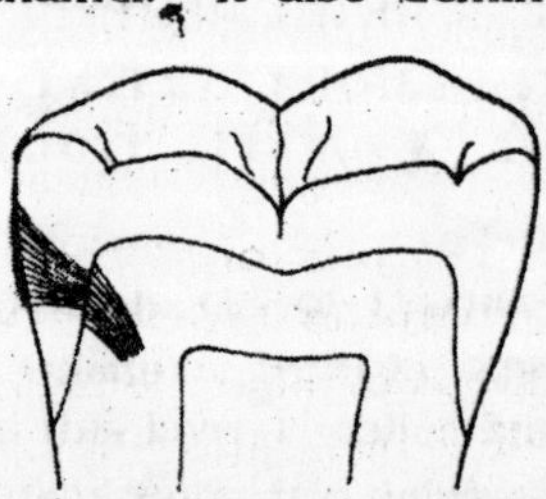

*Fig. 2.4. Dentine caries*

lying dentine, Dentine contains less minerals and consists of numerous dentinal tubles that can transmit microbial acids. Caries spreads faster in dentine than in enamel. However, numerous protective mechanisms are undertaken by the dental pulp and dentine to ward off the damage. Formation of sclerotic dentine, dead tracts and reparative (tertiary) dentine are some of the methods by which dental pulp attempts to protect itself from acids & other microbial products from carious lesion.

**20. WHAT IS SCLEROTIC DENTINE?**

**A :** In slowly advancing carious lesions in a vital tooth, dentine may respond to the initial demineralization by deposition of crystalline material in both the lumen of the tubules and the intertubular dentine, thereby warding off the irritants from the pulp. Such barrier formation reduces dentine penetrability. These hypermineralized areas are known as sclerotic dentine. Clinically sclerotic dentine is usually shiny and darkly coloured but feels hard to the explorer.

**21. WHAT ARE DEAD TRACTS?**

**A :** In moderately advancing carious lesions in a vital tooth, bacterial toxins, acids & hydrolytic enzymes may spread quickly through the dentinal tubules causing degeneration and death of odonotoblasts & their cytoplasmic extensions resulting in mild inflammation of pulp. Groups of dentinal tubules devoid of the cytoplasmic extensions of odontoblasts are called dead tracts. Some authors feel that the dead tracts with terminal calcified ends are protective in nature while others feel that dead tracts are more permeable. Dead tracts are microscopic features.

**22. WHAT IS REPARATIVE DENTINE?**

Odontoblasts are dentine forming cells found in the dentinal end of the pulp. When they are destroyed due to bacterial toxins & other irritants, undifferentiated mesenchymal cells from the pulp may differentiate into odontoblasts and may perform their function. To ward off the irritants reaching through the dentine into the pulp, odontoblasts may lay down, at a faster rate, calcified tissue at the pulpal end of the dentine. This dentine is known as tertiary or reparative dentine. Usually tertiary dentine contains very few irregularly shaped dentinal tubules. Reparative dentine is a very effective barrier to diffusion of materials. The production of reparative dentine will depend upon the regenerative capacity of the tooth & rate of progress of caries. In younger individuals & slowly progressing caries, the chances of reparative dentine formation is higher.

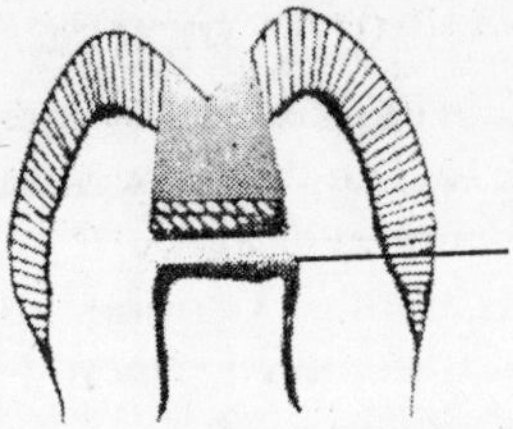


*Fig. 2.5. Reparative dentine*

## 23. WHAT ARE THE VARIOUS CARIOUS LAYER ZONES IN DENTINE?

**A :** Histologically, it is possible to differentiate the various carious zones in dentine in a slowly progressing carious lesion. The outer most zone (dentine closest to the external surface) consists of decomposed dentine with plenty of microorganisms. Removal of this carious infected dentine is a must for all the restorative procedures excepting indirect pulp capping. The next zone seen in the microscope is turbid dentine zone where bacterial invasion with widening and distortion of dentinal tubules are present. The collagen is irreversibly denatured and very little minerals are present. This layer is also not capable of remineralization and should be removed prior to restoration. The zone below (third layer) is transparent dentine. This zone is free from bacteria but there is loss of minerals from intertubular dentine. The collagen cross linking appears intact and this zone is capable of repair, provided the irritants are removed and pulp remains vital. The fourth zone is subtransparent dentine, which is also bacteria free but with demineralization of intertubular dentine. This layer is also capable of remineralization. Below this zone may be normal healthy dentine.

**24. HOW DO DIFFERENTIATE THE VARIOUS CARIOUS ZONES IN DENTINE CLINICALLY?**

**A :** The most superficial carious dentine & turbid dentine (together known as infected dentine) are relatively soft, leathery and stained dark brown or black. When probed they yield to pressure. While excavating (removing with an excavator) there is less hypersensitivity. The transparent and subtransparent zones are slightly harder than carious dentine but softer than normal dentine. The colour may be yellowish or light brown. While excavating there will be more hypersensitivity (expressed as pain). However, the best way of differentiating between affected and infected dentine will be use of disclosing solution.

**25. WHAT IS A CARIES DISCLOSING SOLUTION?**

**A :** 1% solution of acid red 52 (acid rhodamine B or food red 106) in propylene glycol, when used in a cavity, stains the infected dentine red but not the affected dentine. The dye is capable of staining irreversibly denatured dentine collagen and not the reversibly denatured collagen of affected dentine. 0.5% Basic fuchsin in propylane glycol was also used as a disclosing solution earlier.

**26. WHAT IS THE SIGNIFICANCE OF CLINICALLY DIFFERENTIATING AFFECTED AND INFECTED DENTINE?**

**A :** One of the chief aims of conservative dental surgeon is the preservation of the vitality of healthy pulp. It is unwise to introduce microorganism into the pulp during caries removal and restoration. While using rotary instruments under high speed even a slight movement of the instrument may result in an exposure & pushing infected material into pulp. If it is possible to clinically differentiate between infected and affected dentine, careful caries removal without exposure is easy. It is desirable to remove the infected dentine but permissible to leave the affected dentine to undergo remineralization. If infected dentine is permitted to remain in a cavity below a restoration and if that area has communication with oral cavity, the chances of recurrent caries is more. So infected dentine must always be removed prior to restoration excepting while doing indirect pulp capping.

**27. WHAT IS INDIRECT PULP CAPPING?**

**A :** When caries is very deep in a cavity but without involvement of pulp and the pulp is completely healthy, if it is felt that complete caries removal might accidentally expose the pulp with potential risk of bacterial penetration, it is wiser to remove the caries from all areas excepting the pulpal floor and axial walls (places very close to pulp). Some carious infected dentine is left intentionally in some places (for fear of pulp exposure, during caries removal) and by keeping anticarious medicaments & above that a restoration (hoping for arrest of the residual caries). The residual caries is cut off from the oral cavity by an interim restoration with good marginal seal and hence cannot progress further. The healthy pulp is also encouraged to produce more reparative dentine. At a later date, it may be possible to remove the temporary restoration and the underlying carious dentine without fear of carious exposure (because of the thickness of the newly deposited tertiary dentine). This procedure of preservation of pulpal vitality in very deep carious lesions by judicious use of anticarious medicament capping and interim restoration without pulpal exposure is called the indirect pulp capping.

**28. WHAT IS CEMENTAL CARIES?**

**A :** Cemental caries is otherwise called root surface caries. It usually occurs in elderly individuals & is also known as senile caries. The thin cementum offers less resistance to carious attack. In patients with gingival recession, poor oral hygiene and reduced salivation, the chances for cemental caries is higher. Root carious lesions have less well defined margins & tend to be 'U' shaped in cross section (due to parallel progression through dentinal tubules).

**29. WHAT IS NURSING BOTTLE CARIES?**

**A :** In young children fed through a nursing bottle for a prolonged period (eg., Leaving a feeding bottle by the side of the child at night to have a drink as and when desired) or in children who were pacified repeatedly with pacifiers dipped in sweetening agents, a type of rampant caries develop, involving most of their teeth including mandibular anteriors. It is known as Nursing bottle caries. This is due to constant localisation of high carbohydrate & poor oral hygiene.

**30. WHAT IS SENILE CARIES?**

**A :** Carious activity that spurts up during old age is called senile caries. This may be due to either reduction in salivary secretion, exposure of roots following gingival recession, sudden drop in oral maintainance procedures after highly stressful situation or sudden alterations in diet (excessive indulgence in sweets). Usually root caries is associated with the elderly though crown caries might also occur.

**31. WHAT IS PRIMARY CARIES?**

**A :** Caries occuring in an unrestored (unfilled) tooth is known as primary caries.

**32. WHAT IS SECONDARY CARIES?**

**A :** Caries occuring in a restored tooth is known as secondary caries.

**33. WHAT IS RESIDUAL CARIES?**

**A :** While preparing a tooth for restoration, some caries might be left by accident or intention. Such caries is known as residual caries. Leaving caries accidentally might lead to recurrence of caries, while intentionally leaving caries (as in the case of indirect pulp capping), care should be taken that there is no communication between carious lesion and the oral cavity.

**34. HOW CAN CARIES BE PREVENTED?**

**A :** 1) Diet control & reduction of fermentable carbohydrates.

2) Mechanical plaque control measures like brushing, flossing, using interdental sticks.

3) Chemical plaque control measures like chlorhexidine mouth rinses.

4) Use of topical and systemic fluorides to reduce smooth surface caries.

5) Use of pit & fissure sealants for preventing pit and fissure caries.

**35. WHAT IS TRAUMA? WILL IT ALWAYS RESULT IN LOSS OF TOOTH STRUCUTRE?**

**A :** Trauma to tooth means physical injury to the tooth. It can happen following accidents (falls, collisions), playfulness (opening metallic crowns of soft drink bottles with teeth) assault (quarrels, robbery), contact sports (ball games, boxing, atheletics) or wartime injuries. Trauma to tooth need not necessarily result in loss of tooth structure but most of the time it does. It may also render the tooth non-vital (pulp dead). The extent of damage will depend upon the force of the injury, condition of the tooth & its supporting structures.

**36. HOW CAN TRAUMA TO TOOTH CAN BE PREVENTED?**

**A :** While it may not be possible to prevent all accidents, it is wiser to use custom made mouth guards (mouth guards made for that particular individual's oral dimensions) while taking part in any contact sports.

**37. WHAT IS ATTRITION?**

**A :** It is the mechanical wearing away of the incisal & occlusal surface of teeth due to chewing forces. Some extent of

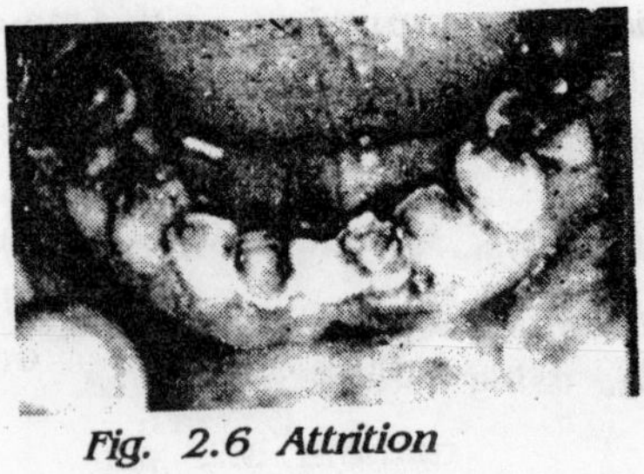

*Fig. 2.6 Attrition*

attrition is unavoidable with age but when the degree of attrition is disproportionate, it may be due to abnormal chewing habits like bruxism (grinding of teeth during sleep). Attrition is usually generalized (affecting all the teeth) and when dentine is exposed, tooth may be hypersensitive.

**38. ARE RESTORATIONS NEEDED FOR ATTRITION DEFECTS?**

A : When the attrition defects are minimal and tooth asympto matic, no treatment is needed. When dentine is exposed with accompanying hypersensitivity, use of tooth paste formulations having formalin, sodium fluoride, strontium fluoride or potassium nitrate for a brief period might give symptomatic relief. Restorative treatment for attrited teeth (most probably onlays or full crowns) are indicated only when there is severe structural loss and/or prolonged symptoms of hypersensitivity. When parafunctional jaw movements like bruxism are present with or without symptoms, efforts should be made to correct the habit.

**39. IS ATTRITION PREVENTABLE?**

**A :** Attrition is not completely preventable as it is the normal wearing away of the occlusal surface due to mastication. However avoiding gritty & grimy food can reduce masticatory wear. Correction of parafunctional jaw movements wlll also reduce attrition.

**40. HOW WILL THE ATTRITED SURFACE LOOK LIKE?**

**A :** It will be smooth, shiny, yellowish and surrounded by a white line of enamel and found only on incisal & occlusal surface of the tooth.

**41. WHAT IS ABRASION?**

**A :** Abrasion is the abnormal tooth loss due to frictional forces between teeth & other objects especially in the presence of abrasive materials. One of the common causes of abrasion is use of a gritty dentifrice (tooth paste or tooth powder) or use of a faulty brushing technique. Usually it is seen as a 'V' shaped cut on the buccal surfaces of posterior teeth - more prominent on the left side for the right handed individuals and vice versa for left handed individuals. The wedge shaped defect is usually seen in the gingival one thirds, but in severe cases extend into the middle third of the tooth also. Abrasional wear can also occur on incisal surfaces of the teeth in people habitually chewing on pipes, pens or pencil. It is also seen as an occupational marker in coblers, carpenters, electricians, seamstresses and tailors who hold nails, needles, wires or pins between their teeth.

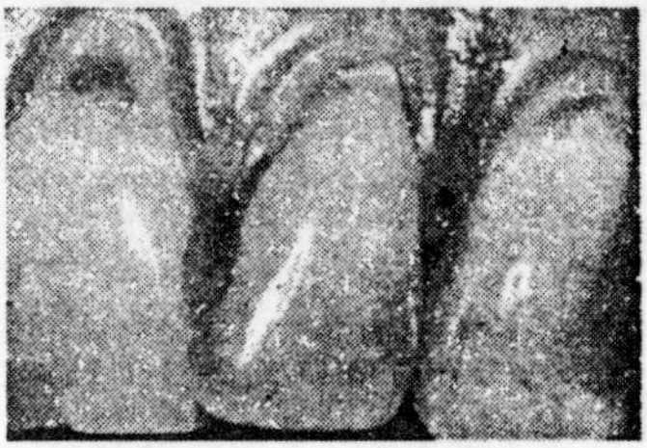

*Fig. 2.7. Abrasion*

**42. WHAT ARE THE SYMPTOMS OF ABRASION?**

In cervical region of the teeth, where the coronal enamel or the radicular cementum is thin, dentine is exposed early. Abraded lesions are usually hypersensitive.

**43. WHAT IS THE TREATMENT FOR ABRADED LESIONS?**

Identifying and eliminating the cause is the primary aim of treatment. Symptomatic relief is obtained with medicated tooth paste. When structural loss is gross, restorations are needed.

**44. HOW CAN ABRASION BE PREVENTED?**

Avoiding faulty habits is the only way of avoiding abrasion defects.

**45. WHAT IS EROSION?**

Erosion is the loss of tooth structure due to acid attacks. The defects are seen in the gingival one third of tooth. They are cresent shaped or saucer shaped with rounded edges. The surfaces are smooth & hypersensitivity is minimal or absent. They may be seen on palatal surfaces when the acids are Hydrochloric acid from gastric juice which are regurgitated to the oral cavity in bulimia and anorexia nervosa patients. They may be seen on labial surfaces when the ingested acid intake is high (example: in lime suckers, people taking more acidulated drinks).

**46. HOW TO PREVENT EROSION?**

Reduction of acidulated drinks intake and correction of eating disorders are the ways of preventing erosion.

**47. WHAT IS MEANT BY RESORPTION OF TEETH?**

**A :** Resorption is a method of loss of tooth tissue due to special cells called odontoclasts. Resorption of tooth affects cementum and dentine. It can be external or internal in nature. Usually in resorption cases, root canal treatment and/or surgery is needed prior to restoring a tooth. Resorption is not such a common cause for loss of tooth structure and usually can not be managed with simple restorations.

**48. WHAT IS HYPOPLASIA?**

Hypoplasia means defective formation of the tooth. Though the normal size & gross shape of the tooth is present, it may be structurally deficient comprising of surface defects like pits, grooves etc., where none naturally exist. This is due to defective formation of teeth.

**49. HOW ARE HYPOPLASTIC TEETH TREATED?**

When the defects are very minor and not aesthetically displeasing, they might be left as such. When the entire crown is grossly hypoplastic, it may be necessary to crown the tooth. If the labial surface alone is affected, it is adequate to fix a labial veneer only.

**50. WHAT ARE MALFORMED TEETH?**

Teeth that are not formed in the proper size and shape are malformed teeth. They may be smaller, larger or mishapen. For aesthetic enhancement and improving functional efficiency, restorations may be needed for malformed teeth.

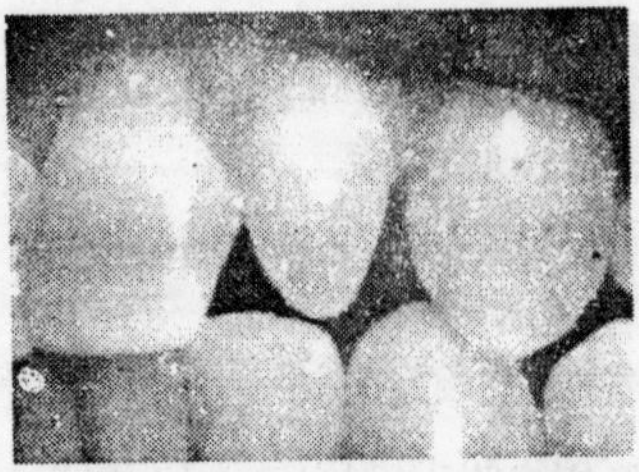

*Fig. 2.8 Malformed tooth*

**51. WHAT ARE THE IATROGENIC CAUSES FOR LOSS OF TOOTH STRUCTURE?**

**A :** For removal of destroyed tooth structure, increasing retention, resistance and appearance of a restoration, a dental surgeon is forced to cut away normal healthy tooth tissue. This is like the action of a surgeon while operating. However, the dental surgeon should ensure that the reduced tooth should be restored to the normal size and shape, for optimum health and function of the supporting structures of the teeth.

# CHAPTER : 3

# NOMENCLATURE

**1. WHAT IS MEANT BY NOMENCLATURE?**

**A :** It is the system of naming things.

**2. WHY IS NOMENCLATURE IMPORTANT?**

**A :** Nomenclature is needed for clarity of thought, unambiguous communication and better understanding.

**3. FOR WHICH ITEMS NOMENCLATURE IS NEEDED?**

**A :** Individual teeth to be identified, different parts of a prepared cavity are to be named for standardized communication.

**4. HOW ARE TEETH SURFACES NAMED?**

**A :** Teeth surfaces are named according to the anatomical structures or landmarks it is closest to. For example, the surface of the tooth closest to the lip (for an anterior tooth) is called labial and that closest to the cheek (for a posterior tooth) is called buccal. The tooth surface diametrically opposite to the buccal that is close to the tongue (for a lower tooth) is called lingual & that close to the palate (for an upper tooth) is called palatal. The surface cioser to the midline is called mesial & the surface away from the midline is called distal. Chewing surfaces are known as occlusal (for posteriors) and incisal (for anteriors). Cervical denotes close to the neck of the tooth & gingival denotes close to the gingiva or gums.

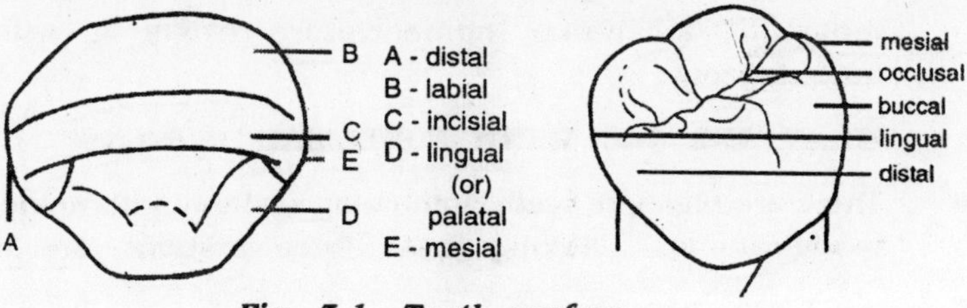


*Fig. 3.1. Tooth surface*

**5. NAME THE SURFACES OF AN UPPER ANTERIOR TOOTH?**

**A :** Labial, palatal, mesial, distal & incisal.

**6. NAME THE SURFACES OF A LOWER ANTERIOR TOOTH?**

**A :** Labial, lingual, mesial, distal & incisal.

**7. NAME THE SURFACES OF A UPPER POSTERIOR TOOTH?**

**A :** Buccal, palatal, mesial, distal & occlusal.

**8. NAME THE SURFACES OF A LOWER POSTERIOR TOOTH?**

**A :** Buccal, lingual, mesial, distal & occlusal.

**9. SOMETIMES WE COME ACROSS ROTATED TEETH WHERE THE SURFACE WE CALL PROXIMAL (MESIAL OR DISTAL) ARE CLOSER TO THE BUCCAL SURFACE. DOES IT CHANGE ITS NAME?**

**A :** Definitely not. While it is true that the surfaces are named after the anatomical structures closest to it, later the anatomical features of that surface are described (e.g. what ridges, pits & grooves are present in that surface) in detail and such anatomical details are used for identifying the surface. This is for avoiding unnecessary confusion. Hence even in a rotated tooth the nomenclature will not change.

**10. WHY ARE INDIVIDUAL TEETH GIVEN A NUMBER OR ALPHABET TO DENOTE IT WHEN THEY HAVE INDIVIDUAL NAME?**

**A :** It is true that every tooth in the oral cavity has its own name but it is too long & cumbersome to pronounce it (e.g. left lower permanent second molar) Hence a shortened number or an alphabet is an easier way of denoting it. Instead of denoting a tooth as left lower permanent second molar, if a shorter nomenclature exists it will be advantageous.

**11. WHAT ARE THE TEETH NUMBERING SYSTEMS?**

**A :** There are plenty of teeth numbering systems with numerous modifications. Among them three systems are more popular. They are (1) ZSIGMONDY PALMER SYSTEM (2) ADA SYSTEM (3) F D I SYSTEM

**12. WHAT IS ZSIGMONDY PALMER SYSTEM?**

**A :** In Zsigmondy Palmer System, permanent teeth are denoted by arabic numerals (numbers) and deciduous teeth are denoted by English upper case alphabets. This system is also known as angular or grid system. In this system, a cross is drawn to denote the patient's four quadrants and the permanent teeth are given numbers from 1 to 8, denoting the tooth's position from the midline. A deciduous tooth is given alphabets A to E, again denoting its closeness to midline.

**Eg PATIENT'S**

| **RIGHT UPPER** | **LEFT UPPER** |
|---|---|
| **RIGHT LOWER** | **LEFT LOWER** |

Eg $\begin{array}{c|c} & \\ \hline 3 & \end{array}$ denotes right lower permanent canine

$\begin{array}{c|c} & \\ \hline & 2 \end{array}$ denotes left lower permanent lateral incisor

$\begin{array}{c|c} & 5 \\ \hline & \end{array}$ denotes left upper second premolar

$\begin{array}{c|c} 6 & \\ \hline & \end{array}$ denotes right upper permanent first molar

Instead of putting the entire cross, the quadrant may also be written as ⌞ ⌝ ⌜ ⌟

eg : $\begin{array}{c|c} 3 & \\ \hline & \end{array}$ is 3⌟ ; $\begin{array}{c|c} \hline & 7 \end{array}$ is ⌜7 ; $\begin{array}{c|c} & 5 \\ \hline & \end{array}$ is ⌞5 ; $\begin{array}{c|c} \hline 1 & \end{array}$ is 1⌝

**13. WHAT ARE THE ADVANTAGES IN THIS SYSTEM?**

(1) Simple to use

2) No confusion between deciduous & permanent teeth

**14. WHAT ARE THE DISADVANTAGES OF ZSIGMONDY PALMER SYSTEM?**

(1) Each tooth does not have a specific number or alphabet. Contralateral as well as antagonistic teeth have the same number or alphabet. During oral communication the side of the tooth or whether it is upper or lower is not known, unless qualified as right

upper 3, left lower D, right lower 6 etc., (Low specificity)

(2) By denoting the number alone, there is a possibility of mistaking with right upper quadrant permanent teeth of A D A system.

(3) By denoting the alphabet alone, there is a possibility of mistaking with right upper quadrant deciduous teeth of A D A system.

(4) Not universally used.

**15. WHAT IS A D A SYSTEM?**

**A :** It is the American Dental Association System of numbering teeth, in which the right upper III molar tooth is numbered 1 and starting from that the permanent teeth are serially numbered in a clockwise direction till the right lower III molar which is tooth NO:32. The deciduous teeth are also serially designated by English Alphabets starting with right upper II deciduous molar as A, progressing in a clockwise direction, till the right lower II deciduous molar is T.

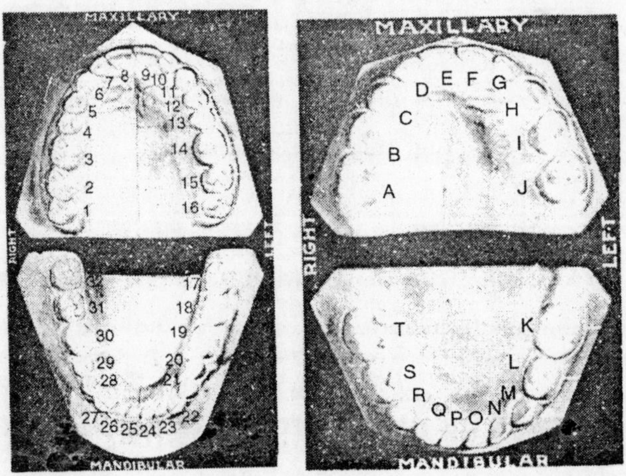


**PERMANENT** **DECIDUOUS**

*Fig. 3.2 A.D.A. System*

**16. WHAT ARE THE ADVANTAGES OF A D A SYSTEM?**

**A :** (1) Each permanent tooth is given a separate number

(2) Each deciduous tooth is given a separate alphabet

(3) From 9-32 and F to T, no possibility of confusing with Zsigmondy Palmer System.

**17. WHAT ARE THE DISADVANTAGES OF A D A SYSTEM?**

**A :** (1) While expressing the number of the right upper quadrant, there is a possibility of mistaking with permanent teeth of zsigmondy palmer system.

(2) While expressing the alphabets of the right upper quadrant, there is a possibility of mistaking with deciduous teeth of zsigmondy palmer system.

(3) Not used in all countries.

**18. IS A D A SYSTEM OTHERWISE CALLED THE UNIVERSAL SYSTEM OF TOOTH NUMBERING?**

**A :** It is true that many American dental books tend to describe the A D A system as Universal system. However, in countries already used to zsigmondy palmer notation, introduction of A D A system may lead to confusion and difficulties because of some overlapping. In Zsigmondy Palmer System Tooth No. 1 indicates permanent central incisor, but in A D A system it denotes right upper third molar. Tooth No. 4 in Zsigmondy Palmer System denotes the I premolar, while in A D A system it means right upper II premolar. So when a system is to be called Universal, if & when it is introduced in all countries, it should be unambiguous with no confusion. A D A system is not fit enough to be called a universal system.

**19. WHAT IS DANE OR HDERUP SYSTEM?**

**A :** This system is popular in scandinavian countries permanent teeth are serially numbered from 1 to 8 from the midline. Right upper teeth are designated with a suffix '+' left upper teeth are designated with a prefix '+'. Right lower teeth are suffixed with '-' and left lower teeth are prefixed with '-'.

Eg., 4+ means upper first premolar of right side

−4 means lower left first premolar.

5+ denotes left upper II premolar.

8− denotes right lower III molar

**20. HOW ARE DECIDUOUS DENOTED IN DANE OR HDERUP SYSTEM?**

**A :** For deciduous teeth, two variants are used. Either roman numerals I to V are used with prefixed or zero is added to arabic numerals 1 to 5 with prefix or suffix of '+' or '-' symbols.

Eg., +03 or + III denotes left upper deciduous canine

− 4 or − IV denotes left lower I deciduous molar

05 − or V− denotes right lower second deciduous molar

02+ or II+ denotes right upper deciduous lateral incisor.

**21. WHAT IS F D I SYSTEM OF NUMBERING TEETH?**

**A :** It is Federation Dentaire International (International federation of Dental Surgeons) system of numbering teeth. It is also known as Two digit system. In this system, each tooth (permanent or deciduous) is given a specific two digit number. The first digit denotes whether the tooth is permanent or deciduous as wells as to which quadrant of the patient, the tooth belongs to. The second digit denotes the position of the tooth from the midline. If the first digit is between 1 & 4, the tooth is permanent. If the first digit is between 5 & 8, the tooth is deciduous. The quadrants, starting from the patients right upper, are serially numbered in a clockwise direction (1 & 5 - right upper 2 & 6 - left upper 3 & 7 - left lower & 4 & 8 - right lower quadrant) The second digit could be 1 to 8 for permanent tooth 1 to 5 for deciduous teeth. The two digits of the number should be pronounced separately eg: If the two digit number of a tooth is 28, it should not be pronounced twenty eight but only as two eight. 13 should not be pronounced as thirteen but only as one three.

**22. WHAT ARE THE ADVANTAGES OF F D I SYSTEM?**

**A :** 1) Each tooth is given a separate number. So specificity is high.

2) No possibility of mistaking for Zsigmondy palmer system or Dane or Hderup system, as each number has two digits.

3) No chance of mistaking with A D A system for teeth No: 11 to 18, 21 to 28, 31 & 32 as the digits are not pronounced together as a single number but only separately.

4) Can be used in all countries without confusing with the existing system.

**23. CAN F D I SYSTEM BE CALLED THE UNIVERSAL SYSTEM OF NUMBERING?**

**A :** Yes. It is different from other systems. When adapted by any country, it is not likely to interfere & cause confusion with the existing system of that country.

**24. WHAT ARE THE DISADVANTAGES OF F D I SYSTEM?**

**A :** Like all other existing systems, there is no provision for supernumerary teeth.

**25. HOW ARE SUPERNUMERARY TEETH DESIGNATED NOW?**

**A :** The symbol 'S' is used to denote the supernumerary tooth, noting the nearest normal adjacent tooth.

**26. WHAT IS THE NECESSITY OF NAMING THE INTERNAL FEATURES IN A CAVITY?**

**A :** Internal features of the cavity are named for better and precise communication between the Teacher and the dental student for suggesting rectification of defects, refinement and modifications in a cavity. It is also useful for better description of the interior of the cavity.

## 27. WHAT ARE THE TYPES OF CAVITIES?

**A :** Most conservative type of cavity could be a pit cavity. It is usually made with a round bur. The pit cavity is usually spherical or spheroidal in nature. It is prepared when the destruction of the tooth structure is minimal and around a pit (May be occlusal, buccal or lingual). Though these cavities were usually made for silver amalgam, the availability of adhesive & acid etched restorations, have made such conservative cavities more common. Generally for non adhesive restorations, conventionally, box like cavities are prepared. Caries attack on teeth does not automatically result in a box like cavity. Only when the dental surgeon is preparing the cavity, does he make it box like for getting better resistance & retention for his restoration. Such box like cavity prepared in the tooth could be single box or multiple boxes connected with each other.

## 28. WHAT ARE SIMPLE, COMPOUND AND COMPLEX CAVITIES?

**A :** In a simple cavity only one surface in affected by caries. In a compound cavity two surfaces of tooth are affected by caries. In a complex cavity three or more surfaces are affected by caries.

## 29. WHAT WILL BE THE INTERNAL FEATURES OF SUCH A BOX?

**A :** The box will consist of walls and floors. Walls are parallel to the long axis of the tooth and floors and seats are

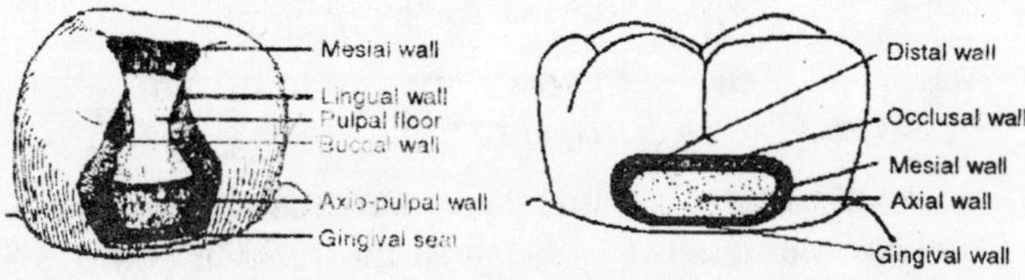


*Fig. 3.3. Walls & Floors*

perpendicular to the long axis of the tooth (exception : occlusal/incisal wall). The walls, floor & seat are named after the surfaces of the tooth, it is closest to or after the anatomical structures nearer to it.

**30. NAME THE WALLS, FLOOR AND SEAT IN A CAVITY?**

**A :** All the following walls, floor and seat may not be present in all the cavities. Depending on the location & complexity of cavities some walls may be absent.

1) Buccal (for posterior)/Labial (for anterior) wall
2) Lingual (for lower)/Palatal (for upper) wall
3) Mesial wall
4) Distal wall
5) Axial wall (parallel to long axis of tooth)
6) Occlusal (for posteriors) / Incisal (for anteriors) wall
7) Pulpal floor
8) Gingival seat

**31. WHAT WALLS ARE PRESENT IN A SIMPLE CLASS I CAVITY WITHOUT EXTENSIONS?**

**A :** Buccal wall, lingual wall, mesial wall, distal wall and pulpal floor.

**32. WHAT WALLS ARE PRESENT IN A CLASS I CAVITY WITH BUCCAL EXTENSION?**

**A :** i) In the occlusal box: Lingual wall, Mesial wall, distal wall, pulpal floor & part of the buccal wall

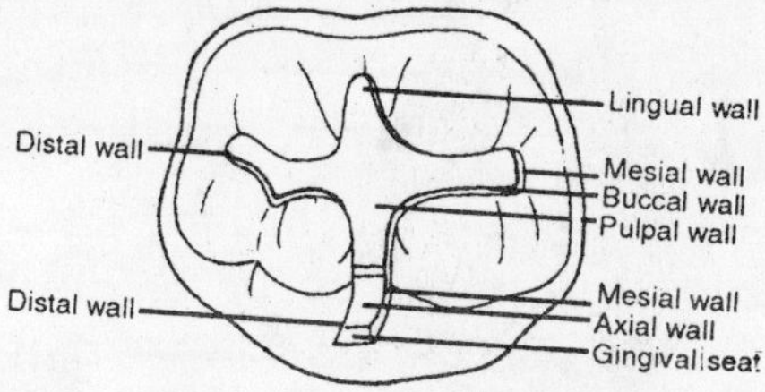


*Fig. 3.4. Class I buccal extension*

ii) In the buccal box: Axial wall, gingival seat & Mesial wall of the buccal box & Distal wall of the buccal box.

**33. WHAT WALLS AND FLOORS ARE PRESENT IN A CLASS I CAVITY WITH LINGUAL EXTENSION?**

**A :** i) In the occlusal box: Buccal wall, Mesial wall, distal wall, pulpal floor & part of lingual wall.

ii) In the lingual box: Axial wall, gingival seat & Mesial wall of the lingual box and distal wall of the lingual box.

**34. WHAT WALLS & FLOORS ARE PRESENT IN A CLASS II CAVITY?**

**A :** In a simple class II cavity without occlusal extension, Buccal wall, lingual wall, gingival seat, axial wall and occlusal walls are present.

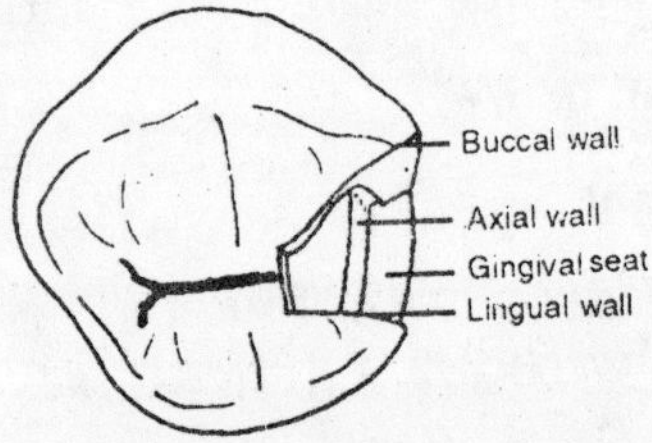


*Fig. 3.5. Class II Without Occlusal extension*

**35. WHAT WALLS & FLOORS ARE PRESENT IN A CLASS II MESIAL CAVITY WITH OCCLUSAL EXTENSION?**

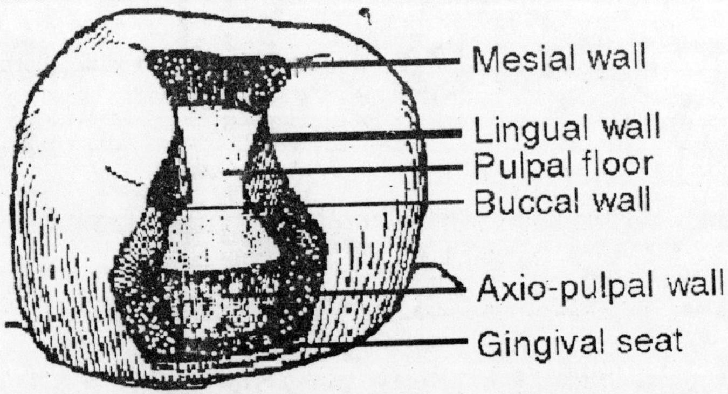


*Fig. 3.6. Class II With Occlusal extension*

**A :** i) **In the occlusal box:** Buccal wall, lingual wall, distal wall and pulpal floor.

ii) **In the Mesial box:** Axial wall, gingival seat, buccal wall of the Mesial box and lingual wall of the mesial box.

**36. WHAT WALLS & FLOORS ARE PRESENT IN A CLASS II DISTAL CAVITY WITH OCCLUSAL EXTENSION?**

**A :** i) **In the occlusal box:** Buccal wall, lingual wall, mesial wall and pulpal floor.

ii) **In the Distal Box:** Axial wall, gingival seat, buccal wall of the distal box and lingual wall of the distal box.

**37. WHAT WALLS & FLOORS ARE PRESENT IN A M.O.D. CAVITY?**

**A :** i) **In the occlusal box** : Buccal wall, lingual wall & pulpal floor

ii) **In the Mesial box:** Axial wall, gingival seat, buccal wall of the mesial box and lingual wall of the mesial box

iii) **In the Distal box:** Axial wall, gingival seat, buccal wall of the distal box and lingual wall of the distal box.

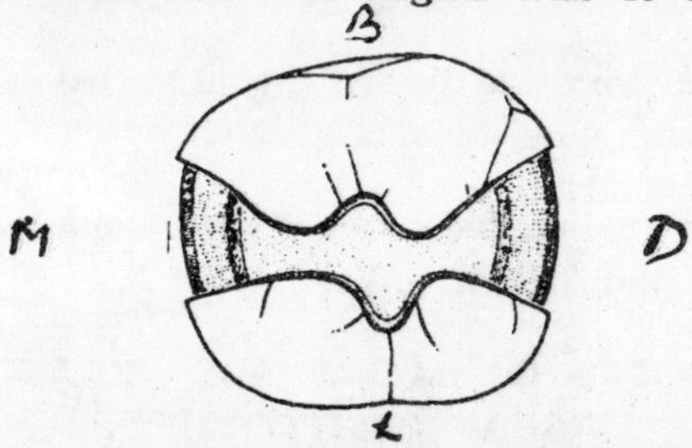


*Fig. 3.7. M O D Cavity*

**38. WHAT WALLS & FLOORS ARE PRESENT IN A CLASS III CAVITY WITHOUT EXTENSIONS?**

**A :** i) **If direct access is available:** Labial, lingual, axial walls & gingival seat

ii) **In Lingual access:** Labial wall, axial wall & gingival seat

iii) **In Labial access :** Lingual wall, axial wall & gingival seat

**39. WHAT WALLS & FLOORS ARE PRESENT IN A CLASS III CAVITY WITH LINGUAL EXTENSION?**

**A :** i) **In the proximal box:** Labial wall, axial wall & gingival seat.

ii) **In the lingual box:** Incisal wall, axial wall, gingival seat and proximal (Mesial or distal) wall.

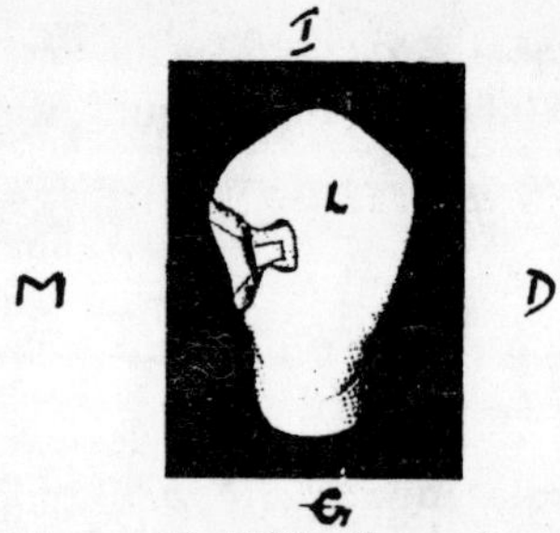


*Fig. 3.8. Class III With lingual extension*

**40. WHAT WALLS & FLOORS ARE PRESENT IN A CLASS IV CAVITY?**

**A :** i) **In the proximal box:** (Lingual access) Labial wall, axial wall and gingival seat.

ii) **In the Incisal box:** Labial wall, lingual wall, pulpal floor & proximal (Mesial/distal) wall

**41. WHAT WALLS & FLOORS ARE PRESENT IN A MESIO OCCLUSO LINGUAL CAVITY?**

**A :** i) **In the Mesial box:** Axial wall, buccal & lingual walls of the mesial box and gingival seat.

ii) **In the occlusal box:** Pulpal floor, Buccal wall, distal wall and part of the lingual wall.

iii) **In the lingual box:** Axial wall, gingival seat, Mesial wall of the lingual box & distal wall of the lingual box.

**42. IS IT NECESSARY TO LEARN THE PREVIOUS TWELVE QUESTIONS BY HEART TO KNOW THE VARIOUS WALLS & FLOORS PRESENT IN DIFFERENT CAVITIES?**

**A :** It will be a real waste of time if you do ! By looking into a cavity you must be able to name the walls & floors by looking at the adjacent surfaces. The previous twelve answers should only serve as a check list for verifying your answers.

**43. WHY SHOULD WE KNOW THE WALLS & FLOORS CORRECTLY?**

**A :** Only when we know the names of walls & floors correctly, can we name the various internal line angles & point angles correctly.

**44. WHAT IS A LINE ANGLE?**

**A :** It is an internal line of a cavity where either two walls or a wall and a floor (seat) meet.

**45. WHAT IS A POINT ANGLE?**

**A :** It is the point where two walls & a floor (seat) or three walls meet.

**46. HOW ARE THE LINE ANGLES NAMED?**

**A :** A line angle (the junction of two walls or a wall and a floor) takes the combined name fo the meeting walls or the wall & a floor

**(eg)**

i) When Mesial wall & buccal wall meet, the line angle is called mesio buccal line angle.

ii) When lingual wall and pulpal floor meet, the formed line angle is linguopulpal line angle.

iii) When axial wall & pulpal floor meet, the line angle formed is axio pulpal line angle.

iv) When buccal wall and axial wall meet, the line angle formed is bucco axial line angle.

v) When axial wall and gingival seat meet, the line angle is named axio gingival line angle.

**47. IS IT ALRIGHT IF THE ABOVE LINE ANGLES ARE CALLED (i) BUCCO MESIAL (ii) PULPO LINGUAL (iii) PULPO AXIAL (iv) AXIO BUCCAL AND (v) GINGIVO AXIAL LINE ANGLES RESPECTIVELY?**

Heavens will not fall if the naming order is reversed, as it is still the combination of the meeting walls or wall & a floor. But conventionally, for uniformity of expression certain rules are followed. When a proximal wall (mesial or distal) formes a line angle with other wall or floor, the proximal wall's, name forms the first part of the line angle. When buccal, lingual (palatal) or occlusal (incisal) wall combines with any other wall (excepting proximal) or floor (seat), buccal, lingual or occlusal wall's name forms the first part of the angle. When axial wall combines with a floor (seat) the axial wall's name forms the first part of the line angle.

So conventionally the order of preference is :

| | | |
|---|---|---|
| FIRST | | Mesial or distal wall |
| SECOND | - | Buccal, lingual or occlusal |
| THIRD | - | Axial wall |
| LAST | - | Pulpal floor & gingival seat. |

**48. DO WE HAVE LINE ANGLES AT THE CAVOSURFACE MARGINS?**

**A :** Cavosurface margin is the junction of the prepared cavity with the inprepared surface of a tooth. By definition a line angle is the junction between two prepared portions of the cavity (two walls or walls & a floor). Hence there are no line angles at the cavosurface margins.

**49. HOW MANY LINE ANGLES ARE PRESENT IN A CLASS I CAVITY WITHOUT EXTENSION?**

**A :** EIGHT : 1) MESIO BUCCAL
2) MESIO LINGUAL

3) DISTO BUCCAL
4) DISTO LINGUAL
5) MESIO PULPAL
6) DISTO PULPAL
7) BUCCO PULPAL &
8) LINGUO PULPAL

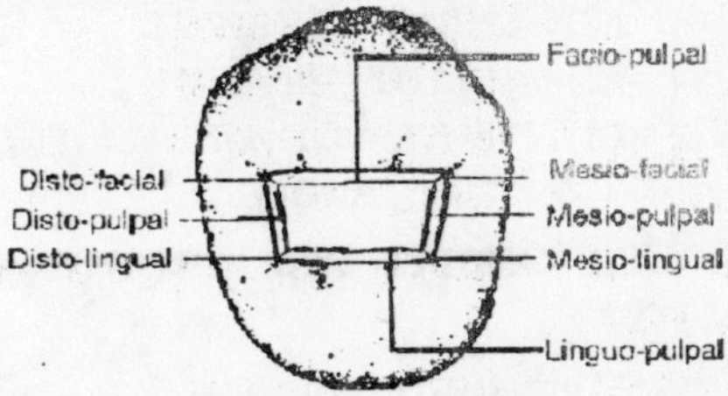


*Fig. 3.9. Class I cavity without extension*

**50. HOW MANY LINE ANGLES ARE PRESENT IN A CLASS I CAVITY WITH BUCCAL EXTENSION?**

**A :** FOURTEEN :
1) MESIO BUCCAL
2) MESIO LINGUAL
3) MESIO PULPAL
4) DISTO BUCCAL
5) DISTO LINGUAL
6) DISTO PULPAL
7) LINGUOPULPAL
8) AXIO PULPAL
9) MESIO AXIAL
10) DISTO AXIAL
11) AXIO GINGIVAL
12) MESIO GINGIVAL
13) DISTO GINGIVAL
14) PARTS OF BUCCOPULPAL LINE ANGLE

**51. HOW MANY LINES ANGLES ARE PRESENT IN A CLASS I CAVITY WITH LINGUAL EXTENSION?**

**A :** FOURTEEN :
1) MESIO BUCCAL
2) MESIO LINGUAL
3) MESIO PULPAL
4) DISTO BUCCAL
5) DISTO LINGUAL

6) DISTO PULPAL
7) BUCCO PULPAL
8) AXIO PULPAL
9) MESIO AXIAL
10) DISTO AXIAL
11) AXIO GINGIVAL
12) MESIO GINGIVAL
13) DISTO GINGIVAL
14) PARTS OF LINGUO PULPAL LINE ANGLE

**52. HOW MANY LINE ANGLES ARE PRESENT IN A CLASS II (M.O) CAVITY?**

**A :** ELEVEN :
1) DISTO BUCCAL
2) DISTO LINGUAL
3) DISTO PULPAL
4) BUCCO PULPAL
5) LINGUO PULPAL
6) AXIO PULPAL
7) BUCCO AXIAL
8) LINGUO AXIAL
9) AXIO GINGIVAL
10) BUCCO GINGIVAL
11) LINGUO GINGIVAL

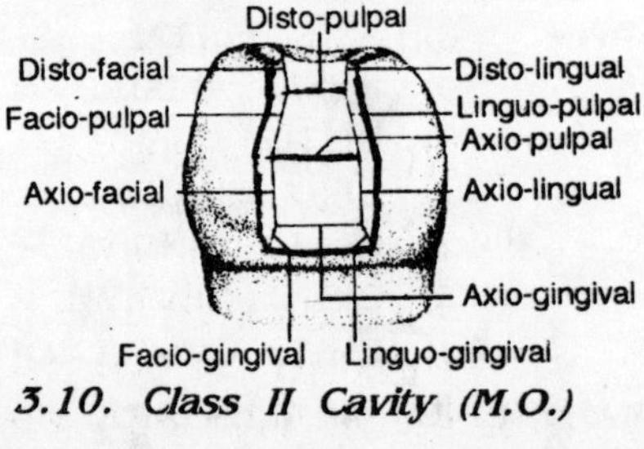


*Fig. 3.10. Class II Cavity (M.O.)*

**53. HOW MANY LINE ANGLES ARE PRESENT IN A CLASS II (D.O) CAVITY?**

**A :** ELEVEN :
1) MESIO BUCCAL
2) MESIO LINGUAL
3) MESIO PULPAL
4) BUCCO PULPAL

5) LINGUO PULPAL
6) AXIO PULPAL
7) BUCCO AXIAL
8) LINGUO AXIAL
9) AXIO GINGIVAL
10) BUCCO GINGIVAL
11) LINGUO GINGIVAL

**54. HOW MANY LINE ANGLES ARE PRESENT IN A CLASS III CAVITY LINGUAL APPROACH (NO LINGUAL WALL) WITHOUT LINGUAL EXTENSION?**

**A :** THREE : 1) AXIO GINGIVAL
2) LABIO GINGIVAL
3) LABIO AXIAL

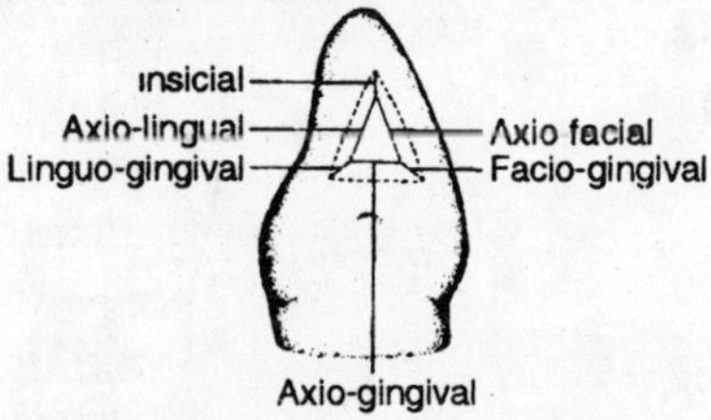


*Fig. 3.11. Class III with lingual approach without lingual exension*

**55. HOW MANY LINE ANGLES ARE PRESENT IN A CLASS III CAVITY LINGUAL APPROACH WITH LINGUAL EXTENSION?**

**A :** SIX : 1) AXIO GINGIVAL
2) LABIO GINGIVAL
3) LABIO AXIAL
4) PULPOGINGIVAL
5) PROXIMO (MESIO OR DISTO) PULPAL
6) INCISO PULPAL

**56. HOW MANY LINE ANGLES ARE PRESENT IN A CLASS IV CAVITY (LINGUAL APPROACH)?**

**A :** SEVEN : 1) AXIO GINGIVAL
2) LABIO GINGIVAL
3) LABIO AXIAL
4) AXIO PULPAL

5) LABIO PULPAL
6) LINGUO PULPAL
7) PROXIMO (MESIO OR DISTO) PULPAL

**57. HOW MANY LINE ANGLES ARE PRESENT IN A CLASS V CAVITY?**

**A :** EIGHT :
1) MESIO AXIAL
2) MESIO OCCLUSAL
3) MESIO GINGIVAL
4) DISTO AXIAL
5) DISTO OCCLUSAL
6) DISTOGINGIVAL
7) OCCLUSO AXIAL
8) AXIO GINGIVAL

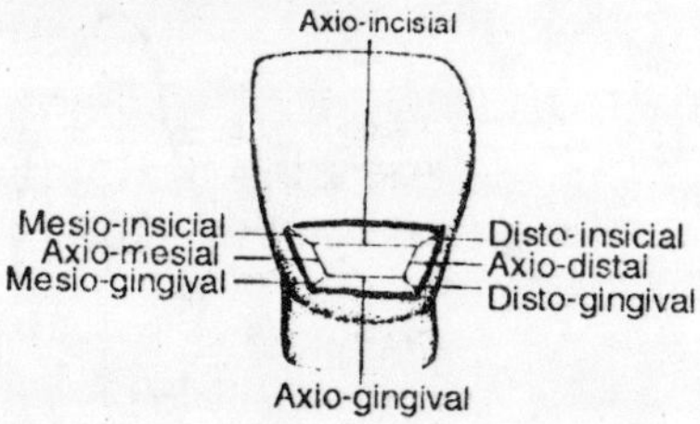


*Fig. 3.12. Class V cavity*

**58. IS IT NECESSARY TO LEARN BY HEART THE PREVIOUS NINE QUESTIONS TO KNOW THE LINE ANGLES PRESENT IN EACH CAVITY?**

**A :** No. It is easier to draw a schematic diagram of the walls & floors present & note down where they meet and name the line angles.

**59. HOW ARE THE POINT ANGLES NAMED?**

**A :** Point angles are named after the three walls or the two walls & a floor that meet at that point. Conventional order of preference in naming is :

| | | |
|---|---|---|
| FIRST | : | Proximal wall (Mesial or distal) |
| SECOND | : | Buccal (labial), Lingual (Palatal) & Occlusal (incisal) wall |
| THIRD | : | Axial |
| LAST | : | Pulpal floor & gingival seat. |

**60. HOW MANY POINT ANGLES ARE THERE IN A CLASS I CAVITY WITHOUT EXTENSION?**

**A :** FOUR : 1) Mesio bucco pulpal
2) Mesio linguo pulpal
3) Disto bucco pulpal
4) Disto linguo pulpal

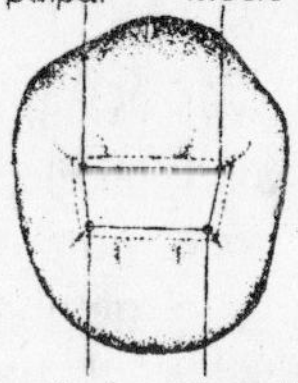


*Fig. 3.13. Class I without extension*

**61. HOW MANY POINT ANGLES ARE THERE IN A CLASS I CAVITY WITH BUCCAL OR LINGUAL EXTENSION?**

**A :** EIGHT : 1) Mesio bucco pulpal
2) Mesio linguo pulpal
3) Disto bucco pulpal
4) Disto linguo pulpal are present in the occulucal box and
5) Mesio axio pulpal
6) Disto axio pulpal
7) Mesio axio gingival and
8) Disto axio gingival are present in the buccal box

**62. HOW MANY POINT ANGLES ARE PRESENT IN A CLASS II MESIO OCCLUSAL OR DISTO OCCLUSAL CAVITY?**

**A :** SIX : 1) Disto bucco pulpal
2) Disto linguo pulpal
3) Bucco axio pulpal
4) Linguo axio pulpal
5) Bucco axio gingival
6) Linguo axio gingival.

In a disto occlusal cavity the first two point angles will be

1) Mesio bucco pulpal

2) Mesio linguo pulpal
3) Bucco axio pulpal
4) Linguo axio pulpal
5) Bucco axio gingival
6) Linguo axio gingival.

**63. HOW MANY POINT ANGLES WILL THERE BE IN A M O D CAVITY?**

**A :** EIGHT:
1) Bucco axio pulpal
2) Bucco axio gingival
3) Linguo axio pulpal
4) Linguo axio gingival.

Point angles of the same name are present in the Mesial & distal boxes.

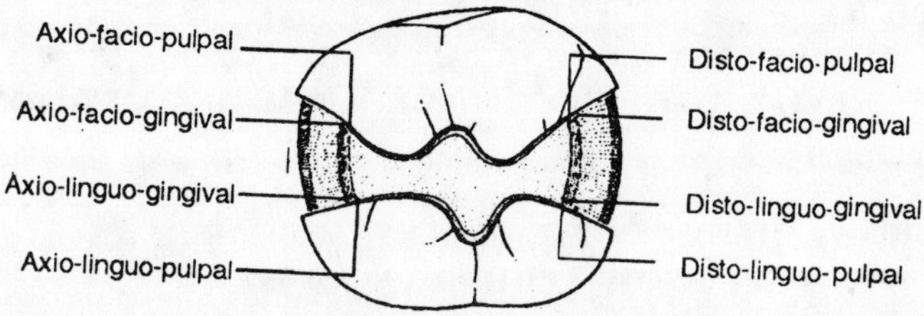


*Fig. 3.14. M.O.D. Cavity*

**64. HOW MANY POINT ANGLES WILL THERE BE IN A CLASS III CAVITY WITHOUT EXTENSION BUT WITH DIRECT ACCESS? (Intact labial & Lingual walls)**

**A :** THREE :
1) Labio axio gingival
2) Linguo axio gingival &
3) Labio linguo axial (commonly called incisal point angle)

**65. HOW MANY POINT ANGLES WILL THERE BE IN A CLASS III CAVITY WITHOUT EXTENSION BUT WITH LINGUAL ACCESS?**

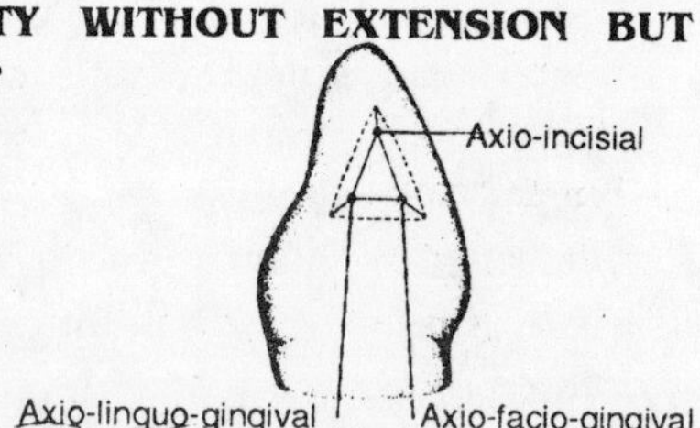


*Fig. 3.15. Cl. III without extension with lingual approach*

A : ONE : 1) Labio axio gingival

**66. HOW MANY POINT ANGLES WILL THERE BE IN A CLASS III CAVITY WITH LINGUAL ACCESS & LINGUAL EXTENSION?**

A : FIVE : 1) Labio axio gingival
2) Inciso axio pulpal
3) Axio Pulpal gingival
4) Proximo (mesio or disto) inciso pulpal
5) Proximo (mesio or disto) pulpo gingival

**67. HOW MANY POINT ANGLES ARE THERE IN A CLASS IV CAVITY WITH DIRECT ACCESS?**

A : SIX : 1) Labio axio gingival
2) Linguo axio gingival
3) Labio axio pulpal
4) Linguo axio pulpal
5) Proximo labio pulpal
6) Proximo linguo pulpal

**68. HOW MANY POINT ANGLES ARE THERE IN A CLASS IV CAVITY WITH LINGUAL ACCESS?**

A : THREE : 1) Labio axio gingival
2) Labio axio pulpal and
3) Proximo labio pulpal

**69. HOW MANY POINT ANGLES ARE THERE IN A CLASS V CAVITY?**

A : FOUR : 1) Mesio occluso axial
2) Disto occluso axial
3) Mesio axio gingival
4) Disto axio gingival

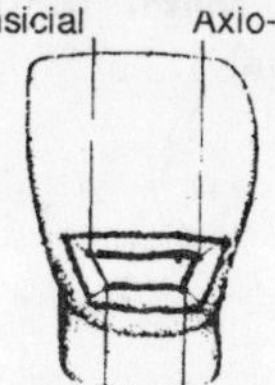


*Fig. 3.16. Class V cavity*

**70. WHAT ARE THE SIGNIFICANCES OF LINE ANGLES AND POINT ANGLES?**

**A :** 1) In olden days, all the line angles and point angles were made sharp especially with very sharp hand instruments called angle formers. Presently sharp line angles and point angles are not made as they tend to concentrate stresses within the restoration. Present concept in cavity preparation is to make definite but not sharp line angles & point angles.

2) Only for direct filling gold restorations, sharp line angles & point angles are needed to wedge & lock the condensed gold.

3) Specific retentive points like pits, coves and grooves are made at point angles and line angles for additional grip of the restoration.

4) Grooves at line angles are sometimes made to provide a single path of insertion for an extra orally made restoration.

5) Line angles and point angles prevent micro-mechanical movements of the restoration within the cavity.

**71. IN WHICH CAVITIES WILL THERE BE A GINGIVAL SEAT?**

**A :** In class I buccal or lingual extension, class II, class III, class IV & V.

**72. BOTH PULPAL FLOOR & AXIAL WALL ARE CLOSE TO THE PULP. WHY ONE IS CALLED PULPAL FLOOR & ANOTHER AXIAL WALL?**

**A :** If both are called pulpal floor, it will lead to confusion. The horizontal one is called pulpal floor and the vertical one is called axial wall.

## CHAPTER : 4

# BLACK'S CLASSIFICATION OF CAVITIES

**1. ON WHAT BASIS CAVITIES ARE CLASSIFIED?**

**A :** Cavities were classified originally based on the frequency of occurrence of Caries on some aspects of teeth.

**2. WHEN DID DR. G.V. BLACK CLASSIFY CAVITIES?**

**A :** More than 100 years ago. Still the same system of classification is followed throughout the world.

**3. INTO HOW MANY CLASSES DID DR. BLACK CLASSIFY CAVITIES?**

**A :** Originally cavities were classified into 5 classes. Class VI was added by later scientists to include cavities not included in the first 5 classes.

**4. WHY IS BLACK'S CLASSIFICATION OF CAVITIES CALLED A THERAPEUTIC CLASSIFICATION?**

**A :** Because Black's classification of cavities took into consideration the restoration designs for the caries affected teeth.

**5. IS BLACK'S CLASSIFICATION OF CAVITIES IMPORTANT FOR THE DENTAL STUDENT?**

**A :** This is one of the common questions asked in the viva voce examination for the dental student. It is expected to be answered *adverbatim* and a student is expected to know it by heart.

**6. WHAT ARE CLASS I CAVITIES?**

**A :** Cavities occurring in the pits and fissures of the occlusal surfaces of the posteriors (molars and premolars), the

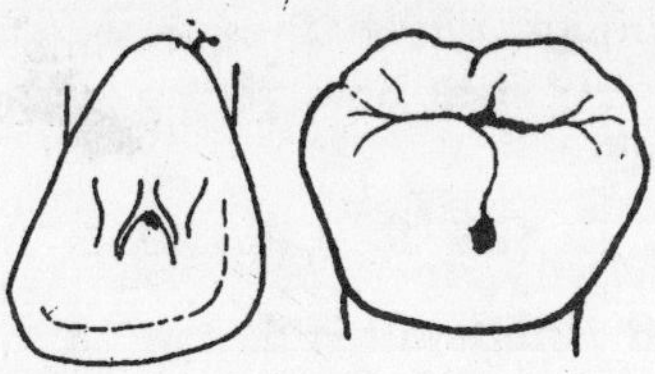

Fig. 4.1. Class I Cavity

occlusal two thirds of the buccal and lingual surfaces of posteriors and the lingual pits of the anteriors.

**7. WHAT DO THE LOCATIONS OF CLASS I CAVITIES SIGNIFY?**

**A :** Class I cavities occur on the pits and fissures that are found normally on the surface of the teeth. Pits & fissures commonly occur on the occlusal surfaces of premolars & molars, occlusal two thirds of buccal & lingual surfaces of molars (buccal & lingual pits) and lingual surface of anteriors (lingual pits). By their structure pits & fissures are potential stagnation areas.

**8. WHAT ARE CLASS II CAVITIES?**

**A :** Cavities occuring on the proximal surfaces of the posteriors (molars & premolars) are class II cavities.

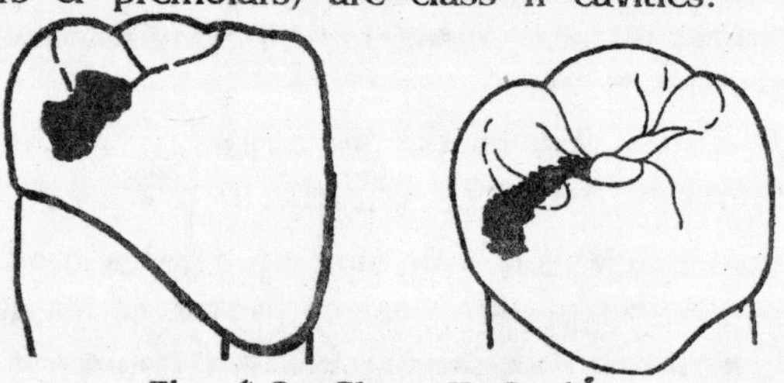

*Fig. 4.2. Class II Cavity*

**9. IF CLASS II CAVITIES INVOLVE ONLY THE PROXIMAL SURFACES, WHY DO WE HAVE AN ADDITIONAL OCCLUSAL BOX IN CLASS II CAVITIES (DISTO OCCLUSAL, MESIO OCCLUSAL)?**

**A :** Though class II cavities are restricted to only proximal surfaces, directly reaching the affected area with a cutting tool is difficult because of the close proximity of the neighbouring tooth. So, many times an occlusal cavity is prepared through which the proximal surface is reached & hence an occlusal box becomes an integral part of the class II cavity.

**10. WHAT ARE CLASS III CAVITIES?**

**A :** Class III cavities are those that occur on the proximal surfaces of anterior teeth without involvement of the incisal edge.

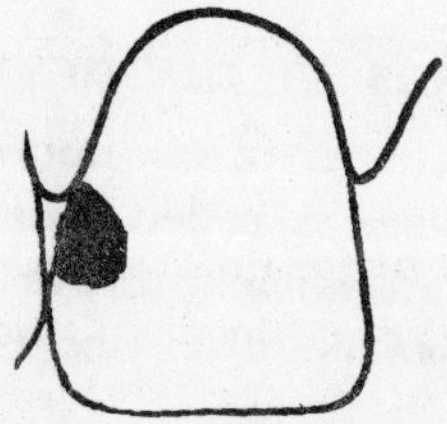

*Fig. 4.3. Class III Cavity*

**11. WHAT ARE CLASS IV CAVITIES?**

**A :** Class IV cavities are those that occur on the proximal surfaces of anterior teeth with the involvement of the incisal edge.

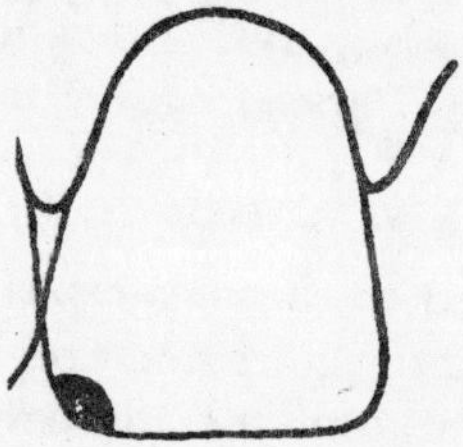

*Fig. 4.4. Class IV Cavity*

**12. IS IT POSSIBLE TO REACH THE PROXIMAL SURFACE OF THE ANTERIOR TEETH EASILY?**

**A :** Unless there is gap between teeth it is very difficult to have direct access to the proximal surface. Usually when the contact with the neighbouring tooth is close, lingual or labial access is taken in anterior teeth.

**13. WHAT ARE CLASS V CAVITIES?**

**A :** Class V cavities occur at the gingival third of the facial and lingual surfaces of all the teeth.

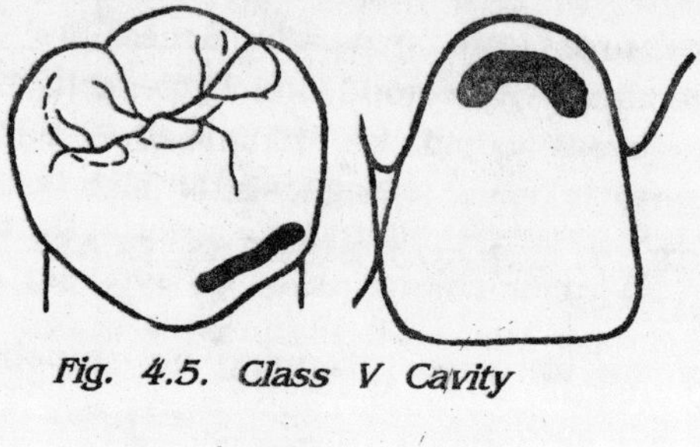

*Fig. 4.5. Class V Cavity*

**14. WHAT ARE CLASS VI CAVITIES?**

**A :** Cavities that occur in areas not covered by any of the previous five classes is called class VI cavities. They may be caries on cusptips, incisal two thirds of anterior teeth or complex cavities like disto occluso lingual, Mesio occluso buccal etc.,

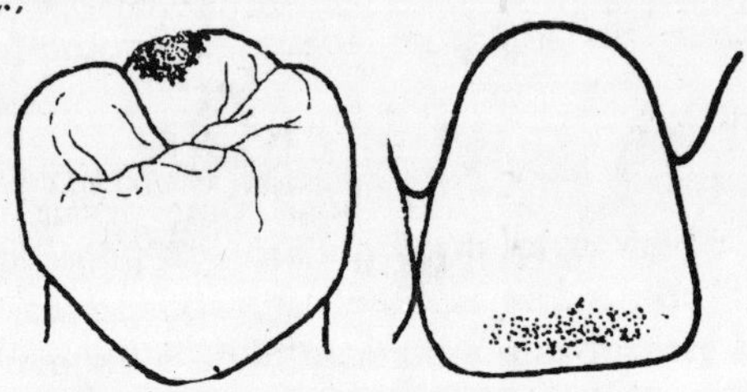

*Fig. 4.6. Class VI Cavity*

**15. WHY IS CLASS VI ADDED TO BLACK'S CLASSIFICATION?**

**A :** G.V. Black tried to classify cavities based on his observations. He tried to find some order and pattern in the caries affected teeth. But the disease need not follow any set pattern or rules. Hence there was a need to include some areas which he thought might not be attacked by caries but in reality, though rarely, might be affected.

**16. WHAT IS COMMON ABOUT CLASS II, III & IV CAVITIES?**

**A :** They are all cavities that occur on proximal surfaces of teeth. These are usually inaccessible areas for cavity preparation. During cavity preparation, most of the time, uninvolved other surface (may be occlusal, lingual or labial) is cut to reach the affected area.

**17. WHAT IS COMMON BETWEEN CLASS I & CLASS V CAVITIES?**

**A :** These areas are generally accessible to oral hygiene procedures. With good oral hygiene procedures, caries in these areas could be minimised. Self assessment of progress is easy. Diagnosis is also easier.

**8. WHAT IS COMMON BETWEEN CLASS II, III, IV & V CAVITIES?**

**A :** They are all caries occurring on smooth surfaces.

**19. IF CARIES OCCUR ON OCCLUSAL PIT AS WELL AS BUCCAL OR LINGUAL PIT OF A MOLAR. UNDER WHAT CLASS WILL IT FALL?**

**A :** It will be a class I with buccal or lingual extension.

**20. IF CARIES OCCURS ON OCCLUSAL AS WELL AS A PROXIMAL SURFACE OF A MOLAR. IS IT CLASS I OR CLASS II?**

**A :** It will be a class II cavity.

**21. IF CARIES OCCURS ON BUCCAL PIT AS WELL AS A PROXIMAL SURFACE OF A MOLAR. IS IT CLASS I OR CLASS II?**

**A :** If the two lesions are small & not interconnected they can be treated as class I cavity (buccal pit) & class II cavity affecting the same tooth. If the decay is gross & needs an interconnected large proximo occluso buccal restoration, it can be treated as a class VI restoration.

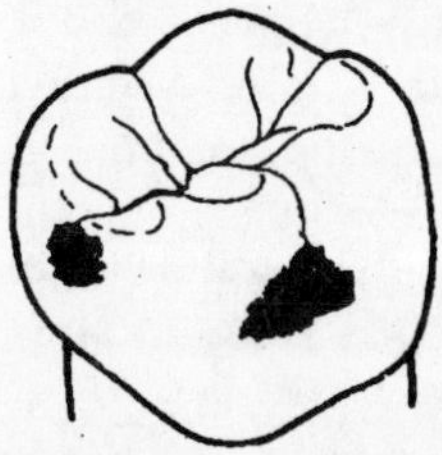

*Fig. 4.7. Caries in buccal pit & proximal surface*

**22. WHEN CARIES AFFECTS THE PROXIMAL SURFACE OF AN ANTERIOR WITHOUT INVOLVING THE INCISAL EDGE AND CARIES IN THE LINGUAL PIT. IS IT A CLASS III OR CLASS I?**

**A :** If the lesions are not interconnected they may be treated as separate class III & class I cavities. If they are to be restored with an inter connected restoration, it may be a class III with lingual extension. If the destruction is too much, it may be a class VI.

## CHAPTER : 5

# PRINCIPLES OF CAVITY PREPARATION

**1. WHAT IS CAVITY PREPARATION?**

**A :** Cavity preparation is a form of bioengineering, wherein the biological considerations supervene and sets the limit to which engineering principles could be used to obtain optimal efficiency of a restoration.

**2. WHAT DOES THE ABOVE DEFINITION MEAN?**

**A :** The purpose of restoring a defective or diseased tooth is to have a durable functional restoration. Many engineering principles are used to obtain optimal efficiency of the restoration by increasing its strength, resistance and grip over the tooth. Because tooth and surrounding structures are living tissues, due weightage and consideration should be given in causing minimal damage to them by the use of the engineering design. There is only a limit to which the engineering principles could be used. For example, if a filling is to be retained by the cavity (to stay within the cavity) the cavity should be as deep as possible. The engineering principle is deeper the cavity, better is the retention. However, in a tooth, there is living pulp tissue on the inner part of the tooth, whose vitality should be preserved whenever possible. The deeper the cavity, more chances of harming the pulp tissue. In this case, the biological consideration of preserving the pulpal vitality limits the sound engineering principle of a deeper cavity for better grip.

**3. HOW IS A CAVITY PREPARED?**

**A :** Cavities are prepared with rotary and hand cutting instruments, usually a series of steps are sequentially followed to prepare a cavity.

**4. CAVITY PREPARATION MEANS REMOVAL OF THE DAMAGED PART OF THE TOOTH, ISN'T IT? WHY A SERIES OF STEPS ARE NEEDED TO DO IT?**

A : Cavity preparation means not only the removal of the damaged portion of the tooth but also to make the tooth fit enough to receive the filling. There are certain requirements for restoring a tooth. They are

(1) Complete removal of damaged tooth tissue

(2) To make the filling as well as the remaining tooth structure strong enough to withstand chewing forces

(3) To ensure the filling stay within the cavity

(4) To remove weakened tooth tissue.

To achieve these aims, a series of steps are followed sequentially to avoid overlooking any objective.

5. **WHO FORMULATED THE STEPS IN CAVITY PREPARATION?**

A : G.V. Black advocated the steps in cavity preparation almost 100 years ago.

6. **ARE THE CENTURY OLD CONCEPTS STILL VALID TODAY?**

A : There are drastic changes in concepts, dramatic improvements in materials and dazzling developments in techniques and they have rendered some of the earlier concepts obsolete. Still, for the non-adhesive restorations, black's principles of cavity preparation provide the basic guidelines and are valid even today.

7. **WHAT ARE THE STEPS IN CAVITY PREPARATION?**

A : (1) Establishment of outline form

(2) Establishment of resistance form

(3) Establishment of retention form

(4) Obtaining the convenience form

(5) Removal of remaining caries

(6) Finishing the enamel margins

(7) Toilet of the cavity

8. **SHOULD THESE STEPS BE PERFORMED IN THE SAME SEQUENCE IN ALL CAVITIES?**

A : Not necessarily. The sequence can be altered depending on the need Moreover, while establishing one form, another form may also be partly or fully established. Some overlapping is inevitable.

## 9. WHAT IS MEANT BY OUTLINE FORM?

**A :** Outline form means the perimeter and dimensions of the cavity. It means where the margins of the cavity are to be located, what should be at various parts of the cavity and what the inner dimensions of the cavity are. The Dental surgeon should have a mental picture of the outline of a cavity before he starts cutting the tooth. In addition to the extent of the disease, there are numerous other factors that affect the extent of outline form.

## 10. LIST THE FACTORS INFLUENCING THE OUTLINE FORM?

**A :**
1) Extent of caries
2) Undermined enamel not supported by dentine
3) Extent of old faulty restoration
4) Extension for prevention - to extend to uninvolved pits & fissures
5) Enameloplasty for deep pits
6) Caries index & O H I - Conservative or Conventional cavity
7) Margins in easily cleansable areas, breaking of contact areas
8) Margin in finishable areas
9) Gingival relationship - location of gingival seat
10) Depth of cavity - location of pulpal floor
11) Maintanance of cuspal contour
12) Curved walls & avoiding sharp margins
13) Convenience for access
14) Stress bearing areas & avoiding them
15) Extension for resistance - cuspal coverage
16) Direction of enamel rods - flare of cavities
17) Type of restorative material and fabrication technique
18) Extension for retention
19) Age of the patient
20) Aesthetics

**11. HOW DOES THE EXTENT OF CARIES AFFECT OUTLINE FORM?**

**A :** Before a tooth is restored, all the caries affected portion should be removed to arrest the progress of the disease. If some caries is left in the cavity, such residual caries will be responsible for secondary caries occuring & spreading around the restoration and purpose of restoration is lost. Removal of caries should be total and the only exception, as already seen, is indirect pulp capping.

**12. HOW DOES UNDERMINED ENAMEL AFFECT THE OUTLINE FORM?**

**A :** Enamel is a very hard but inelastic substance. When supported by dentine it has very good strength. When caries penetrates through enamel up to dentinoenamel junction, there is lateral spread of decay. Though the outer enamel is unaffected, the spread of caries beneath it undermines the enamel, weakening it. One main reason for removing the undermined enamel is to reach and remove the carious dentine. For better access to the carious dentine, the undermined enamel is usually removed. Undermined enamel not supported by dentine, can not withstand masticatory forces. That is another reason why they are removed. However, in case of class III cavities with lingual access, intact labial enamel plate not supported by dentine may be permitted to remain as there is not much masticatory load on the labial surface of anterior tooth.

**13. HOW DOES AN OLD RESTORATION AFFECT THE OUTLINE FORM?**

**A :** When an old faulty restoration is to be replaced with a new restoration, obviously the extent of old restoration will decide the outline form as the old restoration as well as the secondary carries surrounding it are to be removed before refilling.

**14. WHAT IS EXTENSION FOR PREVENTION?**

**A :** It is an old concept advocated by Dr. G.V. Black wherein all the pits and fissures of the tooth are included in the cavity preparation even if they are unaffected by caries.

For example, in molar tooth even if the mesial pit alone is affected by caries and the central pit and the distal pits are completely uninvolved, the cavity is prepared to include the caries free central and distal pits. Such extension of the cavity to the involved, area is done because of the fear of possible involvement of those pits by caries at a later date. This practice is not done presently in every case. If the mesial pit alone is involved a pit cavity only is done without involving the uninvolved pits. If caries occur at a later date, in the uninvolved pits, at that time, separate cavities can be made as per the need. In older days when caries prevention methods like pit and fissue sealents or topical fluoride application were not available, may be such extension for prevention was justified. Presently, with better knowledge of caries, better oral hygiene procedures and better caries preventing techniques, such extensions for prevention (cutting for immunity) are no longer justified.

**15. IS EXTENTION FOR PREVENTION DONE FOR ANY PATIENT?**

**A :** Even now, extension for prevention is done for high caries risk patients who are not capable of maintaining a high degree of oral hygiene (for example, in mentally retanded patients, physically handicapped patients and severely mentally ill patients).

**16. WHAT IS ENAMELOPLASTY? WHERE IS IT DONE?**

**A :** Enameloplasty literally means reshaping of enamel. It is done by selective grinding of enamel. In some teeth, if steep cusps & deep pits are present, the pit might be difficult to clean. In such cases the enamel surrounding the pit are ground away so as to make the area easily cleansable. The area around the pit is made into a saucer shape for easy cleansability and enameloplasty is known as saucerization. While cutting a cavity, if an adjascent uninvolved deep pit is present, instead of extending the cavity into the deep pit, it is possible to selectively grind the enamel & make that area more easily cleansable. Such enameloplasty conserves underlying healthy dentine. A round bur or an egg shaped diamond is used for saucerization after reducing the enamel it should be smoothened with fine diamonds and polished smoothly.

**17. WHAT IS CARIES INDEX ? WHAT IS ORAL HYGIENE INDEX?**

**A :** These are indicies for assessing the status of caries level and oral hygiene level in the mouth. The indicies are supposed to reflect the caries susceptibility of the individual. D M F index means decayed, missing and filled index. In this index a score of 1 is given for any unfilled carious tooth (decayed), filled tooth and teeth extracted due to caries (missing). The sum total reflects the past carious activity. There are many short comings in the D M F index, but it is the one currently available for evaluating carious activity. Past carious activity need not necessarily mean that future caries activity will also be high. However, high caries index is usually supposed to mean a high risk patient. Currently the general trend in cavity preparation is to prepare conservative (minimal extention) cavities. Preparation of conventional (extensive, all pits & fissure including) cavities are done in patients who are prone to develop caries.

**18. IF D M F INDEX IS NOT A SURE METHOD OF PREDICTING FUTURE CARIES, HOW ELSE DO DENTAL SURGEONS RECOGNISE HIGH CARIES RISK PATIENTS?**

**A :** Dental surgeons mainly rely on their clinical judgement for deciding about a conservative or conventional outline. They assess the patient's oral hygiene, evaluate the compliance of the patient to previous caries control measures and decide whether the patient is less likely to develop caries or not. Such dependence on the Dental surgeon's experience rather than elaborate caries activity tests is the current status of predicting future caries activity for the patient.

**19. WHY THERE IS AN EMPHASIS ON CONSERVATIVE CAVITY PREPARATION?**

**A :** In spite of tremendous improvements in dental materials, we still do not have an ideal restorative material. Every dental restorative material has its own shortcoming and hence, it is not equal to normal healthy tooth structure. So while cavity cutting, the emphasis is on complete removal of the diseased tooth structure and minimal necessary removal of normal tooth structure for better resistance & retention.

**20. ARE THE DENTAL STUDENTS CURRENTLY TAUGHT ONLY THE CONSERVATIVE CAVITY PREPARATION?**

**A :** No. The students are asked to make conventional cavity preparation also because there are some special situations where such a cavity is needed. However they are strongly dissuaded against making unnecessary removal of healthy tooth structure. They are cautioned against making very deep or wide cavities.

**21. WHAT IS MEANT BY BREAKING THE CONTACT?**

**A :** For caries in inaccessible regions (class II, class III and class IV cavities) there are always some contact with neighbouring teeth. In those cases, most of the time the caries might be just below the contact & most of the contact area might be caries free. Still, the healthy contact area with the neighbouring tooth is completely broken so that the margin of the cavity is brought just outside the contact area both buccolingually and occluso cervically. The purpose of bringing the margins into the embrassure is easy cleansability. If food stagnation, plaque accumulation and acid production take place, there is a chance for secondary caries formation. To avoid this, the margins of the cavity should be kept meticulously clean and should therefore be in an easily cleansable area. In all class II cavities, the contact area is invariably broken occluso cervically as well as buccolingually and the contact area is entirely replaced with restorative material. However in anterior teeth, because of the inadequacies of anterior restorative materials, healthy contact points, if present are not completely removed but permitted to remain.

**22. IS NOT THE BREAKING OF CONTACT FOR INSERTION OF THE MATRIX BAND?**

**A :** This is the usual wrong answer a novice dental student gives. If the purpose of breaking the contact is only matrix band insertion, then it is totally unwarranted as the matrix band could be inserted easily by using separators rather then cutting the healthy tooth structure. The primary reason for breaking the contact area is to bring all the margins of the cavity in easily cleansable area.

**23. WHAT IS THE DIFFERENCE BETWEEN EASILY CLEANSABLE AREA AND EASILY FINISHABLE AREA?**

**A :** Accessibility of the margins of the cavity to finishing and polishing procedures is important in two ways. If the material is burnishable alloy (stretchable and adaptable plasitcally) then by using rotary instruments the restoration is adapted closer to the margins. This results in reduced marginal leakage. Another point is a rough restoration is more likely to be a potential area for plaque accumulation. Keeping a rough restoration clean is difficult. A rough restoration if closer to gingiva, can mechanically irritiate it also. Rough metallic restorations are more prone for tarmish and corrosion too. For all these reasons, it is absolutely necessary that every restoration should be finished and polished to a high gloss. Aesthetically also a polished restoration is more pleasing to look at. For doing a good burnishing and polishing, the margins of the restoration should be in an easily finishable area. This is another reason for breaking the contact area.

**24. FOR CAVITIES NEAR THE GINGIVAL MARGINS, WHERE SHOULD THE GINGIVAL SEAT BE LOCATED?**

**A :** The tooth - gingival interface is unique. This is one area where the soft tissue has a special attachment, with hard calcified tissue. If any irritant material is present it will not only irritate the soft tissue but may also affect the epithelical attachment. Restorations, barring well polished porcelain and gold are all irritants to gingiva. So, as for as possible, sub-gingival placement of gingiva seat should be avoided. In olden days there was an erroneous notion that sub-gingival area is less caries prone than supragingivial area. It was theoried that the gingival crevicular fluid is alkaline in nature and hence, less conducive for acidic carious activity. While it is true that crevicular fluid is alkaline in healthy gingiva if there is even minimal gingival inflammation, the crevicular fluid is no longer alkaline. Another reason for sub-gingival placement of gingival seat is supposed to be for aesthetics. i.e. even if there is marginal discrepancy, if the margin is sub-gingival, it might not be seen outside. This means there might be a leaky margin below the gingiva which will fail in the long run. So hiding an ill fitting margin below the gingiva and claiming aesthetics is not very sensible. The present concept is to have a supra-gingival margin for easy cleansability (i.e. gingival seat should be coronal to the gingival margin).

**25. DOES IT MEAN SUB-GINGIVAL MARGINS ARE NEVER MADE IN ANY CAVITY? (i.e. IS THE GINGIVAL SEAT NEVER LOCATED BELOW THE MARGINAL GINGIVA?)**

**A :** Sub-gingival margin is permitted when (1) the caries or fracture extends below the gingival level (2) while replacing an old restoration with a sub-gingival margin (3) A well fitting restoration made of biocompatible material might have a sub-gingival margin, for aesthetics.

**26. WHAT SHOULD BE THE IDEAL DEPTH OF THE CAVITY?**

**A :** The ideal depth of the cavity should be 0.5 millimeter below the dentinoenamel junction. This may be the ideal depth for many non adhesive restorations. This is supposed to be the minimal depth required for a restoration. When a cavity is made for an intraorally made incrementally added restoration, the base (bottom) of the cavity is slightly larger than the outer portion of the cavity so that after the incrementally packed restorative material hardens it is locked within the cavity and does not come out. To make a cavity of that shape in enamel alone is difficult as the unsupported enamel rods can fracture from the outer portion resulting in failure of restoration. The inelastic enamel cannot be used for making a retentive cavity. The cavity depth is increased till dentine is reached and into the elastic dentine, undercuts (broadening the bottom of the cavity) are made for locking the restoration. The cavity is not stopped at the level of the dentino enamel junction, because it will be highly sensitive. The reason for the increase in sensitivity of dentine at the dentino enamel junction is attributed to the dichotomy (branching) of dentinal tubules and the cytoplasmic extensions of the odontoblasts. For adhesive and acid etched restorations, such extensions into dentine for retention is superfluous.

**27. WILL THE PULPAL FLOOR IN ALL PARTS OF THE CAVITY BE LOCATED 0.5 MM BELOW THE DENTINO ENAMEL JUNCTION?**

**A :** In an occlusal cavity with cusps and pits, a cross section of the tooth reveals the dentino enamel junction with elevations and depressions. However on smooth surfaces (proximal, buccal & palatal) the Dentino enamel junction is almost straight. So in class I cavities, the pulpal floor is flat & may be only in the central pit or marginal pit areas it is 0.5 mm below the dentino enamel junction but in other areas it is more than 0.5 mm. In other cavities (class II, III, IV, & V) the straight dentino enamel junction permits having an axial wall 0.5 mm below the dentino enamel junction.

**28. CAN THE PULPAL FLOOR BE LOCATED MORE THAN 0.5 MM BELOW THE DENTINO ENAMEL JUNCTION IN A CAVITY?**

**A :** Having the pulpal floor at 0.5 mm below the dentino enamel junction is feasible in minimal carious lesions. However, whenever caries has progressed deeper, removal of such caries result in having atleast parts of the pulpal floor deeper than 0.5 mm from the dentino enamel junction. The ideal location of 0.5 mm below the dentino enamel junction may not be achievable in all the situations.

**29. WHAT IS MEANT BY MAINTENANCE OF CUSPAL CONTOUR?**

**A :** Pulp protection is one of the aims of restorative dentistry. As far as possible, the cavity is not made close to the pulp. This is the reason for keeping the pulpal floor at 0.5 mm below the dentino enamel junction whenever possible and not deeper. Dentine is a very good thermal insulator and the effective thickness of dentine below the cavity help in preserving pulp vitality. Maintenance of cuspal contour is another method of pulp protection. Cusps are conical in shape. Atleast in the younger teeth, pulp horns are expected to be present in the central portion of the cusps. A straight cavity (non-maintenance of cuspal contour) may leave thin dentine in some areas closer to the pulp horns endangering the health of pulp tissue within. Irritants from the restoration, thermal changes, or bacterial penetration might occur more easily. However, if the cuspal contour is maintained atleast equal dentine thickness is present between the wall of the cavity and the pulp horn offering greater protection.

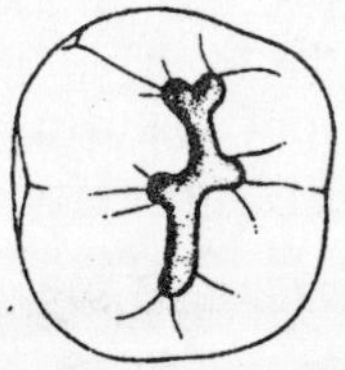

*Fig. 5.1 Maintenance of Cuspal Contour*

**30. WHY SHOULD THE CAVITY OUTLINE BE CURVED AND NOT WITH SHARP ANGLES?**

**A :** The restoration as well as the remaining tooth structure are subjected to masticatory stresses. The constant dynamic stresses on the restoration and the tooth result in development of internal strain on the material & the tooth. Within the elastic modules of the material & the tooth, these strains do not result in plastic deformation. However if the cavity has sharp corners or margins, the stresses tend to concentrate in those area & might result even in fracture of the restoration. To avoid this only, the cavity outline, both buccolingually as well as mesio distally are made of gentle curves & smooth flowing curved walls. Only pulpo occlusally are the walls straight. Junctions between the different parts of the preparation, especially those acting as fulcra, should be rounded to prevent stress concentration in both tooth structure and restoration. Such curved outline is mandatory for avoiding areas of stress concentration.

**31. HOW DOES CONVENIENCE FORM AFFECT OUTLINE FORM?**

**A :** As already seen, caries occurring in proximal surfaces of anterior and posterior teeth have problems of access (reach) to the cavity. If the neighbouring tooth on the affected side is absent, it is possible and permissible to do a cavity completely limited to the proximal side. But in many situations the neighbouring tooth is present and it is almost impossible to reach the affected area without damaging the neighbouring tooth. Hence for obtaining access to the affected area, an unaffected surface (occlusal for class II and labial/palatal for class III & IV) which is accessable is used for reaching the proximal surface. Such modifications in the outline form for convenience of access is justified as otherwise there is no other means of restoring the proximal cavity.

**32. WHAT ARE STRESS BEARING AREAS?**

**A :** It is interesting to know that when the upper and lower teeth are brought in contact, either in centric or eccentric postion, the entire occlusal surface of one tooth does not come into contact with the entire occlusal surface of its antagoinists but only some areas of the occlusal surfaces come against each other. This can be ascertained by keeping an articulating paper between the teeth and closing the jaws in various postions. Markings on the occlusal surface denote the areas of contact and these are the stress bearing areas. The significane of stress bearing areas in relation to outline form is that the margins of the restoration should never end in a stress bearing areas. If the cavity margins end in stress bearing areas, the stresses are met partially by restoration and partially by tooth structure. This can lead to pushing the restoration and tooth away from each other and will result in increased marginal leakage if not fracture of the restoration. It is imperative that in every patient, stress bearing areas should be identified before starting the cavity. If by chance the caries extension ends in a stress bearing area, care should be taken to extend the cavity over healthy tooth structure beyond the stress bearing area. In short, stress bearing areas should be entirely on natural tooth substance or entirely on the restorative material but never at the junction of restoration & tooth. Portions of cusps & ridges are usually stress bearing areas.

**33. WHAT IS MEANT BY EXTENSION FOR RESISTANCE?**

**A :** While establishing the outline form of a cavity when it is found that carious destruction has left a portion of tooth weak and incapable of withstanding masticatory load, cavity outline is extended for reinforcing the weakened area and such extension is called extension for resistance. For example, when caries has destroyed almost half the cusp, the remaining cusp may be weak. In such a situation, the height of the cusp is reduced and restoration covers the cusp, protecting and reinforcing it. Cuspal coverage is an example of extension of outline for better resistance.

**34. HOW DOES THE DIRECTION OF ENAMEL RODS AFFECT THE CAVITY OUTLINE?**

**A :** Enamel consists of enamel rods and they start from the dentino enamel junction and end up on the outer surface of enamel. The enamel rods do not have a straight course from the dentino enamel junction to the outer enamel surface. Usually they have a slightly wavy course which is more marked below cusps and ridges. But the general direction of the enamel rods are perpendicular to the dentino enamel junction. So in a vertical section of a molar tooth, the enamel rods appear to converge towards a pit from the dentino enamel junction and below a cusp, the enamel rods diverge from the Dentino enamel junction towards the cusp tip. In a horizontal cross section, the enamel rods appear to be flaring out from the dentino enamel junction to the outer surface. Because of the direction of the enamel rods, the buccal & lingual walls of the proximal box as well as the mesial and distal walls of buccal & lingual boxes of class I extension & class V cavities invariably flare out externally (The walls diverge from the axial wall to the external surface). If these walls are made to converge towards each other (with the hope of getting extra retention) it will result in lot of unsupported enamel rods (rods without its supporting base at the dentino enamel junction) which are likely to break during mastication leaving spaces between tooth and restoration (more marginal leakage).

**35. WHAT ROLE DOES THE TYPE OF RESTORATION AND THE FABRICATION TECHNIQUE HAVE IN DECIDING OUTLINE FROM?**

**A :** When a non adhesive restoration is done directly in the oral cavity, generally the cavity has a broader base and a narrower outer surface. In other words, the external outline from (outer perimeter of the cavity along the cavosurface margin) is smaller than the internal outline form (inner perimeter of the cavity along the pulpal floor and / or axial wall). This results in better retention (locking of the restoration) within the cavity. However, if the restoration is done outside the mouth, either a wax pattern is made directly in the patient's mouth, or an impression of the prepared cavity is taken to prepare a cast from which (indirectly) a wax pattern can be made. In either case, it is mandatory that the cavity is free from undercuts (areas capable of locking the material) so that the wax pattern or the impression material comes out without distortion (alteration in shape). Moreover, it is necessary for the extra-orally made restoration to be inserted and seated into the cavity without difficulty. For this reason, unlike the cavity for intraorally made non-adhesive restorations, the external outline form should not be smaller than the internal cutline form. For extra-orally made restorations, the external outline form should be slightly larger than the internal outline form (the walls of the cavity should diverge pulpo-occlusally axio proximally or gingivo-occlusally). For adhesive and acid etched restorations, box like cavity may not be necessary. Aprt from this, for burnishable materials like noble metal alloys and direct gold restorations, a cavo surface bevel (slope) is created to have a relatively thin metal margin which is burnished (adapted closely) along the margins for protecting the luting cement (cement used for fixing the restoration in place) and reducing the marginal leakage. But, for amalgam restorations, such bevels are not made along the cavosurface margins as amalgam lacks edge strength and in thin sections likely to break. For composite restorations, enamel bevels are created for having more surface area for etching with acid. While restoring a posterior tooth with composite it is wiser to have smaller occlusal outline form where possible, so that there is minimal exposure of the restorative material to chewing forces. (Micro protection). When the restoration is stronger than the tooth structure, it can protect the tooth structure. If tooth structure is stronger than the restoration, it can protect the restoration. Thus cavity outlines are modified depending on the type of restoration.

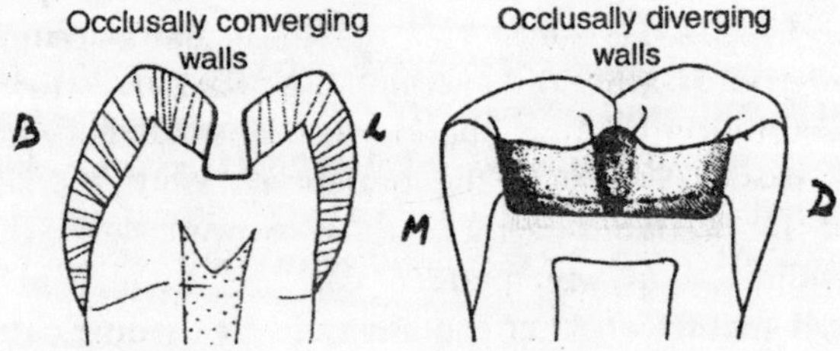


*Fig. 5.2. Taper & inverted truncated shape*

**36. WHAT IS MEANT BY EXTENSION FOR RETENTION?**

**A :** In grossly damaged carious teeth, conventional retention methods may not be enough to get good retention. It may be necessary to creat internal boxes or external retentive flare extension. Such extension for the sake of additional retention are called extension for retention and it affects the outline form. Lingual dovetail in class III restoration in an example of extension for retention.

**37. HOW DOES AGE OF THE PATIENT AFFECT THE OUTLINE FORM?**

**A :** 1) Generally a young patient is more fond of high cariogenic diet than an older patient. So the chances of caries susceptability is higher for the younger patient.

2) An older tooth is supposed to have a higher fluoride content because of the cumulative effect of exposure to fluoride from food, water supply, dentifrices (tooth pastes or powders) etc. An older tooth is likely to be more resistant to caries attack.

3) An older patient is more amenable to oral hygiene instructions and because of his maturity, capable of maintaining good oral hygiene.

4) Interproximal attrition may result in wider contact areas, in older patient.

5) In younger patients, the size of the pulp chamber as well as the pulp horns are likely to be larger, so, extra care is needed in cavity preparations. Deeper cavities in younger patients should be avoided. Generally for an elderly patient, a conservative cavity is indicated. For a younger patient, a conventional cavity is prepared.

**38. HOW DOES AESTHETICS AFFECT OUTLINE FORM?**

**A :** In anterior teeth, aesthetics plays greater role.

1) Preparation margins for restorations are preferably into embrassures (hidden areas)

2) Cavity margins to be parallel to the adjoining surfaces Kidney shaped for class V, and in class III labial approach, parallel cavity margin to proximal surface.

3) Leaving intact unsupported labial enamel for better aesthetics in class III lingual appraoch.

4) Preparation of outline in definite lines without irregularities or abrupt changes in outline.

**39. WHAT IS RESISTANCE FORM?**

It is the shape given to the cavity so that the restoration as well as the remaining tooth structure are able to withstand the masticatory forces without fracturing.

**40. WHAT FACTORS AFFECT RESISTANCE FORM?**

**FACTORS AFFECTING RESISTANCE FORM ARE :**

**A :** 1) Mortise form of a cavity

2) Floor & seat perpendicular to masticatory force

3) Cavity having definite line angles & point angles

4) Avoiding sharp corners in a cavity

5) Having sufficient bulk of restoration

6) Removing unsupported enamel from areas subjected to masticatory load

7) Preservation, where possible or minimal cutting of ridges

8) Joining two cavities if the intervening dentine thickness is less than 0.5 mm.

9) Weaker restoration being protected by tooth structure and stronger restoration protecting tooth structure.

10) Stress bearing areas to be entirely on tooth substance or on restoration.

11) Isthmus of a restoration

**41. WHAT IS MEANT BY THE WORD MORTISE?**

**A :** Mortise is an engineering terminology meaning a box like cavity. Carpenters, while joining two wooden frames cut a hole in one end of wood (mortise) and an appropriate sized projection (Tenon) in the end of another frame to be joined. The hole need not be cubical.

**42. WHAT IS MEANT BY MORTISE FORM IN DENTISTRY?**

**A :** In dentistry, the term mortise from, denotes a box like cavity where each wall and floor is in the form of a flat plane, meeting each other at definite line angles and point angles. On the occlusal surface, for maintenance of cuspal contour and avoiding stress concentration, the walls are curved and smooth flowing.

**43. HOW WILL THE CROSS SECTION OF A MORTISE FORM LOOK LIKE?**

**A :** Cross section of the mortise form could look like a cone, box or an inverted cone (inverted truncated) depending on whether the internal outline form is smaller, equal to or larger than the external outline form.

**44. HOW DOES MORTISE FORM INCREASE RESISTANCE?**

**A :** If the cavity is not box like, but say, hemispherical, forces applied on one end of the cavity can easily dislodge it, as the restoration can rotate within the cavity. A box like form, because of flat pulpal floor tends to resist forces better. In invered truncated shape, maximum amount of resistance is obtained.

**45. WHY SHOULD THE FLOOR OF THE CAVITY BE PERPENDICULAR TO OCCLUSAL FORCES?**

**A :** Whenever masticatory forces are applied to a restoration, it is transmitted to the underlying tooth structure. If the force is applied perpendicular to the floor, there is an equal and opposite force offered by the floor to resist the chewing forces. If the floor is at an angle, under the principle of inclined planes, there will be split up of the occlusal force into two components - one, perpendicular to the floor, resisted effectively by the floor and another a lateral component of force (shearing force) along the surface of the floor. Such lateral forces are harmful to the resistance of the restoration and the remaining tooth substance. Lateral components of forces do not develop when the floors of the cavity are perpendicular to the occlusal forces and walls of the cavity parallel to occlusal forces.

**46. WHAT IS THE DIRECTION OF OCCLUSAL (MASTICATORY) FORCES?**

**A :** In the oral cavity there could be compressive, tensile, shear, torsional and flexural forces because of the occlusal morphology of teeth as well as the diverse possibility of mandibular movements. However, during mastication, it is agreed that the occulusal forces are predominantly compressive in nature and are directed perpendicular to intercuspal plane because of interdigitation of the upper & lower teeth. Inter cuspal plane is an imaginary plane touching all the cusp tips of a tooth. Because occlusal forces are considered to be generally perpendicular to intercuspal plane, the pulpal floor is also made parallel to intercuspal plane.

**47. WILL THE PULPAL FLOOR ALWAYS BE HORIZONTAL?**

**A :** Pulpal floor should always be smooth and flat but it need not be always exactly horizontal. In a lower first premolar, usually the larger buccal cusp tip is at a higher level compared to the smaller lingual cusp. This means that the intercuspal plane will be lingually tilted and hence the pulpal floor will also be sloping lingually. In this case, sloping pulpal floor also permits equal thickness of restorative material bucally & lingually and also protects the larger pulp horn of the buccal cusp.

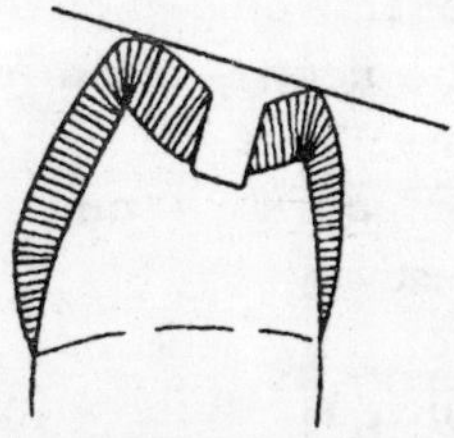

*Fig. 5.3. Pulpal Floor parallel to Occlusal plane*

**48. WHAT IS DIFFERENCE BETWEEN SHARP LINE ANGLES, INDISTINCT LINE ANGLES AND DEFINITE LINE ANGLES?**

A : Sharp line angles were once made in a cavity with angle formers for enhancing the box like structure of the cavity and increase resistance and retention. Sharp margins are found to cause stress concentration, and such cavities are no longer made nowadays, except for direct filling gold. Indistinct line angles and point angles mean the exact demarcation between walls and floors are not clearly seen. i.e, it is not easy to say where the wall ends and a floor starts. In such cases, because of the lack of firm interlocking of the restoration with the tooth, during mastication, micromechanical movement of restoration can occur. This can result in increased marginal leakage, if not in a failure of the restoration. Having a definite line angle means that the line angle is not sharp but slightly round. It is possible to say where the wall ends and the floor starts. There are neither stress concentration nor micro movements of restorations when there are definite line angles.

**49. WHY SHOULD SHARP CORNERS BE AVOIDED IN A CAVITY?**

**A :** As already seen, junctions between different parts of resoration that can act like a fulcrum should be rounded to prevent stress concentration.

**50. WHY SHOULD THE RESTORATION HAVE SUFFICIENT BULK?**

**A :** Every material's strength will vary depending on the thickness of the material. Some malleable and ductile alloys have enough strength even in thin sections. Some brittle materials like amalgam need 2 millimeter uniform thickness or atleast 1.5 milli meter for enough strength. If some restorations do not have adequate thickness, the restoration will have poor resistance.

**51. WHY SHOULD ENAMEL NOT SUPPORTED BY DENTINE BE REMOVED FROM CAVITY?**

A : Underminded enamel not supported by dentine loses 85% of its strength. If it is left on the occlusal surface to withstand masticatory load it is likely to break. So undermined enamel subjected to masticatory load should be removed.

**52. WHAT ARE THE ROLE OF RIDGES IN A TOOTH AND HOW SHOULD THEY BE TREATED DURING CAVITY CUTTING?**

A : Ridges connect cusps. Ridges withstand good amount of stresses and help transmit the occlusal forces through the axial angles to the roots of the teeth. Intact ridges prevent microscopic movements of cusps to cause abstraction (crazing of cervical a cavity, intact ridges should always he preserved. When carries has affected two pits on either side of an intact unaffected crossing ridge, it is advisable to prepare two separate cavities without cutting a large cavity involving the ridge. Experiments conducted by Vale revealed that when a single marginal ridge is cut to 1/4 of its width, about 10% of tooth's iracture resistance is lost. If 1/3 of the width of the marginal ridge is cut, about 30% of the tooth's fracture resistance is lost. If 1/2 of the width of the marginal ridge is cut about 40% of the strength of the tooth is lost. Similarly if a crossing ridge (transverse or oblique) ridge is cut to 1/4 of the inter cuspal distance about 20% of the tooth's fracture resistance is lost. By cutting 1/3 of the inter cuspal distance of a crossing ridge, about 35% of the tooth's fracture resistance is lost. If 1/2 of the inter cuspal distance of a crossing ridge is cut, about 45% of fracture strength is lost. It is advisable therefore to avoid cutting ridges. If, we are forced to cut, minimal thickness (1/4 of intercuspal distance) should be cut. If carious destruction has affected more than 1/2 of the ridge, it is advisable to protect the occlusal surface with stronger onlays. Any ridge left in the cavity should be well supported by healthy dentine. No ridge should remain undermined.

**53. WHEN SHOULD TWO ADJACENT CAVITIES BE JOINED INTO A SINGLE LARGE CAVITY?**

A : Usually it is preferable to make small conservative cavities. If two pits are involved, it is advisable to prepare two separate cavities. However, after preparing two separate adjacent cavities, it is found that the thickness of uninvolved intervening tooth structure between the two cavities is less than 0.5 mm, the intervening tooth structure may be too weak and it is preferable to join the two cavities into a single large cavity. Weakned tooth structure if left between the two cavities might fracture during occlusal loading resulting in failure of restoration.

**54. WILL THE RESISTANCE FORM DEPEND ON THE STRENGTH OF RESTORATION ?**

**A :** Yes. Depending on the strength of the restoration, the extent to which the material could be subjected to occlusal loading should be decided. As already seen, a weaker restoration should not be exposed to masticatory load (macroprotection) and when the remaining tooth structure (after cavity presentation) is weak, it is advisable to protect such weakened tooth structure by stronger restorations (like cuspal coverage).

**55. WHAT IS THE RELATIONSHIP BETWEEN STRESS BEARING AREAS AND RESISTANCE FORM?**

**A :** Stress bearing areas of the occlusal surface bear maximum load during mastication. Such areas should be either entirely on strong restoration or on natural tooth surface. Never should an individual stress bearing area rest partly in tooth and party on restoration.

**56. HAVE NOT SOME OF THE FACTORS AFFECTING RESISTANCE FORM ALREADY BEEN SEEN AS THOSE AFFECTING OUTLINE FORM?**

**A :** Yes. The reason is some factors are interconnected. The resistance form itself is capable of altering the outline form. That is, for reasons of increasing resistance. Certain modifications in cavity outline are made. Some factors that directly affect the resistance form indirectly affect the outline form.

**57. IN ANY COMPOUND CAVITIES (CARIES INVOLVING TWO SURFACES OF TOOTH) OR COMPLEX CAVITIES (CARIES**

**INVOLVING THREE OR MORE SURFACE OF TEETH) WHAT IS THE ROLE OF ISTHUMUS?**

**A :** Isthmus is the junction of two boxes. It is the neck portion of the cavity (or restoration) joining two portions of the cavity (or restoration), clinically many restorations fail in the isthumus areas. Designing the isthmus areas needs careful planning because we should neither weaken the restoration nor the tooth structure. If it is a very braod isthumus, the restoration is strong but the remaining tooth structure is weak. If it is a very narrow isthumus the remaining tooth structure is strong but the restoration is weak. In isthumus areas potentially harmful tensile forces develop under any type of occlusal forces. Photoelastic studies of stress in such restorations have revealed (a) fulcrum of bending at the auxiopulapl line angle (b) stresses increase closer to the surface of restoration & (c) tensile stresses predominate at the marginal ridge area of restoration. To avoid this (1) axio pulpal line angle is rounded or beyeled. (2) axial wall is slanted towards the pulpal floor (this provides greater amalgam bulk in marginal ridge areas) (3) Increasing the depth rather than width of isthumus. By including these features it is possible to increase the resistance of the isthumus area of the restoration to occlusal loading.

**58. WHAT IS MEANT BY RETENTION FORM?**

**A :** Retention form is that shape given to the cavity to prevent dislodgement of the restoration due to masticatory loading.

**59. WHAT ARE THE TYPES OF RETENTION?**

**A :** Retention could be intracoronal or extracoronal in nature. When retention is obtained by modifying the internal anatomy of cavity, it is intracoronal retention. When retention is obtained by modifying the external surface of the tooth it is extra coronal retention.

**60. IS RETENTION CLASSIFIED IN ANY OTHER WAY?**

**A :** Retention is also classified as primary and secondary (principal and auxillary). It is desirable to have atleast one principal mode of retention is every cavity design.

**61. WHAT ARE THE PRINCIPAL MODES OF RETENTION?**

**A :** There are form principal modes of retention. They are (1) Frictional retention (2) Inverted turncated shape (3) Elastic deformation of dentine (4) Specific undercuts (5) Dovetail.

**62. WHAT IS FRICTIONAL RETENTION?**

**A :** When two materials are in close contact, the friction between the two materials itself help in retaining the restoration. While frictional retention plays a siginificant role for all the restoration, it plays a greater role in extraorally made restorations.

**63. WHAT FACTORS INFLUENCE FRICTIONAL RETENTION?**

**A :** (1) The total surface area contact

(2) Presence of opposing walls

(3) Parallelism & near parallelism of walls.

(4) Close proximity between restoration and tooth.

**64. DESCRIBE ABOUT SURFACE AREA CONTACT ?**

**A :** Greater surface area means greater friction. Depending on the length, breadth and depth of the cavity, there could be greater friction and better retention.

**65. HOW DOES OPPOSING WALLS HELP?**

**A :** More the number of opposing walls, better will be retention. In a class I cavity without extension, the buccal and lingual walls form, one set of opposing walls and Mesial and distal walls form another set of opposing walls. If any of these walls is involved by caries and is missing, retention will proportionately be reduced.

**66. WHAT IS MEANT BY PARALLELISM & NEAR PARALLELISM OF WALLS?**

**A :** For good frictional retention, even if large surface area of contact is present & even if all the opposing walls are intact, unless the walls are parallel to each other or atleast as nearly parallel to each other, the frictional retention might be less. This is the reason for having minimal taper for inalys, onlays & crowns. Ideally, having exact parallel walls for an extraorally made restoration provides maximum retention. However, while preparing a cavity with a rotary instrument and the human eye as the evaluator, it is difficult to achieve parallelism. To allow for this human fraility, slight tapering of walls are permitted (2 to 5° for each wall depending on the length of the preparation - Smaller degree of taper for shorter preparations and greater degree of taper for longer preparation) Greater will be frictional retention when the walls are as close to parallelism as possible.

**67. HOW DOES CLOSE PROXIMITY BETWEEN RESTORATION AND TOOTH HELP GAIN RETENTION ?**

**A :** Only when there is close approximation between restoration and tooth, will friction develop. For closer adaptation of restorative material to the tooth, smoothness of the tooth preparation, wetability of the restorative material and the condensation pressure applied over the material are important.

**68. WHAT IS INVERTED TRUNCATED SHAPE OF THE CAVITY?**

**A :** It means the internal outline form (inner dimensions of the cavity) is larger than the external outline form (outer dimensions of the cavity at the cavo surface margins). Inverted truncated shape is a common mode of retention for Intraorally fabricated incrementally added non adhesive restorations. It commonly means pulpo occlusal/gingivo occlusal convergence of the walls. When a cavity has large inner dimensions with a smaller outer dimensions, restoration with material is packed into the cavity and after it hardens and becomes a homogeneous mass it can not come out through the orifice.

**69. IN A CLASS I CAVITY WITHOUT EXTENSION WILL ALL THE WALLS HAVE A PULPO OCCLUSAL CONVERGENCE?**

**A :** In a class I cavity without extensions only the buccal and lingual walls have a pulpoocclusal convergence. If the mesial and distal walls also have a pulpo occlusal convergence, it will no doubt enhance the retention. But such pulpo occlusal convergence of mesial marginal and distal marginal ridges and weaken those stress bearing areas. So the mesial wall and distal walls are either parallel to each other (vertical) or may even have slight pulpo occlusal divergence (to provide a broader base for the marginal ridges). Such pulpo occlusal divergence of mesial and distal walls will not reduce retention as the longer buccal and lingual walls provide sufficient pulpo occlusal convergence for the required retention. While preparing a cavity, a dental surgeon should judiciously evaluate all the factors and selectively apply them without compromising any form of the restoration.

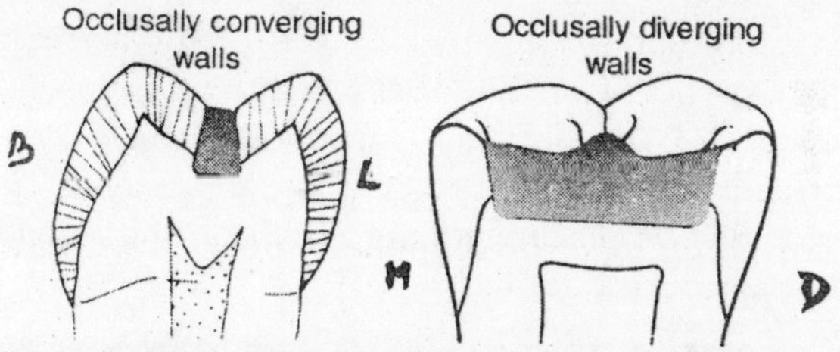


*Fig. 5.4. Amalgam Cavity*

**70. CAN THE INVERTED TRUNCATED SHAPE OF THE CAVITY BE DONE FOR ALL CLASSES OF CAVITY?**

**A :** Inverted truncated shape cannot be made for all cavities for non adhesive intraorally fabricated incrementally added restorations. The reason has nothing to do with the filling material, but with the interfence with resistance features of the cavity. For example, in a class II cavities, in the occlusal box, the buccal and lingual walls can have pulpo occlusal convergence for retention. In the proximal box again, the buccal and lingual walls can have gingivo occlusal convergence to provide retention in an occlusal direction, but there cannot be any axioproximal convergence of buccal and lingual walls from the axial wall to the proximal surface because of the necessity of breaking the contact (to bring the margins of the cavity to easily cleansable and finishable area) and also considering the direction of enamel rods. These reasons negate the possibility of having a inverted truncated shape in the proximal direction to provide retention in a proximal direction.`

**71. IN A CLASS II RESTORATION, WHY IS RETENTION IN A PROXIMAL DIRECTION NEEDED? WON'T THE NEIGHBOURING TOOTH PREVENT THE MOVEMENT OF THE RESTORATION IN A PROXIMAL DIRECTION?**

**A:** Dependence on a neighbouring tooth to retain a proximal restorations is foolish. Every box in a restoration should have its own retention in all directions. A neighbouring tooth has its own physiological movements. To that extent it can permit the proximal restoration to move too. At a later date if the neighbouring tooth is lost due to any reason, what will happen to the proximal restoration that was dependent on this tooth for its retention in a proximal direction? The proximal restoration has to depend on the occlusal interlocking to resist the proximal displacement, which will be placing greater strain on the retentive features of the occlusal box.

**72. IF INVERTED TRUNCATED SHAPE CAN NOT BE MADE IN A PROXIMAL DIRECTION, HOW IS RETENTION GIVEN IN THE PROXIMAL BOX?**

**A:** Inverted truncated shape, through, is an important mode of providing retention, is not the only mode of giving retention. Other ways are used to provide the proximal restoration with retention in a proximal direction.(See Q.83. Ch. V)

**73. CAN'T INVERTED TRUNCATED SHAPE BE USED IN ANY OTHER CAVITY EXCEPT CLASS I AND CLASS II CAVITIES TO PROVIDE RETENTION IN AN OCCLUSAL DIRECTION?**

**A:** It is used in class III cavities, while making a proximal cavity with a lingual or labial access, if sufficient tooth structure is available, the incisal wall is made. From the labial or lingual wall as the case may be the incisal wall & gingival seat converge (Labio lingual convergence or linguo labial convergence) towards the access area. This helps in providing retention in a lingual or labial direction. However, there can not by any axio proximal convergence to provide retention in a proximal direction.

**74. CAN INVERTED TRUNCATED SHAPE BE PROVIDED FOR CLASS V CAVITIES?**

**A:** No. Occlusal wall, gingival seat, Mesial wall & distal wall - all the walls diverge from the axial wall to the outer surface. This is due to the divergence of the enamel rods (their direction from the dentino enamel junction) for retention of a non-adhesive restoration in a class V cavity, other means of retention are provided. (See Q.83, Ch.V)

**75. HOW DOES ELASTIC DEFORMATION OF DENTINE HELP INCREASE RETENTION?**

**A:** Dentine is elastic in nature. While condensing some restoration (like silver amalgam) in dentine, greater condensation energy is applied to microscopically alter the walls of dentine away from each other, resulting in packing more restorative material within the cavity. After the restoration hardens and dentine slowly regains its original position, there is more gripping action & better retention.

**76. WHAT ARE UNDERCUTS?**

**A:** Undercuts are specifically made in some line angles of the cavity to increase the retention when other modes of retention are inadequate. Undercut is different from inverted truncated shape. If inverted truncated shape of the cavity is satisfactory, undercuts may be superfluous.

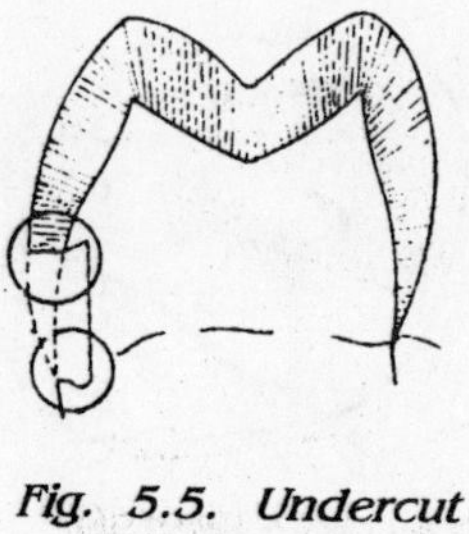

*Fig. 5.5. Undercut*

**77. WITH WHAT INSTRUMENT IS AN UNDERCUT MADE?**

**A:** An inverted cone bur is used for making specific undercuts.

**78. WHAT PRECAUTIONS ARE NECESSARY WHILE PREPARING UNDERCUTS?**

**A :** Care should be taken not to undermine the superficial enamel. Undercuts should always be made in deeper parts of the dentine leaving sufficient dentine above to support the enamel. Moreover, while cutting the undercut along a line angle, the cut is made in the wall & not into the floor. While filling the cavity, care is taken that the base does not fill up the undercut area but only the restorative material is packed into the undercut for obtaining the desired retention.

**79. WHAT IS A DOVETAIL?**

**A:** It is a modification of the outline form for the sake of additional retention. Because the modification looks like the tail of the dove, it is called dovetail preparation. Dovetail shape acts like inverted truncated shape only. Dovetails help in retention in a proximal direction. Cavities where inverted truncated shape in a proximal direction can not be made (class II & class III cavities) dovetail extensions are made in other parts of the cavity to hold the proximal restoration from dislodging proximally. For class II restoration an occlusal dovetail helps restrict proximal movement of the proximal restoration. For class III cavities a lingual dovetail not crossing the middle of the lingual surface enhances retention of the restoration in a proximal direction.

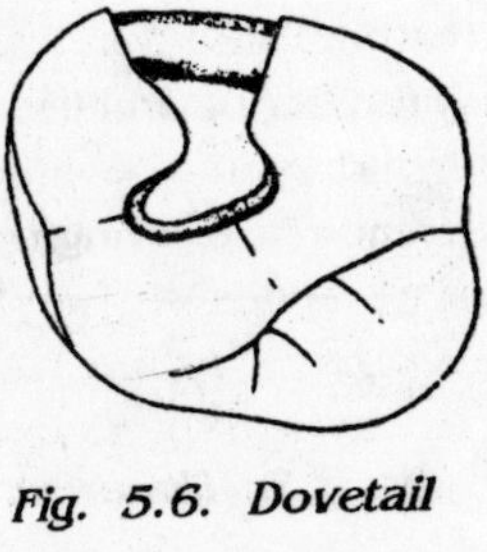

*Fig. 5.6. Dovetail*

**80. ARE THE DOVETAILS ALWAYS INTENTIONALLY PREPARED?**

**A:** The lingual dovetail for a class III restoration is invariably intentionally made. In case of the occlusal dovetail for a class II, most of the time the cavity has to broaden beyond the isthmus area to include the buccal & lingual grooves going from the central pit. Such unintentional formation of an occlusal lock (dovetail) also help in providing retention in a proximal direction for the proximal restoration.

**81. WHAT ARE AUXILLARY (SECONDARY) MODES OF RETENTION?**

**A:**
1. Pits, coves or grooves.
2. Internal boxes
3. Posts for Non-vital teeth
4. Pins
5. Gingival lock
6. Acid etching
7. Adhesive restorations or use of dentine adhesives
8. Luting cements.

**82. IS IT PROPER TO CLASSIFY ACID ETCHING AS WELL AS DIRECT BONDING AS AUXILLARY MODES OF RETENTION WHEN MANY RESTORATIONS PRESENTLY USED DO NOT RELY ON ANY OTHER MODE OF RETENTION?**

**A:** May be it is wrong to classify adhesive restorations and acid etched restorations that depend only on chemical bonding or micromechomical bonding with resin tags as having only secondary mode of retention. Developments in materials science are bringing newer materials solely relying on dentine adhesive bonding agents for retention. It may not be wrong in future to classify acid conditioning and bonding as another principal mode of retention.

## 83. WHAT ARE PITS, COVES AND GROOVES?

**A:** Pits and coves are retentive features made at a point angle while groove is a retentive feature made at a line angle. Pits, coves & grooves could be made with a round bur. Where space is a constraint, a pit or a cove is made and when enough space is available, a groove is made. For example, in a class III cavity, a pit or cove is made in the incisal angle of the cavity and a groove is made at the axiogingival line angle at the expense of gingival seat. A pit is spherical in shape but cove is pouch like in a shape. Depending on the available space either of them is made. The deeper the pit or a cove is made, further away from the pulp should it be. These pits, cove or grooves should be filled with restorations to lock them firmly. If a base enters these groove or pit, then the desired retention for the restoration might not be obtained. For a proximal box of a class II cavity, retentive grooves are made at the buccoaxial line angle at the expense of buccal wall, linguo axial line angle at the expense of lingual wall and gingivo axial line angle at the expense of gingival seat. All these grooves provide retention for the proximal box in a proximal direction. For a class V restoration, retentive grooves are made at occlusoaxial line angle at the expense of occlusal wall & gingivoaxial line angle at the expense of the gingival seat. As already stated, these retentive grooves should be filled with restorative material for locking the restorations.

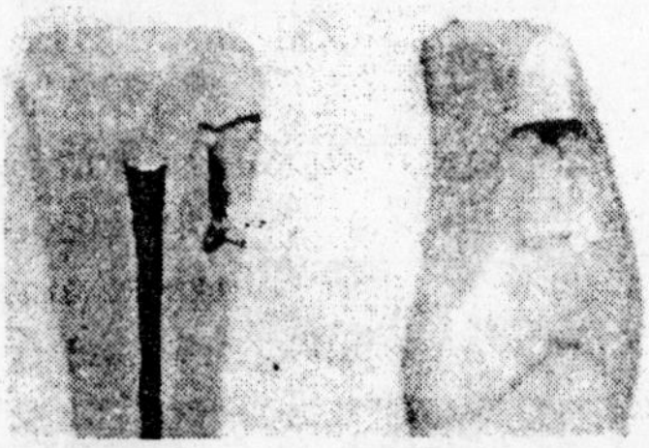

*Fig. 5.7. Pits, Coves and Grooves*

**84. WHAT ARE INTERNAL BOXES? WHERE ARE THEY MADE?**

**A:** In a grossly decayed tooth, when there are not adequate coronal tooth structure for giving other retentive features, internal boxes are made in the dentine in areas less likely to result in pulpal exposures (like gingival seat). Such retentive boxes with walls & floor can provide the desired additional retention. Slots are smaller & narrower boxes.

**85. WHAT ARE POSTS?**

**A:** In root canal treated teeth (endodontically treated nonvital teeth) without enough coronal tooth structure, wrought or cast posts either ready made or custom made are fixed into the root canal & crown portion of the tooth can be built around the posts. While posts are means of retention for building the coronal tooth structure of a non vital tooth, it must be remembered that they do not have any role in vital tooth cavity preparation.

**86. WHAT ARE PINS?**

**A:** Pins are like tiny screws or small thumb tacks. They may be ready made or custom made cast pins. Ready made pins are either cemented, screwed or tapped into tiny pinholes made in dentine with a special drill. A portion of the pin will be buried into the dentine and the portion with a pinhead jutting into the cavity. Restorative materials are packed around the projecting pinhead and below it. After the restoration hardens the larger pinhead will prevent the restoration from slipping over the pin. The pin literally ties the restoration with the tooth. Cast pin will invariably be part of a casting and is cemented along with the restorations.

**87. WHAT IS GINGIVAL LOCK?**

**A:** Gingival lock is also known as reverse bevel. It is a way of increasing the retention in the proximal box of a class II cavity. Usually gingival seat is made horizontal so that it is perpendicular to the occlusal forces to offer good resistance. If the gingival seat is tilted outwards (cervically) there will be development of lateral component of force trying to break the proximal restoration. This is the reason for making the gingival seat horizontal. But, for increasing retention, slight slanting of dentinal portion of the gingival seat inwards (pulpally) is made. This leads to development of a horizontal component of force that tend to force the proximal restorations towards the tooth help retain it. Reverse bevels could be made in the gingival seat be using distal gingival marginal trimmer in the mesial gigival seat and mesial gingival marginal trimmer in the distal gingival seat.

**88. WHAT IS ACID ETCHING TECHNIQUE?**

**A:** Acid etching is an innovating method of providing retention for a composite restoration. In this technique, cleaned enamel surface is isolated from moisture. 30 to 50 percent, usually 37 percent phosphoric acid is applied over the clean polished enamel surface for 15 to 60 seconds. After that, the enamel surface is cleaned with water. During the acid application, enamel would have been attacked by acid with the calcium phosphate minerals of the enamel rods dissolving in the acid. During washing with a water spray the dissolved minerals and the unutilized acids are washed away leaving only the undissolved organic portion network intact. After thoroughly washing for 60 to 90 seconds with water, the tooth is dried with oil free air. The etched enamel surface gives a white frosty appearance. No contamination should occur at this juncture. Enamel bonding agent (resin matrix of the composite resin) liquid is applied gently in the etched area with a brush. The liquid bonding agent flows into the empty rod space. The bonding agent may be chemical or light activated. Once the resin is polymerized, the resin tags that have entered into the tortuous enamel rod space are firmly locked and a composite restoration placed over the bonding agent chemically unites with it and is retained by the resin tags flown into the etched area. Such selective demineralization of enamel by acid & subsequent resin penetrations & resin tag formation forms the basis for acid etched restorations.

**89. WHAT ARE ADHESIVE RESTORATIONS?**

**A:** Currently, there is only one adhesive restoration though there are two adhesive cements. The two adhesive cements are (i) poly carboxylate and (ii) glass ionomer and glass ionomer is the restorative cement. Zinc polycarboxylate is rarely used as a temporary restoration. These adhesive restorations tend to bond chemically with the calcium of the tooth. The bond strength of unmodified glass ionomer is less than that of dentine bonding agents. However, improvements in glass ionomers will yield better adhesive restorations in future. Resin restoration made with dentine bonding agents have good bond strength.

**90. WHAT MODIFICATIONS ARE MADE IN THE CAVITY, FOR ADHESIVE AND ACID ETCHED RESTORATIONS?**

**A:** The conventional box like cavity advocated by G.V. Black is not made. Outline form is very conservative & is limited to removal of diseased tooth structure. Modifications for retention and resistance are minimal. Grossly weakened enamel is removed. When caries is not present, cavity cutting is not done but only preparing the cavity surface is done. In future if these restorations supervene, may be cavity cutting will become obsolete (outdated).

**91. WHAT ARE THE ROLE OF LUTING CEMENT IN RETAINING AN EXTRA ORALLY MADE RESTORATIONS?**

**A:** The luting cements are primarily used to occupy the space between the extra orally made restoration and the and the tooth surface. Non adhesive luting cements provide retention by micro mechanical bonding - the cement flows into the irregularities in the tooth surface and the irregularities on the fitting surface of the restoration. Adhesive cements like glass ionomer and polycarboxylate chemically bond to the tooth surface & only micro mechanically bond with the restoration. For any extraorally made restorations, frictional mode of retention is the primary mode of retentions rather than the retention provided by the luting cement.

**92. WHAT IS MEANT BY CONVENIENCE FORM?**

**A:** Convenience form is the shape given to the cavity for operating convenience for the dental surgeon. It could be convenience for access, convenience for visibility and convenience for instrumentation.

**93. WHAT IS CONVENIENCE FOR ACCESS?**

**A:** As already seen in outline form establishment, proximal cavities are reached from the occlusal for class II, from the lingual or labial side for class III cavities because of inadequate access due to the presence of neighbouring teeth. Such extensions of outline for gaining access to the carious lesion is known as convenience for access.

**94. WHAT IS CONVENIENCE FOR VISIBILITY?**

**A :** It is slight alterations or extention made in the cavity for assessing the internal features of the cavity.

**95. WHAT IS CONVENIENCE FOR INSTRUMENTATION?**

**A:** The inner cavity dimentions should be such as to permit use of instruments for cavity refinement, caries removal, base placement, condensing restorations and finishing the restorations. The instruments must be able to reach into all the parts of a cavity. This does not mean that the cavity should be widened to receive all the large sized instruments a dentist has. The cavity should permit the insertion of small sized instrument for achieving a specific purpose of either caries removal, base placement or condensation. All the dental students are advised to buy only the smallest size of hand instruments and small sized burs.

**96. HOW IMPORTANT IS CONVENIENCE FORM IN CAVITY PREPARATION?**

**A:** Unnecessary cutting of healthy tooth structure only for the sake of convenience is to be discouraged. While extending a cavity for gaining access is inevitable, as for as possible, extention for instrumentation should be avoided by procuring smaller instruments and extentions for better visibility should not be done unless absolutely needed. Regarding the relative important of conveneince from in relation to other steps in cavity preparation, may be this is least important.

**97. WHAT IS MEANT BY "REMOVAL OF REMAINING CARIES"?**

**A:** During establishment of outline form, all enamel caries and dentinal caries upto pulpal floor and/or axial wall level would have already been removed. After establishing the resistance form, retention form, may be some more caries had been removed. At this stage, any caries that remains on the deeper part of the cavity is removed carefully without causing damage to the pulp.

**98. WHY REMOVAL OF ALL CARIES IS NOT THE FIRST STEP IN ANY CAVITY PREPARATION?**

**A:** Caries attack the teeth in an irregular way. If attempts are made for complete caries removal as a first step, there is a tendency for over cutting It might end up in a larger cavity. It is advisable to incorporate the retentive & resistance features as far as possible before complete caries removal is attempted. However in grossly carious badly mutilated tooth, caries removal might be the first step and placement of an interim restoration for arresting the caries & hoping for reparative dentine formation may be the aim. A permanent restoration may be planned, designed and executed later.

**99. SHOULD ALL CARIES BE REMOVED BEFORE DOING A FILLING?**

**A :** Yes, to avoid leaving residual caries that could lead to secondary (recurrent) caries. As already seen, only when it is felt that the removal of caries from pulpal floor or axial wall is likely to cause pulpal exposure jeopardising a healthy pulp, is the carious lesion left and indirect pulp capping done. Otherwise all caries should be removed form the cavity.

L

**100. WHAT INSTRUMENTS ARE USED FOR REMOVING THE DEEP CARIES?**

**A:** Either a large round steel bur (size 4) driven in slow speed (micromotor or airmotor) hand piece or a hand instrument like spoon excavator or a discoid is used for removal of deep caries.

**101. WHY A HIGH SPEED ROTARY INSTRUMENT (AIROTOR) NOT USED FOR REMOVING DEEP CARIES?**

**A:** A hand instrument or a slow speed rotary instrument has greater operator control than a high speed rotary instrument. Chances for over cutting and accidental traumatic exposure of pulp is higher with airotor.

**102. WHY A STEEL BUR IS PREFERRED OVER A DIAMOND POINT OR TUNGSTEN CARBIDE BURS?**

**A:** Steel bur at slow speed cuts dentine better & a steel bur also has more flutes than a carbide bur. Tungsten Carbide bur cuts dentine better at high speed and diamond point cuts enamel better at high speed.

**103. WHY A LARGE STEEL BUR IS USED FOR DEEP CARIES REMOVAL?**

**A:** With a large bur, chances of penetration through the dentine into the underlying pulp is less.

**104. HOW IS THE LARGE STEEL BUR USED IN DEEP CARIOUS LESION?**

**A:** The large steel bur in a slow speed hand piece is moved in brushing strokes from the periphery to the centre. Very light force is used in a wiping motion without any downward pressure towards the pulp. It is preferable to use bur with water coolant spray.

**105. HOW SHOULD THE HAND INSTRUMENT BE USED FOR DEEP CARIES REMOVAL?**

**A:** Either a spoon excavator or a discoid that will conveniently fit into the cavity is selected. The sharp edges are used from the periphery of the carious lesion to the centre used to peel off the layers of soft carious lesions. If the excavator is used from the centre to the periphery, too much pressure might be applied over the thin dentine separating the pulp resulting in its fracture and pulpal exposure.

**106. CAN A TUNGSTEN CARBIDE ROUND BUR BE USED FOR REMOVING DEEP CARIES?**

**A:** Tungsten carbide round burs at high speed may be used for removing hard carious dentine that occur in chronic decay. Use of air coolant directed at the revolving bur help dissipate the frictional heat generated. A tungsten carbide bur with air coolant is a high speed hand piece run at a lesser speed (just above the stall out speed) could be used with minimal pressure pulpally. This gives greater control, better visibility and easy of removal.

**107. CLINICALLY HOW TO DIFFERENTIATE CARIOUS DENTINE IN ACUTE DECAY AND CHRONIC DECAY?**

**A :** 1. Shorter duration (in months) for acute decay. Longer duration (in years) for chronic decay.

2) Acute decay is easily excavated & chronic decay in difficult to remove with an excavator.

3) Colour of chronic decay is dark brown or black. Acute caries is usually straw yellow.

4) No odour in acute decay but it may be foul smelling in chronic decay.

5) Acute decay usually occurs in younger individuals. Chronic decay usually occurs in older individuals.

6) Acute decay is easily penetrated by an explorer but chronic decay is difficult to penetrate

7) Acute decay may be more sensitive than chronic decay.

**108. WHAT IS THE ROLE OF CALCIUM HYDROXIDE IN INDIRECT PULP CAPPING?**

**A:** Calcium hydroxide in highly alkaline in nature. It neutralizes the acids produced in the carious lesion. It alters the pH of the area so that further carious destruction does not occur. Calcium hydroxide is also bactericidal. It destroys the microorganisms in that area. It may also induce formation of reparative dentine by odontoblasts.

**109. AFTER REMOVAL OF REMAINING CARIES, HOW IS THE UNDERLYING PULP PROTECTED?**

**A:** After removal of remaining caries, depending on the thickness of remaining dentine between the cavity and pulp, various pulp protection methods are used. When there is more than two millimeter thickness of remaining dentine only coatings of cavity varnish may be needed. Cavity varnishes are natural or synthetic resins dissolved in a volatile vehicle like chloroform, ether or acetone. The copal resin or couri resin applied over the dentine tend to block the exposed dentinal tubules. When the thickness of remaining dentine is less than two millimeter, application of medicinal liner containing either Zinc Oxide Engenol or Calcium hydroxide help in getting some therapeutic benefit from the application. Slightly inflamed pulp gets sedative benefit from Zinc Oxide Engenol & possible repairative dentine formation might follow application of calcium hydroxide. When the thickness of remaining dentine is less than 0.5 millimeter it is advisable to give a sub base (thicker liner) of calcium hydroxide, glass ionomer or Zinc Oxide Engenol.

**110. WHAT IS MEANT BY FINISHING OF ENAMEL MARGINS?**

**A:** Depending on the type of restoration, the finishing of enamel margins might vary. Some restorations need an obtuse cavo surface margin with enamel. Some restorations need a butt joint with enamel.

**111. WHAT ARE THE THREE POSSIBLE JUNCTIONS BETWEEN ENAMEL AND RESTORATION?**

**A:** i) The enamel may have an acute angle & the restoration has an obtuse angle.

ii) The enamel and the restoration have a butt joint (90° cavo surface angle)

iii) The enamel has an obtuse angle and the restoration has 30 to 40$^{\circ}$ Cavo surface angle (bevelled cavo surface margin)

In no cavity, can the enamel have an acute angle because such unsupported enamel will break soon, leaving a gap in the margins. When the enamel has an obtuse angle, the restoration, if it is malleable and ductile, can be burnished over the bevel and even in thin section have enough strength. Such margins are feasible for stronger noble alloy castings. Sometimes in non stress bearing areas such bevels are done for composite resin restorations also.

Butt joint (90$^{\circ}$ cavo surface margin) is given for most restorations which do not have sufficient edge strength (not enough strength in thin sections)

**112. APART FROM MAINTAINING SUITABLE CAVO SURFACE ENAMEL ANGULATION, SHOULD THE ENAMEL BE FINISHED FOR ANY OTHER REASON?**

**A:** Enamel margins should always be finished to remove any unsupported enamel rods. This is true for all the cavo surface margins. This is the reason for using enamel chisel or hoe or enamel hatchet or gingival marginal trimmer in different areas of cavo surface margins.

**113. WHAT IS MEANT BY UNSUPPORTED ENAMEL RODS?**

**A:** Enamel rods start from the dentino enamel junction and travel outside towards the outer surface of enamel. Though the general direction of enamel rods from the dentino enamel junction is perpendicular to it, the path is curved and tortuous with lot of intermingling of enamel rods. Such tortuosities help strengthen enamel and prevent breakage. If all enamel rods are straight, splitting of enamel along the course of rods may be too easy. Because of the tortuosity of enamel rods, in whatever way cavity is cut, there will always remain some unsupported enamel rods along the cavity margins i.e. some enamel rods present in the margin might have lost their bases in the dentino enamel junction. Such unsupported enamel rods, if permitted to remain in the cavity may fail later during function, leaving tiny gaps between the tooth and the restoration.

**114. IS UNSUPPORTED ENAMEL RODS & UNDERMINED ENAMEL THE SAME?**

**A:** No. Undermined enamel may be large chunk of enamel which lacks dentine support. It is a macroscopic feature. Usually it is included in the outline form of the cavity. In non stress bearing areas, undermined enamel might remain for better aesthetics. Unsupported enamel rods is a microscopic feature. Macroscopically it might appear as a thin sharp ragged edge along the cavo surface margin. It should always be removed with enamel chisel or one of its modifications.

**115. HOW UNSUPPORTED ENAMEL RODS ARE REMOVED?**

**A:** For removing the unsupported enamel rods from the occlusal surface either a straight enamel chisel or a hoe or a hatchet is used. Straight enamel chisel is kept along the cavosurface margin with the bevel of the chisel facing

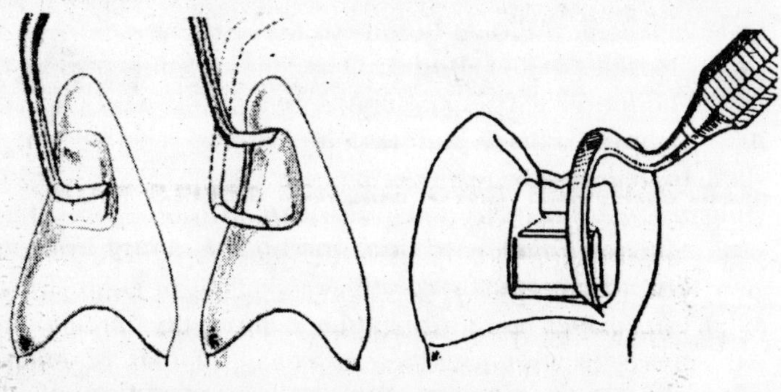

*Fig 5.8. Removal of unsupported enamel rods*

away from the margin and chisel used in a push motion along the cavo surface margin. The sharp cutting edge of the chisel scraps away the unsupported enamel rods which appear like white specks on the bevel. If access does not permit the use of straight enamel chisel a hoe or an enamel hatchet can be used by keeping the instrument with its bevel facing away from the cavity and pressure towards the dentino enamel junction is made to cleave the unsupported enamel rods. For mesial & distal walls hoes may be convenient and for buccal & lingual walls, enamel hatchet may be more convenient. For the gingival cavosurface margin, gingival marginal trimmer has to be used.

**116. SHOULD A GINGIVAL MARGINAL TRIMMER BE USED IN ALL GINGIVAL SEATS?**

**A:** Yes. For any gingival seat a GMT should be used. In the cervical portion of teeth, enamel rods have an apical slant. When a flat gingival seat is made, in the cavosurface margin, unsupported enamel rods remain. They should be removed by using the GMT in a lateral scrapping action. Mesial GMT (both ends) is used for mesial gingival seat are distal GMT (both ends) are used for distal gingival seat.

**117. WHICH GMTs ARE USED FOR BUCCAL AND LINGUAL (PALATAL) GINGIVAL SEATS IN CLASS I WITH EXTENSION?**

**A :** Mesial GMT is used for buccal gingival seat and Distal GMT is used for lingual gingival seat. If access permits, straight enamel chisel can also be used.

**118. HOW ARE CAVO SURFACE BEVELS MADE?**

**A:** Cavosurface bevels are made with rotary instruments held at the proper angle.

**119. WHAT IS TOILET OF THE CAVITY?**

**A:** It means cleaning the cavity preparation of debris and smear layer. If the debris are allowed to remain, they will interfere with the close packing of restorative material with tooth structure & when the debris is sequestrated later, there will be increased leakage around margins, possibility of micromovement of restoration and chances of secondary caries occurrence. In addition to debris, saliva, blood or exudate may contaminate the cavity. Unless all moisture are removed, they will prevent close adhesion of restorative materials with the tooth as well as dilute the cements & interfere and reduce the properties of various restorative materials.

**120. WHAT METHODS ARE USED FOR CLEANING THE CAVITY?**

**A:** Water, air or air water sprays are used for removing detachable debris. Small hand instruments can be used to dislodge any trapped debris. Cavity cleaning solution like 1 to 10% citric acid, ascorbic or acetic acids may be used in shallow cavities, but afterwards the area should be flushed with water jet for at least sixty seconds. Dilute hydrogen peroxide can be used for dislodging debris. 10% Ethylene diamino tetracetic acid can be used for removing smear layer from the cavity.

**121. WHAT IS CAVITY STERILIZATION?**

**A:** G.V. Black advocated a cavity sterilization prior to restoration with the hope of killing any residual bacteria deep in the dentinal tubules. In olden days antiseptics like silver nitrate, phenol, thymol, creosote and alcohol were used for such sterlization. How efficient these medicaments are in achieving sterilization of the cavity is not known, but they are definite pulp irritants. So these drugs are not used currently.

**22. WHAT IS SMEAR LAYER? SHOULD IT OR NOT BE REMOVED THE TOOTH FROM A CAVITY BEFORE RESTORATION?**

**A:** When the tooth surface is cut or scraped, an amorphous layer of denatured collagen, hydroxy apatite and cutting debris is formed and this layer is called smear layer. Some of these cut debris might enter the dentinal tubules forming smear plugs, blocking it. Smear layer is a few micrometer thick and it interferes with close adaptation of restoration with tooth structure. So it is advisable to remove smear layer. But smear plugs help in blocking dentinal tubules and prevent penetration of bacteria, their chemicals, toxins leaching out of bases & restorations into the pulp through the dentinal tubules. So it is wiser to permit smear plugs to remain in place. The current trend is to remove smear layer but permit smear plugs remain in place. This might be achieved by using mild acids for shorter duration.

**123. SHOULD THE CAVITY BE ABSOLUTELY DRY BEFORE RESTORING IT?**

**A:** A moisture contaminated cavity is not suitable for receiving the restoration. Proper isolation and drying the cavity with dry cotton pellets will be adequate. Use of compressed air for drying the cavity should be for few seconds only. Excessive drying (dessication) of the usually moist dentine can lead to pulpal damage.

**124. WHAT MODIFICATIONS HAVE OCCURED IN BLACK'S STEPS IN CAVITY PREPARATION DUE TO SCIENTIFIC ADVANCE?**

**A:**

1. OUTLINE FORM : Mainly Conservative : No extension for prevention : Emphasis on pulp protection.
2. RETENTION FORM : For small adhesive and acid etched restorations, this form may be skipped.
3. RESISTANCE FORM : For small adhesive & acid etched restorations, minimal preparation for resistance need be made.
4. CONVENIENCE FORM : Minimally observed
5. REMOVAL OF REMAINING CARIES : Unless communicating with oral cavity, caries closest to pulp might be treated with calcium hydroxide with no necessity of reentry later & removal of the left caries.
6. FINISHING THE ENAMEL WALL : Except for occlusal stress bearing areas, unsupported enamel might be left in situ for better aesthetics.
7. TOILET OF CAVITY : Avoiding caustic antiseptics : Used of air water spray mechanical cleaning. : Selective removal of smear layer.

# CHAPTER : 6

# INSTRUMENTS USED IN CONSERVATIVE DENTISTRY

**1. WHAT IS AN INSTRUMENT? WHAT IS AN EQUIPMENT?**

**A:** Instruments are generally small, hand held and used for treating a patient. Equipments are generally larger, they are accessories for treating a patient. Examples of instruments are mouth mirrors, probes, tweezer, various chisels, excavators, carvers, condensers, separators & knives. Equipments are Dental unit, operating stools, dental chair, X-ray unit, sterilizer, amalgamator, duplicating machine, porcelain furnace, casting machine, model trimmer, CADCAM machine etc.

**2. HOW ARE INSTRUMENTS CLASSIFIED?**

**A:** Instruments can be classified as hand instruments (manually used) rotary instruments (engine driven) and ultrasonic instruments. Instruments may also be classified as cutting instruments, Condensing instruments, finishing and polishing instruments, isolation instruments and miscellaneous instruments. Instruments are also classified as per the alloy used for manufacturing it either completely or atleast the working part. They may be made of stainless steel, carbon steel, tungsten carbide, anodized aluminium titanium or plastic. Commonly instruments are made of stainless steel. Instruments are also classified as excavators, chisels, knives etc.

**3. ARE HAND CUTTING INSTRUMENTS INDISPENSABLE IN CAVITY CUTTING?**

**A:** Once upon a time, before the invention of rotary cutting instrument, the entire cavity used to be cut with hand instruments. The early hand instruments were bulky, heavy handled and were difficult to use. Presently most of the hand cutting instruments are outdated and no longer used in cavity preparation. Availability of high speed instrumentations has rendered the hand cutting instruments obsolete. May be spoon excavator is the only hand cutting instrument commonly used even now. However basic knowledge of the earlier instruments is necessary at least for the historical value.

**4. WHO CLASSIFIED THE HAND INSTRUMENTS?**

**A:** The original acceptable classification was by Dr. G.V. Black. He gave the nomenclature of the instruments as well as the instrument formula.

**5. DR. G.V. BLACK'S NAME APPEARS TOO FREQUENTLY. DID NO OTHER DENTAL SURGEON CONTRIBUTE ANY THING IN THE FIELD OF CONSERVATIVE DENTISTRY?**

**A:** In conservative Dentistry, like in any other field of science, numerous scientists would have contributed to the growth and development of the speciality but few would have matched the broad outlook, diverse interest and pioneering spirit of Dr. G.V. Black who lived a hundred years ago. That is why he is called father of conservative dentistry.

**6. WHAT IS BLACK'S SYSTEM OF INSTRUMENT NOMENCLATURE?**

**A:** Instruments are classified into order, suborder, class & subclass and the instrument's full name will denote its order, sub order, class & sub class.

1. Order denotes its functions - eg: excavator, scaler, chisel, knife.
2. Suborder denotes position or manner of use - push, pull, lateral cutting.
3. Class denotes design of working end - eg: spoon, hoe, hatchet, cleoid, discoid, sickle.
4. Subclass denotes the shape of the shank - eg: Monoangle binangle, triple angled, contra angle - etc. The instrument's name starts with sub class, class, sub order and ends with order eg: Binangle hatchet push excavator. The manner of use in many situation is non specific

and is omitted. For practical purposes, only the working end and the shape of shank are described.

**7. WHAT ARE THE PARTS OF A HAND INSTRUMENT?**

**A:** A hand instrument consists of a shaft or handle, shank or neck and blade, nib or tine.

1. Handle or shaft is usually straight. It may be hexagonal or octagonal in cross section. If it is serrated its increases friction for gripping. If the handle has blade & shank on both ends, it is a double ended instrument. Advantage of a double ended instrument is greater operator convenience and less frequent instrument change. Instrument handle will contain the instrument formula.

2. The working portion (functional part) of the instrument known as blade (in a cutting instrument) begins at the last angle of the shank and ends in the cutting edge. Blade will have a single bevel or two bevels to end in a cutting edge. For non cutting instruments the working part is called a nib and the nib may end in a face (eg: amalgam condenser). If the blade has only one bevel, it is unibeveled and if there are two bevels, it is a bibeveled instrument. Bevel or bevels end in a cutting edge and excepting in gingival marginal trimmers and angle formers, the cuttingedge is at a right angle to the long axis of the blade.

3. Shank or neck is the portion of the instrument that connects the handle with blade. Shank is usually narrower than the shaft and tapering shank may also have one or more angulations to bring the working part of the instrument as close to the long axis of the handle as possible to balance the instrument (to allow for concentration of force on the blade without rotation of the instrument in the grasp). This is also known as contra angling the instrument. The angulations in the shank also help in better access to the cavity. Depending on the number of angles in the shank, an instrument could be monoangled, biangled or triple angled. Shorter blades

& a small blade angle needs bin angling while longer blades & greater blade angle need triple angling.

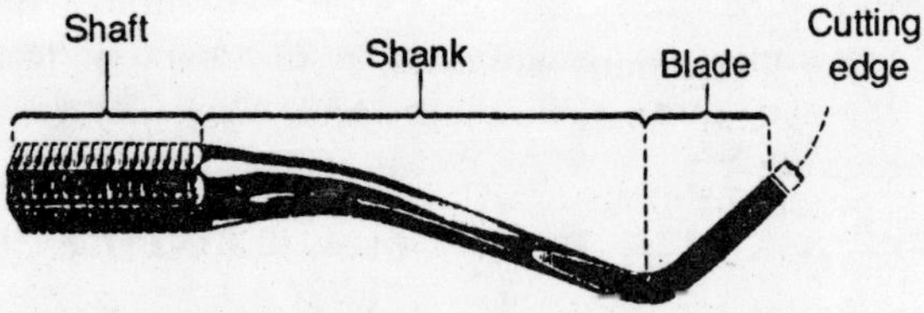


*Fig. 6.1. Parts of a hand instrument*

**8. WHAT IS BLACK'S INSTRUMENT FORMULA?**

**A:** Black's instrument formula expressed in a series of numbers gives the idea about the instrument's dimensions. It can be either a three numbered formula or a four numbered formula. Most of the hand cutting instruments have only three numbered formula. Only instruments like gingivial marginal trimmers, angle formers and some vareities of offset chisels, whose cutting edge is other than a right angle to its blade have a four numbered formula. A three number formula could be 10-4-8 and a four number formula could be 12-85-8-15.

**9. WHAT TO DO THESE NUMBERS SIGNIFY IN THE INSTRUMENT FORMULA?**

**A:** In a three numbered formula, the first number denoted the width of the blade in one tenth of a millimeter. i.e, if the first number is 15, it means the width of the blade is 1.5mm. If the first number is 8, the width of the blade is 0.8 mm. The second number in a three number formula denoted the length of the blade in millimeters. If the second number is 4, it means the length of blade is 4 millimeters and if the second number is 12, it means the length of the blade in 1.2 centimeters (12mm). The third number denotes the angle the balde forms with the long axis of the instrument in centigrades.

10. **ARE NOT CENTIGRADES THE UNITS USED FOR MEASURING TEMPERATURE?**

A : It is true, centigrades are one of the units for measuring temperature. It is also true that centigrades are the units of measuring the angulation in one system where a circle is divided into 100 parts and each degree will be a centigrade.

11. **ISN'T A CIRCLE DIVIDED USUALLY INTO 360 PARTS?**

A : In the Astronomical system of dividing a circle, it is divided into 360 parts and that is what most of us have studies in school. So when somebody says a right angle, the immediate correlation is $90^0$. An acute angle conjures up memory of any angle less than $90^0$ and an obtuse angle, between $90^0$ and $180^0$ . However in the centric system of dividing a circle, a right angle means $25^0$ and acute angle is less than $25^0$ and obtuse angle is between $25^0$ & $50^0$. Excepting with reference to hand instruments, angles expressed in any other portion of this book refers only to astronomical angle.

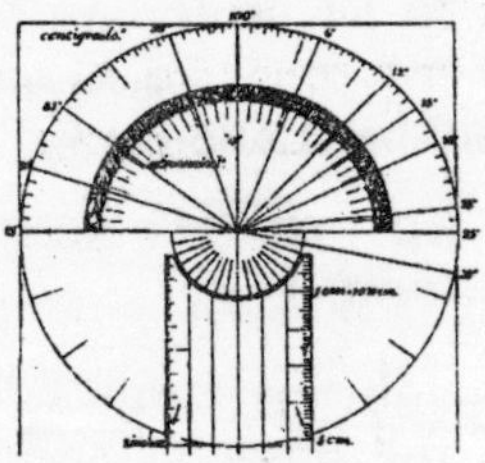

Fig. 6.2. Centigrade System

12. **EVERYBODY KNOWS A RIGHT ANGLE MEANS 90 DEGREES. WHY CREATE CONFUSION BY INTRODUCING ANOTHER SYSTEM?**

A: It is true that most of us were taught only about astronomical system of dividing a circle into $360^0$ But that doesn't make the other system wrong. It is the metric system where a circle is divided into 100 parts. May be during G.V. Black's time it was very popular. Or, may be

Dr. Black wanted all the units to be in metric system. So the third number denotes the blade angulations to the long axis of the instrument in centigrades.

**13. WHAT IS 14$^0$ IN CENTRIGRADES EQUAL TO IN ASTRONOMICAL DEGREE?**

**A:** It is equal to 54$^0$ in astronomical scale.

**14. WHY CAN'T WE SUBSTITUTE THE ASTRONOMICAL DEGREE TO THE CENTIGRADE DEGREE ATLEAST NOW?**

**A:** Even if it is sensible, such unilateral decision will only lead to confusion. Universal scientific bodies should take note of such discrepancies and suggest coordinated corrective action throughout the world.

**15. WHAT DO THE NUMBERS IN A FOUR NUMBER INSTRUMENT FORMULA STAND FOR?**

**A:** It must be remembered that in a four number formula, the fourth number (angle of the cutting edge to the long axis the instrument) is kept in the second position of the sequence.

**16. DOES IT MEAN THE SECOND NUMBER IN THREE NUMBER FORMULA AND A FOUR NUMBER FORMULA STAND FOR DIFFERENT THINGS?**

**A:** Unfortunately, yes. In a three number sequence, it stands for the length of the blade in millimeters. In a four number formula, the second number denotes the angle the cutting edge forms with the long axis of the instrument.

**17. WHAT IS THE ADVANTAGE GAINED BY KEEPING THE FOURTH NUMBER IN THE SECOND POSITION OF A FOUR NUMBER INSTRUMENT FORMULA?**

**A:** Absolutely none. May be Professor Black wanted to confuse his dental students. Logically this fourth number could as well have been kept in the fourth place without giving any room for confusion. Any how changing this disparity too needs concerted action by world dental governing bodies.

**18. HOW IS A DENTAL STUDENT SUPPOSED TO ANSWER THE QUESTION ABOUT THE NUMBERS IN A FOUR NUMBER INSTRUMENT FORMULA?**

**A:** The dental student's expected answer is :

1. The first number denotes the width of the instrument in one tenth of a millimeter.
2. The fourth number kept in the second position denotes the angle in centigrade the cutting edge forms with the long axis of the instrument.
3. The second number denotes the length of the blade in millimeters.
4. The third number denotes the angle the blade forms with the long axis of the instrument.

**19. IS THERE A DEVICE FOR MEASURING THE DIMENSIONS IN PARTS OF MILLIMETERS & ANGULATIONS IN CENTIGRADES OF AN INSTRUMENT?**

**A:** Yes. The Boley gauge. While positioning the instrument, the blade should be kept in such a way that the blade angle is less than $50^0$ centigrade.

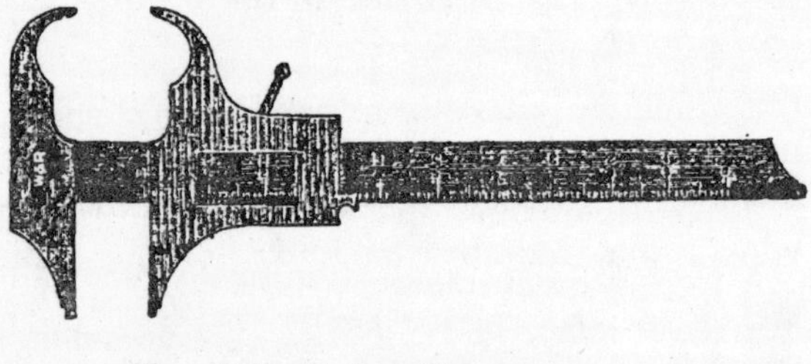

*Fig. 6.3. Boley Guage*

**20. IS BLACK'S CLASSIFICATION OF HAND INSTRUMENTS VALID TODAY?**

**A:** With the evolution of rotary cutting instruments, the use of hand cutting instruments for cavity cutting has become obsolete. Presently, out of the numerous hand cutting instruments may be the spoon excavator is the only one commonly used for removing carious dentine. Straight enamel chisel and its modifications are used for finishing the enamel margins. Apart from these instruments mainly filling & finishing instruments are used. As hundreds of hand cutting instruments have become obsolete now, they may be omitted. For example, Hoe excavators and Hatchet excavators were cutting instruments which are not used now. Reading about them will only lead to confusion with enamel hatchet and hoe chisel which are still used for finishing enamel margins. So only a few selected instruments which are in common use now will be described in detail in this book.

**21. WHAT IS A SINGLE PLANE INSTRUMENT? WHICH IS A DOUBLE PLANE INSTRUMENT?**

**A:** A single plane instrument has all the angles in the shank, and the blade in one plane only. A double plane instrument is one where all the angles in the shank, and the blade are not in the same plane. One easy way of identifying a double plane instrument will be by the curved blade.

**22. WHAT IS A MOUTH MIRROR?**

**A:** A mouth mirror is an instrument having a mirror head top and a detachable handle. The mirror could be plain or concave. Plain mirror is superior because of the undistorted image. Concave mirror is rarely used except for seeing enlarged internal details of the cavity.

A front surface mirror is one where the reflecting surface is on the top of the glass piece. This gives better visibility and because of the absence of intervening glass, there are no double image. However the mercury coating on the top (front surface) is likely to be easily lost due to scratching. In a back surface mirror (which is the commonest & cheaper one) there is a possibility of double image because of the thickness of glass before the reflecting surface.

## 23. WHAT ARE THE USES OF MOUTH MIRROR?

**A:** 1. Vision - The reflected image of the teeth and oral tissues especially in inaccessible areas of the oral cavity enhances the visibility. The mouth mirror should be dry for good reflection. However, in the oral cavity, because of the breath of the patient, the mirror surface tend to get fogged and this fogging could be removed by blowing warm air over it or by dipping the mirror top in antifogging solution.

2. Retraction - Mouth mirror is useful for retracting the lip, check or tongue from the field of operations. This is not only increases visibility on the field of operation but also protects the mobile tissues from any inury from rotary or hand cutting instruments.

3. Illumination : When direct light on any area is in adequate, mouth mirror could be held at an angle to reflect the light on to the working area.

4. Guard : While using a sharp hand instrument a guard should be kept distal to the field of operation alongwith the working axis of the instrument to protect against accidental slippage & sort tissue injury. The back of the mirror top will serve as a good war.

## 24. WHAT INSTRUMENTS ARE USED TO EXPLORE A LESION?

**A:** A Probe or an explorer is used for exploring a lesion. It is used for detecting & assessing carious lesion in the tooth. It is useful in detecting demineralised dentine. It is useful for releasing debris from the tooth. It is useful for removing cotton kept within the cavity. It is used in removing slight excess fill up around carosurface margins. It is used for identifying hypersensitive areas in a tooth. It is used for assessing marginal fit of a restoration. All probes are single ended or double ended instruments.

## 25. WHAT ARE THE TYPES OF PROBES/EXPLORERS?

**A:** 1. It could be a straight explorer that has a smooth straight shank with a slight curvature near the tine (trip of the probe)

2. It could be a right angled explorer having a shank with a right angle and the exploring tip that is at right angle to the handle.
3. The cowhorn or sickle explorer is also known as the arch explorer, has a curved shank with a semi circle like an arch ending in a tip.
4. The Briault's probe is also known as interproximal explorer is usually triple angled and its tine (tip) is towards the handle. It is useful for detecting proximal caries.

**26. WHAT ARE DENTAL TWEEZERS?**

**A:** Dental tweezers (also known as cottonpliers) consists of two arms joined at one end. The other ends of the two arms of tweezers usually remain apart. When the arms are held and pressed together, the two beaks come and approximate against each other.

**27. WHAT ARE THE USES OF TWEEZERS?**

A : Tweezers are useful in carrying things to and from the mouth. They are used for carrying cotton rolls, cotton pledgets, sponge pellets to and around the cavity. They are also useful in carrying salvia soaked cotton rolls from the oral cavity to the waste disposal unit.

**28. WHAT ARE THE LOCKING TWEEZERS?**

A : They are similar to the ordinary tweezers except that there is a lock in the middle. When the two arms of the locking tweezers are pressed against each other, the lock clips into position and keeps the two beaks firmly against each other, holding firmly whatever is held in between. This avoids the unneccessary anxiety of the operator about the possibility of slippage of whatever is carried by the tweezer. To release the lock, the locking head is slipped away from the notch manually.

**29. WHAT ARE DIAGNOSTIC INSTRUMENTS?**

A : A mouth mirror, probe and tweezer are together used known as diagnostic instruments. Tweezer is used for carying & keeping cotton rolls in the vestibules & lingual sulcus for isolation. Cotton pledgets are taken in the tweezer for drying the tooth. Mouth mirror is taken inside to visualize all the surfaces of the teeth, one after another with probes used to check the integrity of tooth and test the vulnerable areas. Because these instruments primarily help in diagnosing diseased oral structures, they are known as diagnostic instruments.

**30. WHAT IS THE SPOON EXCAVATOR?**

**A :** Spoon excavators are instruments and double ended. One blade is curved to right and another curved to left. The thin cutting edge is along the periphery of the circular blade. Spoon excavators are double planned instrument because of curved blades. They are lateral cutting instruments (used in scrapping action like how a laddle is used to scrap the food sticking to the side of a vessel.) The shank is biangled or tripled angled for better accessibillity. Spoon excavators are also modified hatchets. While hatchet has a straight cutting edge, the spoon excavator has a circular cutting edge. Spoon excavators are also known as scoops because of the scooping action used.

**31. WHAT IS MEANT BY RIGHT AND LEFT OF THE INSTRUMENT?**

**A :** Unibevelled handcutting instruments with their cutting edge parallel to the long axis of the instrument (eg., Enamel hatchet, GMTs, spoon excavators, angle formers) come as paired instruments. Some of them have one or more angles in the shank and some have the cutting edge not at a right angle to the blade. The paired instruments are known as the right and left instruments.

**32. HOW TO IDENTIFY THE RIGHT AND LEFT OF THE PAIR?**

**A :** Manufacturer of the instrument should have placed identifying ring for the right of the pair. Sometimes they also add the letter 'L' or 'R' after the instruments formula marked on the shaft of the instrument.

**33. IF THE MANUFACTURER HAS NOT PROVIDED ANY RING OR MARKING IN THE HANDLE OF THE INSTRUMENT, HOW TO IDENTIFY THE RIGHT AND LEFT OF THE INSTRUMENTS?**

**A :** When the manufacturer hasn't provided a indented ring in the shaft of letter 'R' or 'L' after one instrument formula, the operator should hold the instrument in front of him, with the blade facing away from him and the cutting edge facing down. (This is similar to the instruments working position in a lower tooth). In this position the operator should see whether the bevel in the blade is to his right or left. If the bevel is to his right it is the right of the pair and if the bevel is to his left it is the left of the pair.

**34. DOES THE RIGHT INSTRUMENT MEAN THAT IT CAN BE USED ONLY FOR THE RIGHT SIDE TEETH AND LEFT INSTRUMENT IS TO BE USED FOR LEFT SIDE TEETH?**

**A :** That is the wrong idea most dental students commonly have. Both the instruments can be used in the same cavity and in any tooth of the mouth. If the instrument is used in lateral scrapping motion then the right instrument is used from (operations) right to left and the left instrument is used for operations left to right. For example, in a class II mesio occlusal cavity in tooth No. Four Six (46) the right of the mesial GMT could be used along the gingival cavosurface margin from right to left (Lingual to buccal) and the left of the mesial GMT could be used from left to right (buccal to lingual). The same instruments, if used in a similar cavity in tooth No. 36 (Three Six), the left of GMT is used from lingual to buccal and right GMT is used from buccal to lingual.

**35. HOW ARE THE GMTs USED IN A MESIO OCCLUSAL CAVITY IN TOOTH NUMBERS 16 (ONE SIX) AND 26 (TWO SIX)?**

**A :** In the gingival cavosurave margin of masial box of 16, the right GMT will be used from buccal to palatal and the left GMT will be used from palatal to buccal. In mesial box of 26 right GMT will be used from palatal to buccal and left GMT will be used from buccal to palatal.

**36. WHILE USING IN THE UPPER TEETH, THE RIGHT GMT IS USED FROM LEFT TO RIGHT AND THE LEFT GMT IS USED FROM RIGHT TO LEFT. IS IT NOT CONFUSING BECAUSE FROM RIGHT INSTRUMENT IS SUPPOSED TO BE USED FROM RIGHT TO LEFT?**

**A :** By classifying unibevelled paired instruments into right and left, professor Black has contributed to confusion. He could have simply classified them into 1 & 2 or A & B. Afterall the nomenclature is for differenciating the two instruments. Both can be used in the same cavity, except the direction of movement will vary from tooth to tooth. By looking at the curved blade and/or bevel the operator can find out the best method of use of the instrument. We must also remember that while identifying the instrument, are kept blade away from us and the cutting edge down. While working in an upper tooth, the cutting edge facing upwards and obviously there is a reversal in direction of use. The only thing a student should remember is that both right and left instrument could be used in any tooth. They could also used both in the same tooth, though in different places of the same cavity (if used in laternal scrapping) motion or in different places of the same cavity (if used in downward push motions).

**37. WHAT IS STRAIGHT ENAMEL CHISEL?**

**A :** The shank connecting the enamel chisel blade with the handle is straight and it is known as straight enamel chisel. It is used for planning (smoothening) enamel or cleaning (splitting) undermined enamel. Straight enamel chisel is a single ended single plane instrument. The blade is unibevelled and has a sharp cutting edge. When it is used for planning, the bevel should be facing away from the cavity. The instrument issued in push motion (straight thrust). Sometimes along with a single bevel on the blade there may be creating secondary bevels edges. This provides lateral cutting efficiency for the blade. Such lateral cutting may be useful in refining the internal line angles.

**38. IS THERE A RIGHT AND LEFT STRAIGHT ENAMEL CHISEL?**

**A:** No. Straight enamel chisel is not a paired instrument. The same chisel by turning it along its long axis can be used on both buccal and lingual cavosurfaces for removing the unsupported. Enamel rod.

**39. ARE THERE ANGLED CHISELS?**

**A:** Yes there are monoangled, binangled & triple angled chisels, depending on whether there is a single, double or triple angles in the shank of the instrument.

**40. WHY SOME CHISELS HAVE ANGLES IN THE SHANK?**

**A:** To have better access to the cavity.

**41. IN ANGLED CHISELS HOW IS THE CUTTING EDGE TO THE LONG AXIS OF THE INSTRUMENT?**

**A:** The cutting edge of an angled chisel is at a right angle to the long axis of the instrument.

**42. ON WHICH SIDE IS THE BEVEL IN ANGLED CHISELS?**

**A:** The bevel could be on the side of the blade nearer to the shaft of the instrument and it is known as mesial bevel. The bevel could be on the side of the blade farther to the shaft and may be known as distal beveled, reverse beveled or contra beveled. In unibeveled instruments having their cutting edge perpendicular to the long axis of the instrument, manufacturer puts an indented ring in the shaft.

**43. WHAT IS WEDLSTAEDT CHISEL?**

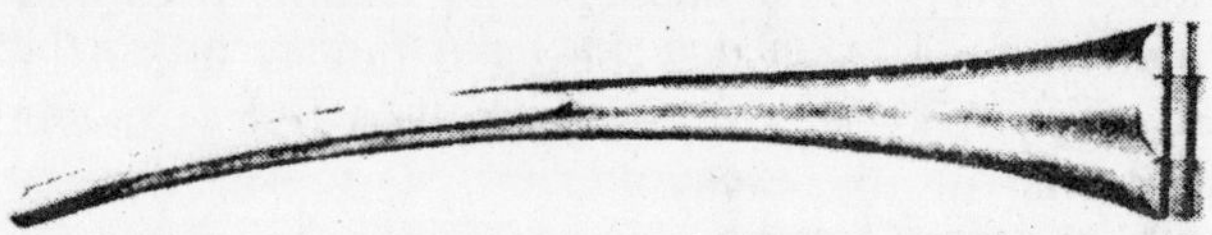

*Fig. 6.4. Wedlstaedt Chisel*

A: It is a chisel with a slightly curved blade for use especially in proximal surface of anterior teeth. The angulation will be around $3^0$ centigrade.

**44. WHERE WILL TRIPLE ANGLED CHISELS BE MORE USEFUL?**

A: In the incisal portion of a proximal anterior cavity.

**45. WHAT IS HOE?**

A: There are hoe excavator and hoe chisel. Hoe excavator is not used currently. Hoe chisel is similar to hoe excavator but hoe chisel blade is sturdier. Hoe chisel is a modification of straight enamel chisel.

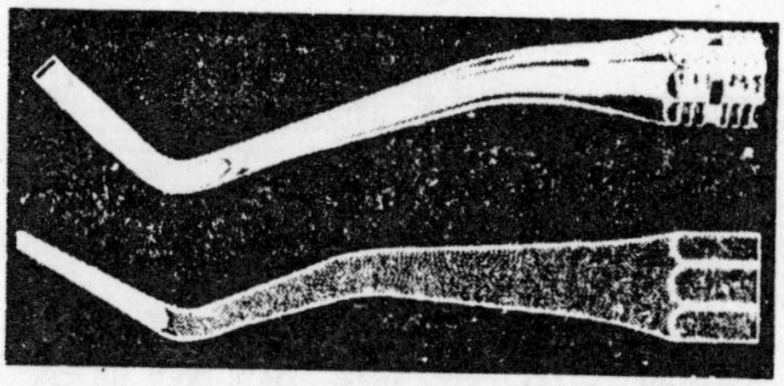

*Fig. 6.5. Hoe & Hatchet*

**46. HOW IS HOE A MODIFICATION OF STRAIGHT ENAMEL CHISEL?**

A : Hoe is a modified enamel chisel in which the cutting edge is perpendicular to the long axis of the instrument.

**47. HOW DOES HOE DIFFER FROM A CURVED CHISEL?**

A: When the blade angle to the long axis of the shaft is less than 12.5 degrees it is a curved chisel. If the blade angle is more than 12.5 degrees, it is a hoe. A hoe chisel is used for removing unsupported enamel rods and undermined enamel. A distally bevelled hoe is useful in mesial wall of a cavity & a mesially beveled hoe is useful in the distal wall of the cavity.

**48. HOW IS HOE USED?**

A: Either in a downward cutting motion or push (for mesially beveled hoe) or pull (for distally beveled hoe) for smoothening floors (compare with the method of use of garden hoe)

**49. WHAT IS HATCHET?**

**A:** Like hoe, there is a hatchet excavator and an enamel hatchet. Hatchet excavator is a bibeveled (beveled on both sides of the blade) instrument (like on osteotome) Enamel hatchet is a modified form of a straight enamel chisel & its cutting edge is parallel to the long axis of the shaft. Enamel hatchet is a paired instrument with a right and left instrument. Hatchet excavator is not used currently and enamel hatchet is useful in removing the unsupported enamel rods & undermined enamel.

**50. HOW IS AN ENAMEL HATCHET USED?**

**A:** Enamel hatchets are used in a downward cutting motion on the buccal & lingual walls of the cavity. They can also be used for breaking thinned out proximal enamel wall in a class II cavity, while breaking contact. Enamel hatchets are single planed double ended instruments.

**51. WHAT ARE OFFSET HATCHETS?**

**A:** They are like regular enamel hatchets except that the whole blade is rotated a quarter of turn forward or backward. They are single planed paired instruments. They are useful in areas of difficult access.

**52. WHAT IS A GINGIVAL MARGINAL TRIMMER?**

**A:** As the name implies, it is an instrument used to trim the gingival cavosurface margin.

**53. WHY SHOULD THE GINGIVAL CAVOSURFACE MARGIN BE TRIMMED?**

**A:** Gingival seat is usually located at the cervical one third of the teeth. The enamel rods in the cervical one third of the teeth are apically directed from dentino enamel junction to the outer enamel surface. In the enamel portion of a flat gingival seat, there will always be some unsupported enamel rods (rods without their bases at the dentino enamel junction). If they are not removed and the tooth restored, there is a possibility of these tooth restored, there is a possibility of these structures breaking away leading to marginal leakage. This is the reason for planing the gingival cavosurface margins.

**54. FROM WHICH INSTRUMENT HAS THE GMT EVOLVED?**

**A:** The gingival marginal trimmer has evolved from the enamel hatchet. It is a modified enamel natchet.

**55. WHAT ARE THE DIFFERENCES BETWEEN AN ENAMEL HATCHET AND A GINGIVAL MARGINAL TRIMMER?**

**A:**
1. Enamel hatchet has a straight blade & is a single plane instrument while gingival marginal trimmer has a curved blade and in a double planed instrument.
2. In enamel hatchet the cutting edge is at a right angle to the blade of the instrument & has only a three numbered formula. In a Gingival marginal trimmer the cutting edge is not at a right angle to the blade and hence has a four number formula.

**56. HOW MANY GINGIVAL MARGINAL TRIMMERS ARE THERE?**

**A:** If they are single ended instruments, there are four. If they are double ended instruments then they are two. Thus there will be a mesial gingival marginal trimmer with two blades and a distal gingival marginal trimmer with two

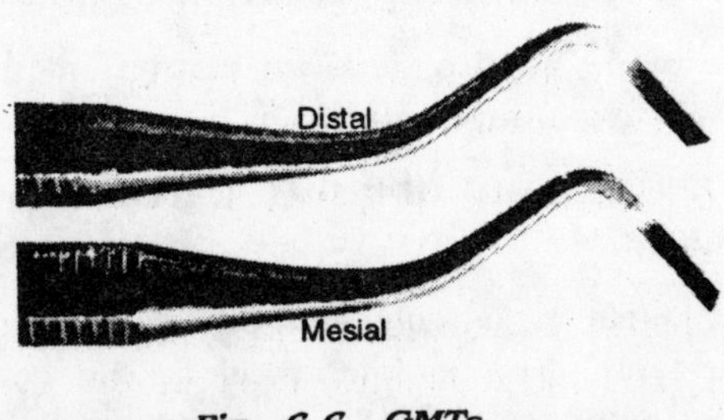


*Fig. 6.6. GMTs*

blades. A mesial GMT is used for removing the unsupported enamel rods from the gingival cavosurface margin of any mesial cavity. A distal GMT is used for removing the unsupported enamel rods from the gingival cavosurface margin of any distal cavity. In addition, a mesial GMT can be used on the gingival cavosurface margin of a buccal box & distal GMT can be used on the gingival cavosurface margin of a lingual or palatal box.

**57. IS GMT USED FOR ANY OTHER PURPOSE?**

**A:** It is also used for roundening the axio pulpal line angle. This reduces chances for stress concentration. Some authors suggest the use of GMT for placement of gingival lock (a retentive feature) in dentine. A mesial GMT is used to create a gingival lock (reverse bevel) in the dentinal portion of the gingival seat in the distal box. A distal GMT is used to create a gingival lock (reverse bevel) in the dentinal portion of the gingival seat in the mesial box.

**58. HOW TO DIFFERENTIATE THE MESIAL PAIR OF GMT WITH THE DISTAL PAIR OF GMT?**

**A:**

1. Look at the acute angle tip in the blade of GMT. If it is closer to the shaft, it is the mesial GMT. If the acute angle tip of the blade is away from the shaft it is the distal GMT.
2. Examine the blade. It has a nearer end (nearer to the shaft) a cutting edge and farther end (farther to the shaft). If the nearer end forms an acute angle with the cutting edge, it is a mesial GMT. If the farther end of the blade forms an acute angle with the cutting edge, it is a distal GMT.

**59. ARE THERE RIGHT AND LEFT GMTS?**

**A:** Mesial pair has one right and left and distal pair also has a right and left. There should either be an indented ring or marking 'R' in the shaft to denote it is the right of the instruments.

**60. HOW TO IDENTIFY THE RIGHT AND LEFT GMTS?**

**A:** The GMT is held with the blade facing away from the operator & cutting edge facing down (position of use in a lower tooth). In this position, if the bevel is to the operators right, it is the right of the instrument. If the bevel is to the operator's left, it is the left of the instrument.

**61. HOW IS THE GMT USED?**

**A:** GMT is used in a lateral scrapping motion.

**62. NAME ANY OTHER INSTRUMENT USED IN A LATERAL SCRAPPING ACTION?**

**A:** Spoon excavator, discoid.

**63. WHAT ARE ANGLE FORMERS?**

**A:** They are instruments used for accentuating the line angles and point angles in a cavity. These instruments also have fourth number formula because the cutting edge of the instruments is not at a right angle with the blade of the instrument. The cutting edge angle to the long axis of the shaft will be $80^0$ centigrade. They are paired instruments with a right and a left.

**64. ARE ANGLE FORMERS COMMONLY USED NOW?**

**A:** No. Except for gold foil (direct filling gold) restorations, in no cavity are the internal line angles and point angles supposed to be sharp. The internal line and point angles are expected to be removed to avoid stress concentration.

**65. WHAT ARE DISCOIDS & CLEOIDS?**

A: The discoid is a hand cutting instrument with a disc like blade. The blade to shaft angle is like that of a mono

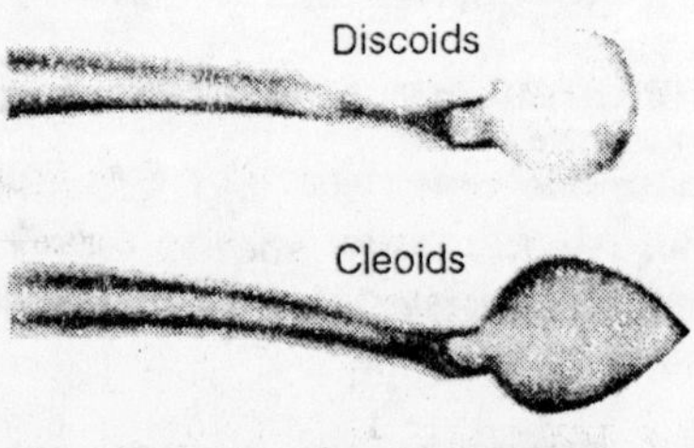


*Fig. 6.7. Discoids & Cleoids*

angle chisel and the blades are longer than a spoon excavator. Cleoid has a claw like cutting blade. The cutting edges are sharp for both these instruments. The instruments were originally used for cavity cutting and caries removal. The instruments may be single ended instruments or a single instrument with discoid at one end and cleoid at another end.

**66. ARE CLEOIDS & DISCOID STILL USED NOW?**

**A:** Yes. But they are not used for cutting cavities but they are used for carving amalgam and wax patterns.

**67. WHAT IS A CEMENT SPATULA?**

**A:** Cement spatula is double ended instrument with stiff flat wide blade used for manually mixing cements supplied as powder & liquid. It is also used for mixing chemically activated composite resin supplied as base & catalyst pastes. It is also used for mixing two pastes of Zinc Oxide Eugenol impression material.

**68. FROM WHAT MATERIAL A CEMENT SPATULA MADE OF?**

**A:** Cement spatula may be made of stainless steel, agate or plastic

**69. WHY CAN'T STAINLESS STEEL SPATULAS BE USED FOR MIXING ALL CEMENTS?**

**A:** Powders of silicate cement and glass ionomer contain glasses that can abrade the spatula during mixing of cements and the abraded steel particles might become part of these tooth coloured restorations. Cements like polycarboxylate & glass ionomer tend to stick to a stainless steel spatula tenaciously and cleaning them is difficult.

**70. WHAT IS AGATE?**

**A:** Agate is a naturally occuring mineral. It is a hard type of quartz usually with streaks. Its abrasive resistance enables it to be used for mixing silicate cement, without damage. However, presently cheaper plastic spatulas are available, which are disposable. They do not get abraded by glass particles of silicate or glass ionomer or quartz fillers of composite resin. If the plastic spatula is to be resued, it is easy to clean the spatula of the set cement.

**71. OVER WHAT SURFACE THE CEMENTS ARE MIXED?**

**A:** Cements are mixed over a thick glass slab or over a waxed paper mixing pad.

**72. WHAT ARE THE ADVANTAGES OF MIXING OVER A GLASS SLAB?**

**A:**
1. A glass slab can be cleaned & reused.
2. A glass slab can be cooled in a refridgerator to lower the mixing temperature to prolong the working time of a cement. A glass slab retains the coolness for longer period than a paper pad.
3. A glass slab does not absorb any constituent of the cement (like water from the liquid of the cement).

**73. WHAT ARE THE ADVANTAGES OF A PAPER PAD?**

**A:**
1. Paper pad is disposable. There are no possibility of contamination with an older mix cement.
2. Waxed paper pad is nonabsorbable.
3. Paper pads could also be cooled, but not as effectively, as a glass slab.
4. Paper pads provide the resilient support while contouring a matrix band with a burnisher.

**74. CAN A GLASS PLATE BE USED INSTEAD OF A GLASS SLAB?**

**A:** Apart from the possibility of easy breakage only a thick glass slab can absorb the evolved exothermic heat from cements like zinc phosphate effectively.

**75. WHAT IS A PLASTIC INSTRUMENT?**

**A:** It is an instrument used for carrying the mixed base cement or the restorative cement from a cement spatula to the cavity. Usually one end of the plastic instrument is flat and other end is cylindrical. The flat end is used for carrying the cement and the cylindrical end is used for positioning and manipulating the cement into the cavity.

**76. WHAT MATERIAL IS A PLASTIC INSTRUMENT MADE OF?**

**A:** A plastic instrument is made of stainless steel. It is useful for placement of zinc oxide eugenol, zinc phosphate, silicophosphate, copper and silicate cements. However, composites, glass ionomer & poly carboxylate tend to stick to stainless steel. For these restorations, a plastic instrument made of anodized aluminium titanium nitride coated are used, to which, these materials do not tenaciously stick.

**77. WHY AN INSTRUMENT MADE OF STAINLESS STEEL IS KNOWN AS A "PLASTIC INSTRUMENT"?**

**A:** Because the instrument usually carries unset materials which are in soft (plastic) stage the instrument is called a plastic instrument.

**78. WHAT IS AN AMALGAM CARRIER?**

**A:** Amalgam carrier is a stainless steel instrument used for carrying mixed amalgam to the cavity. Its usefulness lies in convenience of delivery to inaccessible cavities as well as not touching the amalgam with bare fingers (avoiding moisture contamination of a Zinc containing alloy as well as avoiding possible mercury absorption through skin).

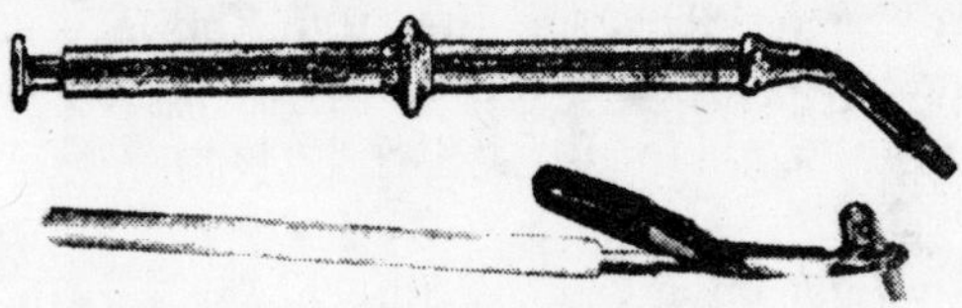

*Fig. 6.8. Amalgam carrier*

**79. HOW IS AN AMALGAM CARRIER USED?**

**A:** The hollow tip of the amalgam carrier is inserted into the mixed amalgam four or five times to pack the carrier with amalgam. It is then carried into the mouth and the tip is kept into the cavity & plunger is pressed ejecting cylindrical pellets of amalgam.

**80. HOW MANY TYPES OF AMALGAM CARRIERS ARE AVAILABLE?**

**A:** Two or three varieties are available. The differences are minor and designs are modifications to improve access. Modified amalgam carriers are available for retrograde fillings after apicectomy. They are Hill carrier, Messing carrier & Dimashkieh carrier.

**81. WHAT ARE AMALGAM CONDENSERS?**

**A:** Amalgam condensers are either hand condensers or mechanical condensers. If it is a mechanical condenser, it consist of a hand piece like device with changeable tips for different types of cavities and different areas of the same cavity. Hand condensers are double ended instruments with the nibs (condensing tips) coming in different sizes and shapes. The nibs may be round, elliptical, triangular, trapezoidal or rectangular to fit different parts of a cavity. Their sizes may also vary considerably. Most condenser faces are flat but may be anguiar or concave to facilitate contouring buccal or lingual surfaces. The condenser face could also be smooth or serrated.

**82. WHAT IS THE ADVANTAGE OF SERRATIONS ON THE CONDENSER FACE?**

**A:**

1. Serrations increases the total surface area of the condenser tip and the amalgam condensed will be of the same shape for better locking with next layer of amalgam.
2. Serrations impart lateral forces, forcing the amalgam to be better adapted to the cavity
3. Serrations prevent slippage of amalgam.

**83. ARE THERE ANY OTHER CONDENSERS?**

**A:** Gold foil condensers are available in different sizes & shapes.

**84. WHAT ARE AMALGAM CARVERS?**

**A:** Amalgam carvers are double ended instruments with sharp blades for removing the excess amalgam and shaping the amalgam to the natural contour. Examples of amalgam carvers are Frahm's carver (diamond carver) Wards 'c' carver, or Hollenback's carver. In these carvers one blade is parallel to the long axis of the instrument and the other blade is perpendicular to the long axis of the handle. Cleoid discoid instrument can also be used for carving amalgam.

*Fig. 6.9. Amalgam Carvers*

**85. WHAT ARE AMALGAM BURNISHERS?**

**A:** Burnishers are double ended instruments whose nibs are spherical, conical or shaped like beaver tail. The nibs are smooth and help adapt the metallic restorations to the margins of the cavity. Sprateley burnishers are useful for adapting proximal metallic restoration.

**86. WHAT KNIVES ARE USED IN DENTISTRY?**

**A:** Bod Parker (B.P) knives are commonly used in making incisions, creating drainage etc. They come in two sizes of handles with detachable and disposable blades of different sizes and shapes. It can also be used for removing excess direct gold restorations. Black's knives come as a pair with one blade at a right angle to the handle with cutting edge away from the handle & another towards the angle. Wilson's knife can be used interproximally to remove excess restorative material. Stein's knife with a trapezoidal nib and Fish Knives are also used for removing excess direct filling gold along the cavo surface margins.

**87. WHAT FILES ARE USED IN OPERATIVE DENTISTRY?**

**A:** Gold foil files are used to trim away the marginal excess of direct filling gold. The tips of the files may be foot shaped, hatchet shaped or parallelogram shaped. The serration on the surface of the face of the nib could be directed away from the handle or towards the handle enabling the file to be used in a push or pull motion.

**88. WHAT ARE THE ADVANTAGES AND DISADVANTAGES OF STAINLESS STEEL INSTRUMENTS?**

**A:** Stainless steel instruments

1) remain bright for a long period
2) absence of rusting & corrosion
3) can be repeatedly autoclaved or sterilized in hot air oven. But stainless steel instruments lose their sharpness of the cutting edge quickly than carbon steel or carbide instruments. They are also not as hard as carbon steel.

**89. WHAT ARE THE ADVANTAGES AND DISADVANTAGES OF CARBON STEEL INSTRUMENTS?**

**A:** Carbon steel instruments are

1) harder than stainless steel instruments
2) having durable sharp cutting edges but carbon steel instruments tend to rust and corrode and if autoclaved, should be protected properly.

**90. WHAT ARE THE ADVANTAGES OF INSTRUMENTS WITH TUNGSTEN CARBIDE TIPS?**

**A:** Some hand held cutting instruments are made with tungsten carbide blades welded to a stainless steel handles. Tungsten carbide tips are

1) harder than stainless steel
2) better resistant to heat. But tungsten carbide tips are brittle & the instrument is likely to fracture in case of accidental fall.

**91. WHY INSTRUMENTS ARE MADE OF ANODIZED ALUMINIUM?**

**A:** Insertion instruments for composite resin are made of anodized aluminium to prevent the composite sticking to it. Instruments coated with titanium nitride also prevent the sticking of composite.

**92. WHY ARE HAND CUTTING INSTRUMENTS SHARPENED?**

**A:** For cutting effectively, the cutting edge of an instrument should be thin. With repeated use the sharp cutting edge becomes thick and dull. To restore the keenness of the cutting edge, the instrument should be sharpened once the cutting edge becomes dull & thick. Care should be taken while sharpening to have the same angulation of bevel.

**93. HOW ARE HAND CUTTING INSTRUMENTS SHARPENED?**

**A:** Sharpening is done by reducing the thickness of the metal at the cutting edge, while maintaining the angle and shape of bevel. Sharpening can be done manually by having a fixed sharpening Arkansas stone over which the instrun.ent is moved in one direction with the bevel in contact with the oil lubricated stone surface. Sharpening can also be done for instruments with curved blades, with a Cylindrical rotary stone in a hand piece held at the proper angle over the bevel. These free hand techniques are not highly dependable to maintain the original bevel shape & chances of errors are high. Sharpening machines are available with moving sharpening stones in a reciprocating (to and fro) movement. The instrument to be sharpened is held fixed and supported by an angle guide that maintain the angle of the bevel. Circular sharpening & polishing wheels may also be available with clockwise and anticlockwise movements. The instrument will be held in positon by the angle guide.

**94. WHAT ARE ROTARY INSTRUMENTS?**

**A:** Rotary instruments are engine diven instruments revolving around their long axis.

## 95. WHAT ARE THE USES OF ROTARY INSTRUMENTS?

**A:** Rotary instruments are used for cavity cutting, trimming extra orally made restorations, polishing restorations and pin channel preparation.

## 96. HOW ARE ROTARY INSTRUMENTS CLASSIFIED?

**A:** Rotary instruments are classified either according to the speed for rotation, their usage or depending on the holding device.

## 97. HOW ROTARY INSTRUMENTS ARE CLASSIFIED ACCORDING TO THE SPEED OF ROTATION?

**A:** There are no consensus regarding the classification of rotary instruments according to the speed of rotation. Instruments are classified generally into low speed and high speed. Some authors include medium speed, ultra low speed and high speed. Some authors include medium speed, ultra low speed and ultra high speed.

| NAME | SPEED IN RPM (REVOLUTIONS PER MINUTE) | | |
|---|---|---|---|
| | Classification I | Classification II | Classification III |
| 1. ULTRA LOW SPEED | 300 - 3,000 | | |
| 2. LOW SPEED | 3,000 - 6,000 | Below 12,000 | 500 - 15,000 |
| 3. MEDIUM SPEED | 20,000 - 45,000 | 12000 - 2,00,000 | |
| 4. HIGH SPEED | 45,000 - 1,00,000 | ABOVE 2,00,000 | 1,00,000 - 3,00,000 |
| 5. ULTA HIGH SPEED | ABOVE 1,00,000 | | |

## 98. WHICH ONE OF THE ABOVE CLASSIFICATION IS RIGHT?

**A:** There is no universally accepted classification. It is safer for a preclinical student to answer that rotary instruments are classified as high speed (bet. 1,00,000 & 5,00,000 rpm) and low speed (up to 20,000 rpm) instruments.

## 99. HOW ARE ROTARY INSTRUMENTS CLASSIFIED ACCORDING TO USAGE?

**A:** 1. Cutting instruments - These instruments cut into the tooth tissue remove it. Examples are steel or tungsten carbide dental burs.

2) Abrading instruments : These instruments abrade against the tooth tissue and remove it. Examples are diamond points, mounted and unmounted stones and discs made of carborundum, aluminium oxide, garnet, sand, cuttle, emery, (silicon carbide), diamond etc.

3) Polishing instruments : These instruments are used to polish tooth surface and restoration surfaces. Examples are bristle brushes, bristle cups, abrasive impregnated rubber cups & wheels.

**100. HOW ARE ROTARY INSTRUMENTS CLASSIFIED ACCORDING TO THE HOLDING DEVICES?**

**A:** 1) Slow speed instruments - burs and diamond points, trimming and polishing instruments.

2) High speed (airotor) instruments - Tungsten carbide burs and diamond points.

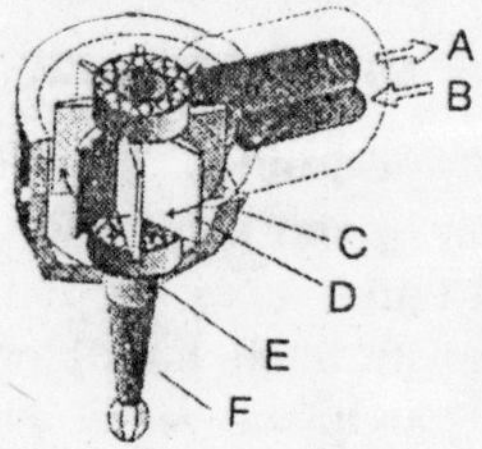


A - Exhaust air out
B - Drive air in
C - Head casing
D - Turbine
E - Ball - race bearing
F - Bur

*Fig. 6.10. High Speed cartridge*

**101. WHAT IS A HOLDING DEVICE?**

**A:** A dental hand piece is a holding device. It holds the rotating instrument (bur, point, trimming stone etc) in position during function. The dental hand piece could be a slow speed hand piece or a high speed hand piece.

**102. HOW DOES THE HIGH SPEED HANDPIECE WORK?**

**A:** The high speed handpiece is driven by compressed air. The head of the handpiece contains a cartridge which contain the air turbine with a central chuck. The turbine is held in position by two sets of ball bearings on the upper & lower ends. When air pressure turns the turbine, the central chuck also rotates along with it. The bur is attached to the central chuck. Bearings ensure that while the turbine rotates, the cartridge doesn't.

**103. HOW DOES THE BUR STAY IN THE CENTRAL CHUCK?**

**A:** Chuck is hollow. One end of the chuck is split into three or four leaves that can be released or tightened by turning the bur chuck anticlockwise or by pressing the spring activated top in some hand pieces. While inserting or removing the bur, the central chuck should be open (the end leaves released) and the bur chuck is turned in a clockwise direction to tighten the central chuck (or the pressure on the spring activated top on the head of hand piece is released).

**104. WHAT IS BUR CHUCK?**

**A:** A bur chuck is a device used to loosen or tighten the central collect chuck to insert or remove a bur.

**105. WHAT ARE THE TYPES OF HANDPIECES?**

**A:** Handpieces are generally classified into 1. High speed airotor handpieces 2. Slow speed conventional hand pieces. Slow speed conventional handpieces are further subdivided into a straight handpiece right angle handpiece, contra angle handpiece. Highspeed handpiece were available only in contra angle design so far but recently straight hand piece designs are also available.

**106. HOW DOES THE SLOW SPEED HANDPIECE WORK?**

**A:** A motor is needed to turn the central shaft which will be coupled to the drive spindle of the handpiece. In a straight handpiece, the drive spindle ends in a collect chuck for receiving the bur. In a right angle handpiece the drive is turned through $90^0$ by gears so that better access in the oral cavity is achieved. However, right angling tends to convert the bur into a lever arm and when bur is activated, the hand piece tend to rotate the hand making it unstable and needing greater hand control. But by contra angling the hand piece, this rotation of hand piece can be avoided. By providing a crown wheel gear box between two drive shafts such contra angling is achieved. In the head of the hand piece, the crown wheel gearing is attached to drive pinion which has the bur tube for placing the bur. The two bearings (upper & lower) hold the bur tube and pinion in place.

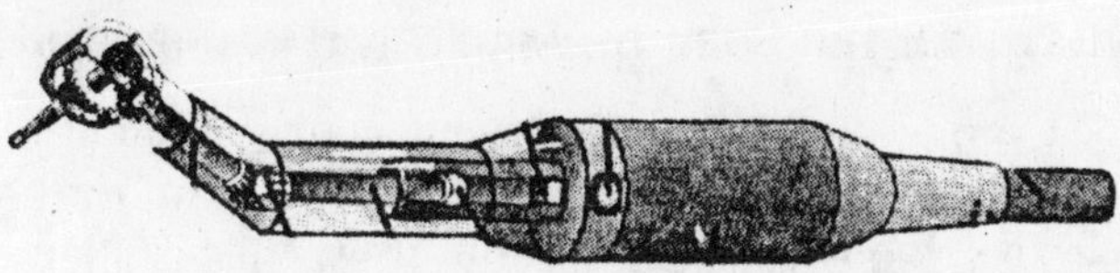

*Fig. 6.11. Slow speed HP*

**107. WHAT MOTOR IS NEEDED TO DRIVE A SLOW SPEED HANDPIECE?**

**A:** Either an air driven motor (air motor) or a electrically driven miniature motor (micromotor) can be used for driving the handpiece. However, the same slow speed handpiece can be used for both air motor and micromotor.

**108. DO ALL THE HANDPIECES HAVE COLLET CHUCK MECHANISM FOR HOLDING BUR?**

**A:** No. Only airotor handpieces and slow speed straight hand pieces use the collet chuck mechanism.

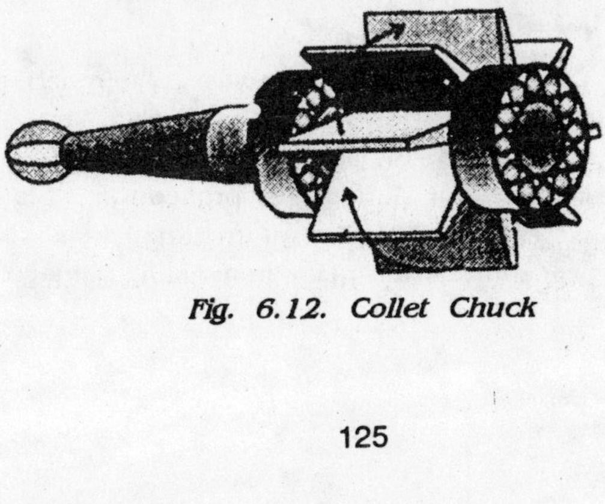

*Fig. 6.12. Collet Chuck*

**109. HOW IS THE BUR USED IN A SLOW SPEED CONVENTIONAL CONTRA ANGLE HANDPIECE?**

**A:** The bur is held by a latch in the handpiece. For inserting the bur, the latch is released (latch can move only in one direction) the bur inserted into the bur tube and the latch is closed. The 'D' shaped cut in the top of the bur engages the corresponding projection in the bur tube and the bur rotates when hand piece is activated. This latch type attachment is also called a ratchet attachment.

**110. WHAT ARE THE USES OF AIROTOR HANDPIECE & BURS?**

**A:** They are useful for gross cavity cutting, removal of old restorations, removal of gross excess from restorations, selective tooth grinding for occlusal rehabilitation.

**111. WHERE ARE RIGHT ANGLED HANDPIECES USED?**

**A:** They have limited use in some oral surgery procedures because of better access.

**112. WHERE ARE STRAIGHT HANDPIECE USEFUL?**

**A:** They have very little use in the oral cavity for cavity cutting or tooth reduction, because of access. They are currently, used in the oral cavity for smoothing procedures. Their main use is in the dental laboratories and extra oral use in the dental clinics for trimming and polishing extra orally made restorations. The laboratory straight hand piece is bulkier and sturdier than the lighter dental operatory handpiece.

**113. WHERE ARE THE CONTRA ANGLE SLOW SPEED HAND PIECES USED?**

**A:** They are used intra orally for cavity refinement, retentive groove placement, caries removal and intra oral polishing of restorations. The slow speed of the revolving instrument gives greater control during the procedure. Slow speed also means less development of frictional heat during the polishing procedure and it helps in avoiding damage to pulp.

**114. ARE THERE DIFFERENT TYPES OF SLOW SPEED CONTRA ANGLE HAND PIECES?**

**A:** Yes. Commonly used slow speed contra angle handpiece is 1:1 handpiece where the output is equal to the input. This handpiece is identified by a blue colour band on the shank of the hand piece, and a blue dot on the head of the handpiece. (Speed 5,000 to 40,000.) It is used for cavity refinement & groove placement. A speed reducing hand piece of 7:1 ratio is available & the speed is between 500 to 5,500 rpm. This is useful for pin channel preparation and caries removal. Such speed reducing hand pieces (reduction gear handpieces) have a green band around the shank and a green dot in the head of the hand piece. Speed increasing handpieces are also available in 1:4 ratio (speeds between 16,000 rpm to 1,60,000 rpm). Such hand pieces have a red band in the shank and a red dot on the head of the hand piece. Two red rings may indicate 1:10 increase in speed.

**115. ARE HANDPIECES AVAILABLE ONLY IN ONE SIZE?**

**A:** Handpieces are available in normal head (adult) size and miniature head (peadiatric) sizes. The smaller head hand pieces are to be used in children and adults with limited mouth opening.

**116. ARE THERE ANY OTHER ATTACHMENTS IN THE HAND PIECES?**

**A:** Some handpieces come with fibre optic light attachments. Such illumination is bright, with no possibility of any shadows because the light being on the under surface of the hand piece. This illumination is better than the conventional operating light of the dental chair because of the proximity to the field of operation. All the handpieces have provision for a coolant system. All the revolving burs generate frictional heat which may rise very rapidly and unless disipated, can harm the pulp. The coolant system could be concealed within the handpiece or may be external. At high speed an aerosol spray of water and air cool the bur better than plain air or water alone. The outlets for water are positioned and angulated in the head of handpiece in such an way that the aerosol jet is directed at the cutting portion of the revolving bur heads. Some handpieces have only one coolant outlet while some have three outlets equidistant from one another. The advantage of multiple coolant spray is, even if one spray is blocked by a portion of tooth being cut, the other sprays might reach the revolving bur head.

**117. IN WHICH DIRECTION WILL THE BUR ROTATE IN A HAND PIECE?**

**A:** In airotor hand pieces, the burs will rotate only in the clockwise direction. In slow speed handpieces (both straight hand piece & contra angle handpieces) it is possible to choose the direction of rotation between clockwise and anticlockwise directions.

**118. WHAT ARE THE DIFFERENCES BETWEEN HIGH SPEED AND LOW SPEED HAND PIECES?**

**A:**

1. High speed handpieces rotate at very high speed. Usually calculated in lakhs of revolutions per minute. Slow speed will be in thousands of rpm.
2. Within limits, it is possible to vary the speed of the bur in a slow speed handpiece and it is not possible in a high speed handpiece.
3. It is possible to change the direction of rotation in a slow speed handpiece while it is not possible in a airotor handpiece.
4. Airotor handpiece & burs are to be used in feather touch brushing strokes. Pressure on high speed hand pieces stall the bur & it will stop rotation. Slow speed handpieces definitely need more pressure.
5. Airotor handpieces have very low torque and slow speed handpieces have high torque.
6. Airotor handpieces use smaller sized, friction grip burs or diamond points. Slow speed, contra angle hand

pieces use larger latch type burs while slow speed straight hand pieces use long shank burs or point.

7. The coolant system in a high speed handpiece is always internal whereas in slow speed hand pieces the coolant system could be either internal or external.

**119. WHAT IS TORQUE?**

**A:** Torque is turning movement of the instrument. Torque is the ability to withstand lateral pressure on the revolving tool, without decreasing its speed or reducing its cutting efficiency. Torque depends on the type of bearing and the amount of energy applied to the handpiece. Higher the speed, lesser the torque. Hence when pressure is applied on the airotor handpiece the bur stops rotating. Conventional hand pieces have greater torque.

**120. WHAT ARE THE ADVANTAGES OF HIGH SPEED CAVITY CUTTING?**

**A:** 1. Ease of cutting 2. Greater patient comfort 3. Less operator fatigue 4. When sufficient coolant is used no pulpal irritation 5. Less time consuming 6. Less vibration of the instrument

**121. WHAT ARE DISADVANTAGES OF HIGH SPEED CAVITY CUTTING?**

**A:** 1. Lack of feel & tendency for overcutting 2. Reduced visibility due to copious coolant flow 3. Possible aerosol spread of infection 4. Possible ear damage due to high whining noise of aerotor 5. Possible discharge of broken bur tips, broken tooth structure or old restoration at high speed to the operator's/assistants' eye and possible damage.

**122. HOW SHOULD THE HANDPIECES BE MAINTAINED?**

**A:** 1. Daily lubrication of the handpiece with the lubricant suggested by the manufacturer, is mandatory.

2. Lubrication before sterlization is necessary.

3. Always running the handpiece, only with a bur, point or blank in the chuck.

4. Never dropping the handpiece for fear of damaging the bearings or cartridge

5. Avoiding entry of saliva or blood into the cartridge of handpiece.

6. Periodical cleaning of the water inlets & outlets to maintain effective coolant spray in the proper direction.

7. Thorough external cleaning of handpiece before sterilization.

**123. HOW ARE HAND PIECES STERILIZED?**

**A:** Presently available hand pieces are autoclavable. Oil sterlization of handpieces is obsolete.

**124. WHAT ARE BURS?**

**A:** Burs are blade cutting instruments used in handpiece. Dental burs are commonly made from steel or tungsten carbide. Steel burs are single piece of tempered tungsten vanadium alloy steel and the blades are machined out of steel blank. Tungsten carbide burs have a stainless steel shank to which is welded a tungsten carbide Cobalt Composite tip, which is then ground with diamond to produce the cutting edges.

**125. WHAT ARE DIAMOND POINTS?**

**A:** Diamond coated points are another rotary cutting tool. It consists of an inner steel blank over which industrial diamonds of different girt are either electroplated with Nickel or are sintered with a metal matrix.

**126. WHERE ARE DIAMOND POINTS USED?**

**A:** At high speeds, diamond points cut enamel, amalgam, composite porcelain effectively.

**127. WHERE ARE TUNGSTEN CARBIDE BURS USED?**

**A:** At high speed, tungsten carbide burs cut dentine, amalgam, composite and cast metal effectively.

**128. WHERE ARE STEEL BURS EFFECTIVE?**

**A:** At slow speed, steel burs cut carious dentine effectively.

**129. CAN A DIAMOND POINT BE CALLED A DIAMOND BUR?**

**A:** Technically no. But in common usage, many dentist and text books call a diamond point as a diamond bur. Though burs and points are used as cutting tools, due to difference in manufacturing techniques, a diamond point can not be called a bur.

**130. WHAT ARE THE PARTS OF A BUR?**

**A:** A bur or a point consists of 3 parts. There is no consensus in naming the three parts. While every body agrees that the working part is known as the head, there are differences of opinion about naming the other two parts. They are named either as shank and neck. Attachment and neck or shank and shaft:

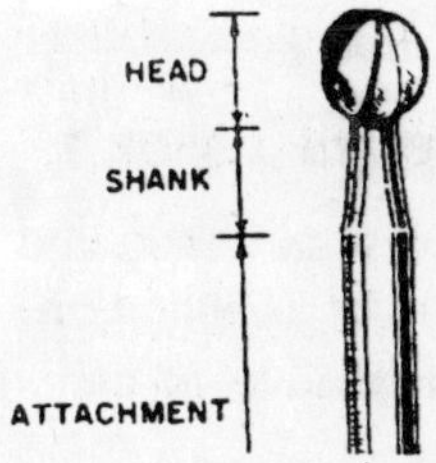


*Fig. 6.13. Parts of a Bur*

**131. WHY CAN'T THE BUR BE DIVIDED INTO A SHAFT SHANK AND BLADE LIKE A HAND INSTRUMENT, TO AVOID CONFUSION?**

**A:** A sensible suggestion, but has to be accepted by the international scientific community

**132. WHAT TERMINOLOGY IS TO BE FOLLOWED IN THIS BOOK?**

**A:** The terminology will be shank, neck and head.

**133. HOW ARE BURS CLASSIFIED?**

**A:** 1. Depending on their mode of attachment to hand piece

a. friction grip b. latch type

2. Depending on which hand piece it will be used a) slow speed contra angle bur b) straight handpiece bur & c) airotor bur.

3. Depending on the direction of rotation: a) Right cutting (clockwise rotation b) Left cutting (anticlockwise rotation. Common types are right cutting burs.

4. Depending on the shape of the burs : a) round b) wheel c) inverted cone d) plain cylindrical fissure burs e) crosscut cylindrical fissure bur f) plain tapered fissure burs g) cross cut tapered fissure burs h) pear shaped burs i) end cutting burs j) flame shaped burs k) bud shaped burs l) torpedo shaped bur m) beaver bur n) Baker Curzon bur.

**134. HOW ARE ROUND BURS USED?**

**A:** Round burs are spherical in shape and are used for enamel penetration, extension of preparation, placement of retentive grooves, pits and removal of carious dentine from deep cavities.

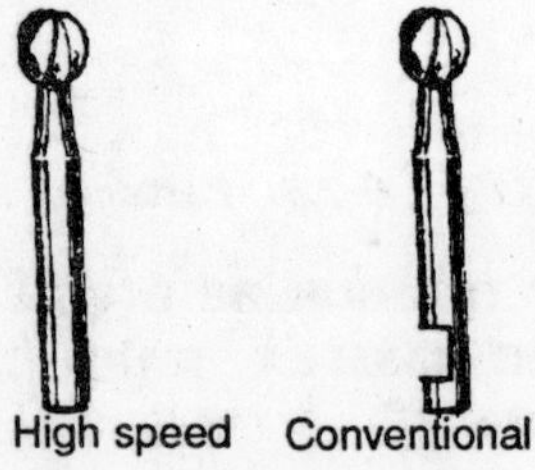


*Fig. 6.14. Round Bur*

**135. WHERE ARE WHEEL BURS USED?**

**A:** Wheel burs are used for placing grooves and for gross removal of tooth structure.

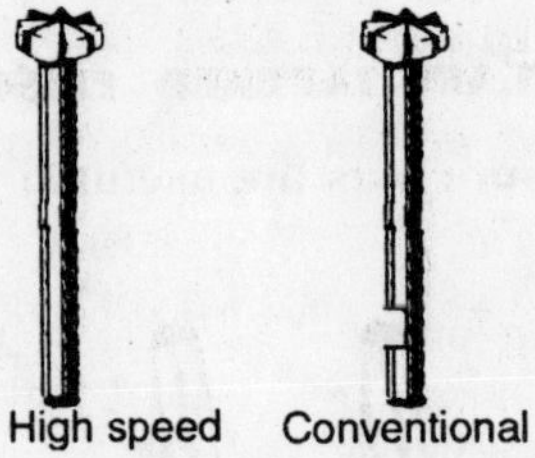


*Fig. 6.15. Wheel Bur*

**136. WHERE ARE INVERTED CONE BURS USED?**

**A:** Inverted cone burs are used for placing undercuts in dentine. They can also be used for cavity extensions and smoothening floors.

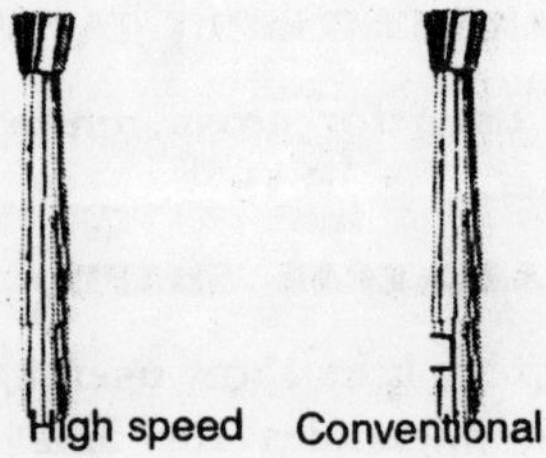


*Fig. 6.16. Inverted Cone Bur*

**137. WHERE ARE PLAIN CYLINDRICAL FISSURE BURS USED?**

**A:** Plain fissure bur is used for extending the cavity.

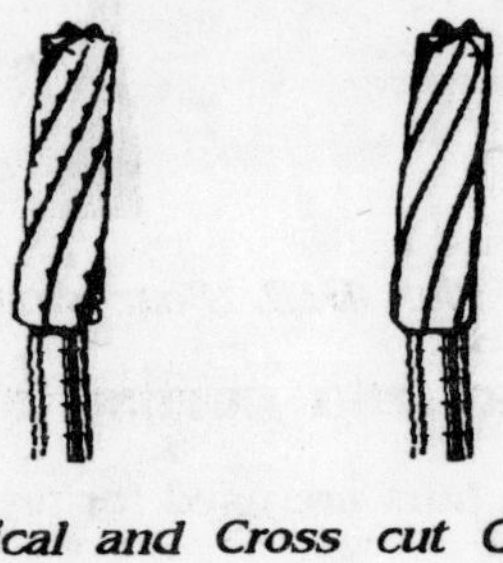

*Fig. 6.17. Plain cylindrical and Cross cut Cylindrical burs*

**138. WHAT IS THE ADVANTAGE OF CROSS CUT IN A FISSURE BUR?**

**A:** Cross cutting increases the cutting efficiency in low and medium speeds. Ref. Fig. 6.17

**139. WHERE ARE PLAIN TAPERED FISSURE BURS USED?**

**A:** Plain tapered fissure burs are useful in preparing inlay cavity preparations.

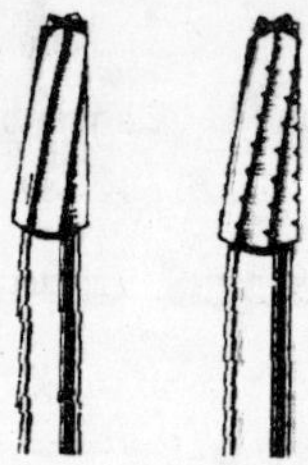

*Fig. 6.18. Plain tapered and Crosscut tapered burs*

**140. WHERE ARE CROSSCUT TAPERED FISSURE BURS USED?**

**A:** They are used for gross removal of tooth tissue at lower speeds. Ref. Fig. 6.18

**141. WHERE ARE PEAR SHAPED BURS USED?**

**A:** Pear shaped burs are useful in preparing cavities with roundered lineangles for amalgam.

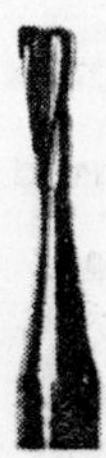

*Fig. 6.19. Pear shaped Bur*

**142. WHERE ARE END CUTTING BURS USED?**

**A:** End cutting burs are used for preparing shoulders for Jacket crown preparations. The advantage of end cutting bur is it cuts, only apically and not axially.

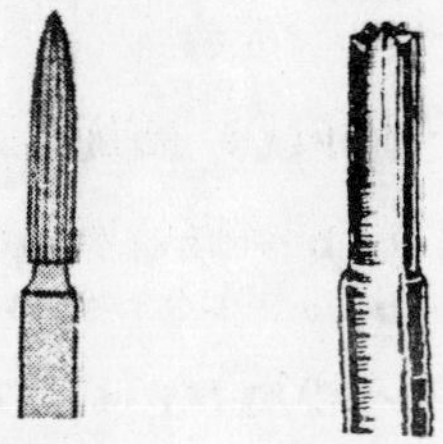

*Fig. 6.20. End cutting Bur & Flame shaped bur*

**143. WHERE ARE FLAME SHAPED BURS USED?**

**A:** They are useful in placing secondary bevels in the prorimal walls and refining gingival margins. Ref. 6.20

**144. WHERE ARE BUD SHAPED BURS USED?**

**A:** Bud shaped (egg shaped) burs are used mainly to reduce the lingual and occlusal surfaces of teeth during crown preparation.

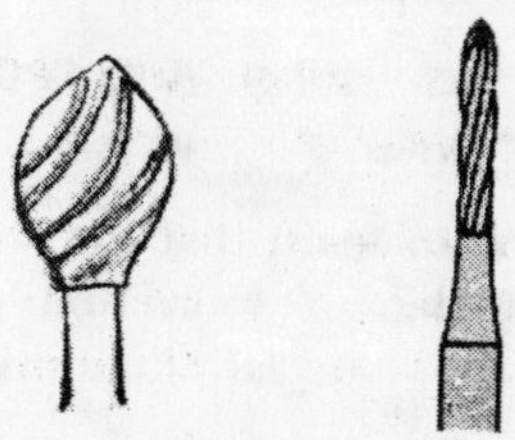

*Fig. 6.21. Bud shaped Bur & Torpedo shaped Bur*

**145. WHERE ARE TORPEDO SHAPED BURS USED?**

**A:** Torpedo shaped burs are also known as chamfer burs. They help giving a chamfer finish margin for cast metal restorations. Ref. Fig. 6.21

**146. WHAT IS A BEAVER BUR?**

**A:** It is a fine cross cut bur used to cut cast metal in the month.

**147. WHAT IS A BAKER CURZON BUR?**

**A:** It is a bladeless tungsten carbide cobalt composite tip brazed to a steel shank for finishing preparation and restorations.

**148. WHERE ARE TWELVE BLADED CARBIDE BURS USED?**

**A:** They are used for bevelling & smoothening enamel margins. They can also be used for smoothening composite fillings.

**149. WHAT ARE SPECIALITY CUTTERS?**

**A:** They are instruments used in some special situations rather than in routine cavity cutting (eg: Twist drills for pin channel preparation, Peeso reamers for post space preparation and GatesGlidden drills for root canal preparation in coronal two thirds of straight canals.

**150. DO DIAMOND POINTS ALSO COME IN THESE SHAPES?**

**A:** The shapes described are not exhaustive but only examples. Burs are available in other shapes also. Diamond points are also coming in the above shapes & other shapes also.

**151. WILL ALL THE BURS AND POINTS BE NEEDED FOR CAVITY CUTTING?**

**A:** It is surprising to learn that for preparing a cavity, few burs may be sufficient. Individual preferences and specific requirements for special situations might necessitate more burs.

**152. WHAT ARE THE PARTS OF THE HEAD OF A BUR?**

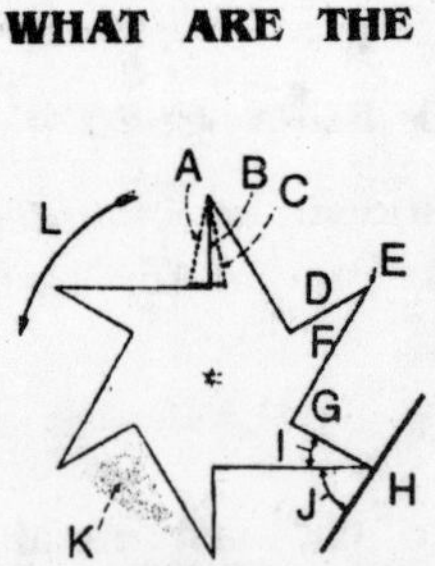


A - Negative rake angle B - Radial rake angle
C - Positive rake angle D - Face
E - Cutting edge F - Tooth
G - Back (flank) H - Work
I - Tooth angle J - Clearance angle
K - Flute or chip space L - Rotation

*Fig. 6.22. Parts of Head of a Bur*

**A:** A dental bur has bur teeth. The spaces between bur teeth are called flute or chip space. Bur tooth's one side is known as face and the other side is back. In some burs there may be land between face and back. Each bur tooth has a blade angle.

**153. DESCRIBE A BUR TOOTH?**

**A:** Bur tooth has a face (leading side of the bur tooth towards the direction of rotation) and a back (trailing side of the bur tooth towards the direction of rotation). The face and back may meet at the cutting edge or blade. Sometimes a plane surface may be present between face & back and it is known as land.

**154. WHAT IS FLUTE OR CHIP SPACE?**

**A:** Flute is the space between two successive bur teeth.

**155. WHAT IS A RAKE ANGLE?**

**A:** Rake angle is the angle that the face of a bur tooth makes with the raidal line from the centre of the bur to the blade. Rake angle is said to be negative, if the face leads (is in front of) the radial line. If the face trails (is in back of) the radial line, the rake angle is said to be positive. If the face coincides with the radial line, it is supposed to be a radial rake angle.

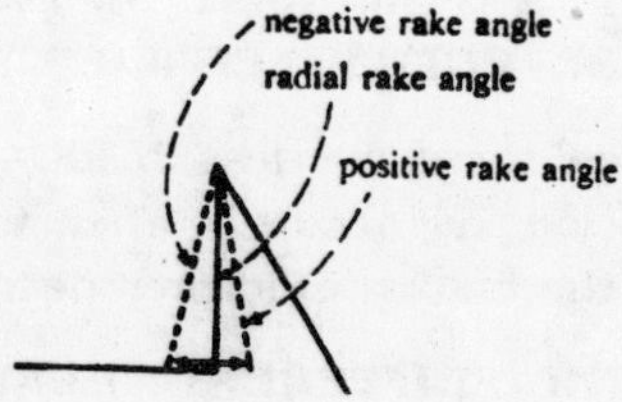


*Fig. 6.23. Rake angle*

**156. WHAT ARE THE ADVANTAGES AND DISADVANTAGES OF A POSITIVE RAKE ANGLE?**

**A:** A positive rake angle means a thin bur tooth. The advantage is greater cutting efficiency. Disadvantage is more possibility of bending and possibility of fracture of bur tooth.

**157. WHAT ARE THE ADVANTAGES AND DISADVANTAGES OF A NEGATIVE RAKE ANGLE?**

**A:** A negative rake angle means a thick bur tooth. The advantages are longer bur life and less clogging. Disadvantages will be less cutting efficiency compared to a positive rake angle.

**158. WHAT RAKE ANGLES DO MOST BURS HAVE?**

**A:** Most burs are made with negative rake angle.

**159. GENERALLY HOW MANY BUR TEETH DOES A CUTTING BUR HAVE?**

**A:** A cutting bur has 6 to 8 bur teeth ( and six to eight flutes in between) and are known as 6 fluted or 8 fluted burs.

**160. WHAT ARE FINISHING BURS?**

**A:** Finishing burs are multifluted burs used for smoothening a restoration.

**161. HOW MANY BUR TEETH DOES A FINISHING BUR HAVE?**

**A:** A finishing bur has 12 to 40 blades (bur teeth and corresponding flutes)

**162. DOESN'T AN INCREASE IN NUMBER OF BUR TEETH INCREASE CUTTING EFFICIENCY?**

**A:** No. When there are less blades, the chip space is more & less clogging occurs. When there are more number of blades, the cutting efficiency decreases with more clogging.

**163. ARE THE DIFFERENT BURS INTERCHANGEABLE BETWEEN DIFFERENT HANDPIECES?**

**A:** A slow speed straight handpiece bur can not be used in a slow speed contrangle handpiece Slow speed contra angle bur can not be used in an airotor hand piece nor an airotor bur be used in a conventional contra angle hand piece. The reason is not only because of the difference in mode of attachment, but also the differences in dimensions of the shank (the portion entering into the hand piece) of the bur.

**164. WHAT ARE THE DIMENSIONS OF THE BURS USED FOR DIFFERENT HAND PIECES?**

**A:** The diameter of a laboratory straight hand piece bur is 3/32 inch (2.35 m.m.). The diameter of a conventional contra angle bur is 3/32 inch (2.35 m.m). The diameter of an airotor bur is 1/16 inch 1.6 m.m.) special laboratory straight hand piece burs of 3 millimeter (2/16 inch) diameter are also available. This means an airotor bur will be too loose inside the slow speed contra angle hand piece and it can not be latched into place either, due to absence of latch recess in the bur shank. Though some practitioners try to use a conventional contra angle bur in a straight hand piece, it is advisable to use appropriate burs for the appropriate hand pieces. 3 millimeter diameter burs can be used only on special 3 millimeter laboratory hand pieces.

**165. IN WHAT SIZES ARE THE BURS AVAILABLE?**

**A:** The burs are available in different sizes to suit the needs of the individual operator.

**166. IS THERE ANY DIFFERENCE IN THE LENGTH OF THE BURS?**

**A:** Usually the shank length of a straight hand piece is 1.25 inch (32 millimeters). The shank length of a conventional latch type (ratchet type) bur is 0.520 inch (15 millimeter) and the shank length of an airotor bur is 0.5 inch (12.5 millimeter). Though these are the standard dimensions, long shank and short shank burs are available. A short shank bur is useful in peadiatric cases and patients with microstomia (small mouth) or inability to open the mouth fully due to any disease. A long shank bur is useful in some endodontic treatment like pulpotomy.

**167. ARE THESE BURS WITH LONGER OR SHORTER NECKS?**

A: No. The neck size is constant even if the length of shank varies.

**168. WHY THERE IS USUALLY A TAPER IN THE NECK?**

A: The taper in the neck of the bur is to permit greater visibility of the cutting head while preparing a cavity.

**169 ARE THERE VARIATIONS IN THE LENGTH OF THE HEAD?**

A: Yes. Burs with longer heads are available. They are available mainly in fissure burs especially tape ring fissure burs. Longer burs are given the letter 'L' after their number.

**170. WHAT ARE THE NUMBERING SYSTEMS FOR THE BURS?**

A: Manufacturers used to have their own numbering systems. There were no standardization. Different countries have their own arbitary way of numbering burs. This has led to the possibility of similar burs from different manufacturers being given different numbers and different burs from different manufacturers being given the same number.

**171. CAN'T THE BUR NUMBERS BE STANDARDIZED INTERNATIONALLY?**

A: International standardization has been attempted in 1986. This numbering system is supposed to identify any bur about 1. The material with which the bur head is made of 2. For use in which hand piece the bur is intended to be 3. The shape and length of the head of the bur 4. The grit size (surface finish) if the material is diamond 5 the maximum diameter of the bur in one tenth of a millimeter.

**172. HOW IS IT POSSIBLE TO KNOW SO MANY DETAILS FROM A SINGLE NUMBER?**

A: If the number is large enough all the details will be known. The ISO number has 15 (fifteen) digits! Every three numbers provide the details of the materials with which the head is made of, the type of shank, shape of cutting head, grit size and the diameter of the head. For example if the ISO number is 807314107534018, it has to be divided into sets of three digits. 807 denotes it is diamond, 314 denotes it is friction grip airotor bur 107 denoting it is a cylindrical bur 534 denotes it is coarse grit diameter and 018 denotes the bur size is 1.8 m.m.

**173. BUT, FROM THE NUMBER 807, HOW IS IT POSSIBLE TO KNOW THAT IT IS DIAMOND?**

**A:** If the first three digits are 310, or 330 it is steel If the first three digits are 500, it is tungstencarbide. If the first three digits are 615,625,635 it is Aluminium Oxide. If the first three digits are 806 or 807 it is diamond.

**174. HOW DOES THE SECOND SET OF THREE NUMBERS DENOTE THE SHANK FORM?**

**A:** If the second three digits are 103, 104 & 105 it is for use in a standard straight hand piece. If the second three digits are 124, it is for special heavy duty laboratory hand piece that requires a special hand piece chuck for fixing this special 3 millimeter diameter bur. If the second set of 3 digits are 202,204, 205 & 206, the bur is for conventional (slow speed) contra angle hand piece. If the second set of 3 digits are 313, 314, 315 & 316, the bur is for airotor hand piece. If the second set of numbers is 900, it denotes unmounted stones set requiring a carrying mandrel to be used in a hand piece.

**175. HOW WILL THE THIRD SETS OF THREE DIGITS REVEAL THE SHAPE OF BUR HEAD?**

**A:** If the third set of 3 digits are 001 and 002, it has round head. If the third set of 3 digits are between 010-020 it has inverted cone head. If the third set of 3 digits are between 030-039 it has double cone head.

If third set of 3 digits are between 040 - 099 it has a wheel head. If the third set of 3 digits are between 100-150, it has cylinder head (straight fissure). If the third set of 3 digits are between 160-229, it has cone (Tapering fissure) head. If the third set of 3 digits 230-237 it has pear shaped head. If the third set of 3 digits are 243, it has flame shaped head. If the third set of 3 digits are 260, it has bud shaped head. If the third set of 3 digits are 284, it has torpedo shaped head. If the third set of 3 digits are between 320-329, they are discs.

**176. WHAT DOES THE FOURTH SET OF 3 DIGITS STAND FOR?**

**A:** The fourth set of three digits will denote the surface finish to the abrasive points with and dental burs. These three digits, for abrasive points specify the grain coarseness. If the fourth set of 3 digits are 494, it is superfine with an average grain size of 15 microns. If the number is 504, it is extra fine with grain size of 30 microns. If the number is 514 it is extra fine with grain size of 50 microns. If the number is 524, it is medium with grain size of 100-120 microns. If the number is 534, it is coarse with grain size 135-140 microns. If the number is 544, it is extra coarse with grain size of 180 microns. In case of machine cut steel or tungsten carbide bur, 001 means straight bur tooth, 006 means right hand twist, 007 denoting crosscut twist, 019 means double diagonal, 071 meaning coarse flute, 072 means fine flute, 140 means fine diamond cut, 175 means medium tooth lab bur. 215 coarse tooth lab bur etc.

**177. WHAT DOES THE FIFTH SET OF 3 DIGITS STAND FOR?**

**A:** The fifth set of 3 digits denote the maximum diameter (thickness) of the bur head in one tenth of a millimeter.

**78. IS THE ABOVE LIST COMPLETE?**

**A:** No. The complete list is too exhaustive. There are too many designs, shapes & sizes of burs.

**179. IS THE ISO SYSTEM OF NUMBERING BURS EASY TO USE?**

**A:** It is easy to use once all the data are fed into a computer. Then it will be very easy to describe the bur from a given ISO number or to find out the ISO number from a description of the bur

**180. BUT WITHOUT AN EXHAUSTIVE AND COMPREHENSIVE DATA SHEET, IT IS DIFFICULT TO DECIPHER THE FIRST FOUR SETS OF 3 DIGIT NUMBERS. IS THERE ANY WAY**

**OF USING THE LAST 3 DIGIT NUMBERS ALONE TO EXPRESS WHAT WE NEED?**

A: That is what many practitioners are currently doing. They just ask for a long shank tapering fissure fine diamond No. 010 or short shank tungsten carbide round No. 008 and that solves the problem of rattling out a fifteen digit number.

181. **WHAT DO THE COLOUR BANDS IN SOME DIAMOND POINTS INDICATE?**

A: It is the colour coding to identify the surface finish of the diamond point. Yellow colour band in the shank denote superfine. Red colour denotes fine grit. Absence of colour band means medium grit and green band indicate coarse grit.

182. **HOW ARE BURS NUMBERED IN A.D.A. SYSTEM?**

A: ¼, ½, 1,2,3,4,5,6,7,8,9,10 & 11 are round burs. 33½ to 40 are inverted cones. 55 ¼ to 62 are straight fissures. 700 to 703 are tapering fissure burs. 957 to 959 are end cutting burs. 200,201,218,219,230,231,242 to 246 are finishing burs.

183. **WHAT ARE STONES AND TRIMMERS?**

A: Stones and trimmers are abrasive instruments intended for reducing extraorally made restorations. They are larger than burs & points. They may come as mounted or unmounted stones.

184. **WHAT IS A MOUNTED STONE/TRIMMER?**

A: They are abrasive instruments of different shapes available mounted rigidly to shafts that can fit either a straight hand piece, conventional contra angle handpiece or rarely a airotor handpiece.

185. **WHAT ARE COMMON ABRASIVE MOUNTED STONES?**

A: Aluminium oxide (Alundum) is bonded in ceramic and it is available as white or pink stones. Silicon Carbide (Carborundum) is bonded in ceramic and is available as black or green stones. Aluminium Oxide is used for cutting porcelain & Acrylic resin Silicon Carbide or Aluminium Oxide are used for cutting gold.

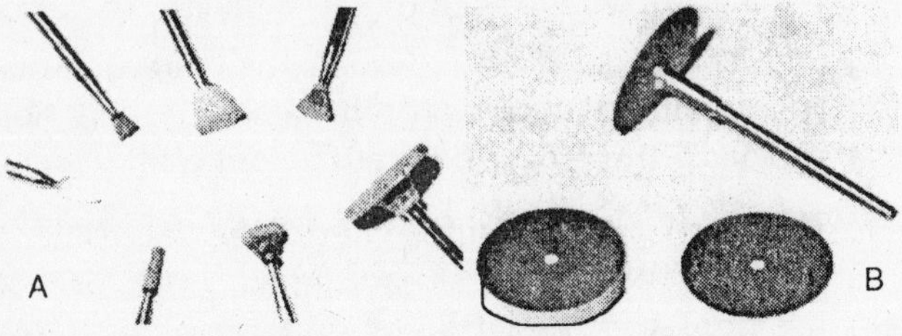


*Fig. 6.24. Mounted and Unmounted stones*

**186. WHAT ARE UNMOUNTED STONES?**

**A:** These abrasive instruments are not supplied as mounted to a rigid shaft. They are supplied as circular wheel stones with a hole in the centre. The shape might vary, but all the stones have a hole in the centre. These stones are to be mounted on screw type mandrels and used. Instead of thick stones, thin discs are also available. Fig. 6.24

**187. GIVE SOME EXAMPLES OF UNMOUNTED STONES?**

**A :**

1. Heatless stone is a coarse stone for grinding metal or porcelain. The thickness ranges between 3/32" to 3/16". The diameter could be1/2" to 1".

2. Busch silent stone is a very fine grit stone used exclusively for grinding porcelain. Its thickness is 2 milli meters & diameter 5/8".

3. Carborudum disc - It is flat, circular with a diameter of 7/8" and thickness between 0.5 & 0.6 mm. It has coarse or fine silicon carbide (Carborundum) particles. It is used for cutting, disking or grinding and they fracture readily.

4. Ultra thin separating disc - diameter 7/8" and thickness 0.25 mm. It is fragile & it should be mounted on a large headed mandrel. It is used for separating metal or porcelain.

5. Safe sided disc - It is a disc on which the abrsine in coated only one side. They may be used for proximal reduction of tooth without damage to neighbouring tooth.

6. Diamond discs - diamond particles are mounted in metal discs.

7. Flexible abrasive strips have the abrasive materials impregnated on one side of paper, nylon or cloth. They are for inter proximal smoothening of a restoration. They are to be used manually and are available in different widths.

**188. WHAT ARE RUBBER ABRASIVE WHEELS & POINTS?**

**A:** Abrasives are impregnated in rubber polishing wheels and points during manufacture. They are mostly supplied as mounted rubber wheels, points, cups etc. or unmounted wheels, discs etc. Their thickness varies between 1/16" to 1/8" & diameter could be 3/8" to 1". They are used for eliminating coarse, grooves and ditches in metals before polishing. Wheels are used to smoothen flat or convex surfaces. Cone shaped points are useful in smoothening concave surfaces, grooves and occlusal surfaces of restoration.

**189. WHAT ARE FLEXIBLE ABRASIVE DISCS AND STRIPS?**

**A:** A rigid abrasive or polishing disc can be used for selective gross trimming. A flexible abrasive or polishing disc is able to maintain the contour of the structure (tooth or restoration) being reduced. Silicon carbide, Aluminium Oxide, garnet, flint (sand) cuttle (powdered calcified sheel of a Mollusk), rouge (ferric oxide), Crocus (impure ferric oxide are the abrasives which are coated on paper, cloth or resins and are flexible. They are to be mounted on either screw type mandrels or snap on mandrels. These flexible abrasive and polishing discs are available in different circular sizes ranging from 1/4" to 7/8" diameter. These flexible discs usually have the abrasive coating only on one side.

**190. WHAT IS THE DIFFERENCE BETWEEN SNAP ON MANDRELS AND SCREW TYPE MANDRELS?**

**A:** For a screw type mandrels, the screw has to be removed, from the mandrel & screw inserted into the pinhole in the centre of the disc and screwed on to the shaft of the mandrel again. The abrading surface can be facing towards the handpiece or away from the handpiece or even two discs could be fixed on a single mandrel with their non abrasive surfaces against each other. This can enable the operator to use either the front or back of the disc depending on the accessability of the surface to be abraded.

**191. WHAT ARE THE ADVANTAGES AND DISADVANTAGES OF DIFFERENT TYPES OF MANDRELS?**

**A:** In a screw type mandrel, the advantage is two pinhole discs with their abrading surfaces away from each other could be mounted together to trim either with the front or back surfaces depending on the operator's convenience. The back mounted flexible abrasive disc can be used conveniently on lingual surface of anterior teeth. The disadvantages of screw type mandrel is (1) it can be used only is one direction - either clockwise or anticlockwise depending on the direction of the threads in the screw. If the mandrel is to be operated in the same direction as the thread of screw, it will result in the screw becoming loose. (2) The screw head, will not be in the same level as the disc. This can interfere with abrasive & polishing procedure as the elevated revolving screw head can touch a convex restorative surface and alter the contour.

**192. WHAT ARE THE ADVANTAGES OF A SNAP ON MANDREL?**

**A :** 1. The projection on the head of the snap on or pop on mandrel will be flush, with the level of the flexible disc and will not be interfering with working areas. The thin flat heads may be square or circular, which hold the appropriate discs by friction grip.

2. As no screw is holding the disc, the mandrel can be operated, either in forward or backward (clockwise or anticlockwise) direction. The disadvantage is two single sided flexible discs can not be mounted back to back for convenient use in different areas as only one disc can be mounted on a snap on mandrel at a time. The disc may have to be mounted reverse if better access is needed in some areas.

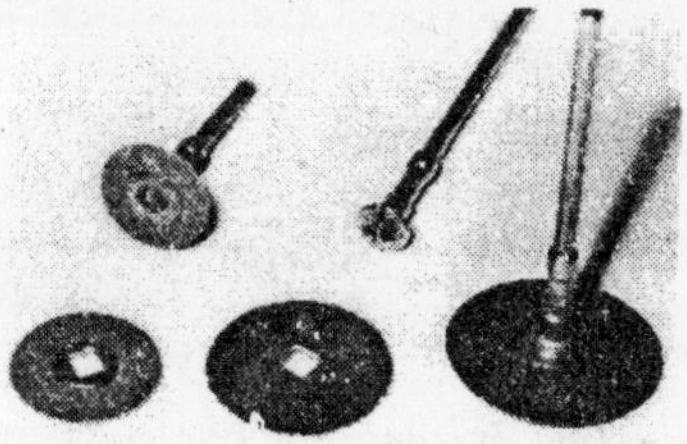

*Fig. 6.25. Snap on mandrels*

**193. HOW DOES THE SNAP ON MANDREL HOLD ON TO THE DISCS?**

**A:** The snap on or pop on mandrel head (the projecting part) has one or two partial vertical splits. This means that it is compressible. The metallic central portion of the disc has as lightly smaller dimension than the split head of the mandrel. When the disc is snapped on to the mandrel the split is compressed & the disc slips in. Once in position, the compressed split head holds the snap on disc.

**194. ARE MANDRELS AVAILABLE ONLY FOR STRAIGHT HAND PIECES?**

**A:** Mandrels are available for both straight hand piece and slow speed contra angle hand piece (Latch or ratchet type attachment).

**195. WHAT ARE POLISHING INSTRUMENTS?**

**A:** Unmounted rubber cups and wheels, mounted bristle brushes for straight as well as contra angle hand pieces and thin rag wheels are available for polishing. For use in the dental lathe, felt cones, cloth wheels, polishing buffs are available.

**196. WHAT POLISHING MATERIALS ARE COMMONLY USED?**

A : 1. Calcium carbonate (whiting, precipitated chalk)

2. Zinc Oxide

3. Tin Oxide

4. Iron Oxide

5. Chromium Oxide

**197. HOW ARE THE POLISHING MATERIALS SUPPLIED?**

A: 1. As a slurry (powders mixed in water or alcohol)

2. As pastes (polishing pastes)

3. As soft bricks (rouge - iron oxide)

**198. IS THERE A POLISHING BUR?**

A: A round blank made of steel is used for polishing amalgam. The spherical blank is smooth and has no cutting edges. It is passed over a set amalgam restoration to smoothen and polish it.

**199. WHAT ARE ALTERNATIVE METHODS OF CUTTING TOOTH STRUCTURE?**

A: Airbrasive technique (use of abrasive particles directed at the tooth surface under pressure) was introduced in the early fifties but it never became popular, as the depth of cutting could not be kept under control. Nowadays attempts are made to use laser beam for cavity cutting. Enamieloplasty and coalasing deep grooves have been successfully accomplished with laser bearns. Research is on for regular use of laser beams for cavity cutting.

# CHAPTER - 7

# CLINICAL SIGNIFICANCE OF ANATOMY AND HISTOLOGY OF DENTAL TISSUES

**1. WHAT IS THE ADVANTAGE OF KNOWING ABOUT THE ANATOMY AND HISTOLOGY OF DENTAL TISSUES?**

**A:** Knowledge of macroscopic and microscopic structure of the tooth is essential during cavity cutting to take maximum advantage, mechanically and biologically.

**2. DESCRIBE ABOUT MACROSCOPIC STRUCTURE OF ENAMEL?**

**A:** Enamel is formed by ameloblasts which do not survive after enamel is formed. The clinical significance of this is that there is no possibility of re-formation of enamel once it is lost. Structural loss of enamel, if symptomatic or causes aesthetic impairment, should be restored.

**3. WHERE IS ENAMEL PRESENT IN THE TOOTH?**

**A:** Enamel covers the entire surface of the crown, though in varying thickness in various regions & different teeth. It may be like a knife edge cervically or have a maximum thickness of 2 millimeter at incisal ridge of an incisor or 2.3 to 2.5 mm at the cusp of premolar and 2.5 to 3 milli meter at the cusp of a molar. The clinical significance of this is that the amout of enamel to be cut before reaching dentine will vary from area to area of tooth. In cervical areas dentine is reached quicker than occlusal areas, so the width of the occlusal wall of a class V cavity is always greater than the width of the gingival seat of the cavity. Similarly, in the class III cavities, the incisal wall thickness is more than the cervical (gingival seat) wall thickness.

**4. IS ENAMEL TRANSLUCENT?**

**A:** Yes. Because normal enamel is translucent, it transmits the yellowish colour of dentine through and tooth is seen yellowish white in colour. The clinical significance of this is while preparing a cavity, the pulpal floor or axial wall might appear yellow, but it may be wrong to conclude that dentine has been reached because of the possibility of a thin layer of enamel being present above the dentine. The enamel presence could be confirmed by the absence of sensitivity (as experienced by the patient) and the metallic sound heard while passing the probe over enamel. Another clinical significance is enamel looses its translucency and appears more opaque when subjected to drying. Hence it is important to do the colour matching for restoration before isolating the tooth from saliva. Isolation of tooth from moisture can lead to a temporary loss of loosely bound water from enamel and may appear a little opaque. If shade matching is done islolating and drying a tooth, the selected shade might appear more opaque than normal, wet oral conditions.

**5. WHAT IS THE CHEMICAL COMPOSITION OF ENAMEL?**

**A:** Enamel consits of inorganic substances, mainly hydroxypatite (calcium phosphate crystals) for upto 94% by volume (98% by weight). The organic portion and water constitute 6% by volume (and 2% by weight). The clinical significance of this high mineral content is the ease with which glass ionomer can bond to enamel because of the higher calcium content.

**6. WHAT ARE THE HISTOLOGICAL FEATURES OF ENAMEL?**

**A:** Enamel consits of enamel rods that extend from the dentino enamel junction to the external surface of the tooth. The enamel rods are densely packed and interwined in a wavy course. The wavy course of enamel rods and their intermingling, permits the selective demineralization of enamel rods and use of enamel bonding agent to permeate the demineralized areas, solidify and form the enamel tags. The number of enamel rods can vary from 50 lakhs for a mandibular incisor to about 1.2 crores for an upper molar. The length of the enamel rods could be slightly greater than the thickness of enamel in a given area (greater length is due to wavy course of enamel rods). The wavy course of enamel rods is the reason for occurence of unsupporterd enamel rods along the cavity margin in whichever way the cavity is cut. The general direction of enamel rods is considered to be prependicular to the dentino enamel junction except in the cervical regions of permanent teeth, where the enamel rods are apically tilted. The general direction of enamel rods is of great significance in deciding about the cavity margins to avoid weak enamel structure. The outward apical slanting of enamel rods in gingival seat area always necessitates use of gingival marginal trimmers.

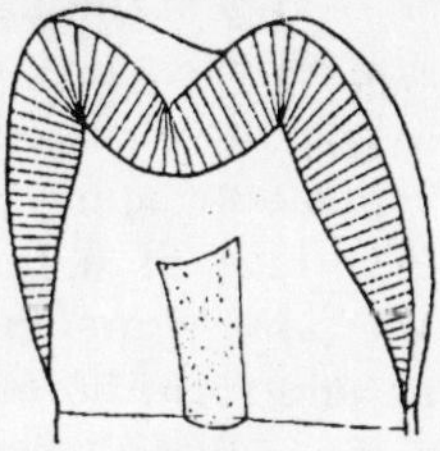

*Fig. 7.1 Enamel rods*

**7. HOW STRONG IS ENAMEL?**

**A:** Enamel is the hardest substance in the human body. But enamel is a rigid (unyielding, inelastic) substance which is highly brittle, having a high elastic modules and low tensile strength. When it is supported by dentine, which is highly elastic, enamel is capable of withstanding masticatory pressure. The clinical significance is that undermined enamel not supported by dentine and which is likely to be subjected to masticatory forces, is to beremoved during cavity prepation.

**8. WHAT IS GNARLED ENAMEL?**

**A:** Gnarled enamel occurs more commonly in occlusal & incisal areas and near cervical areas. Here, there are greater entwining of enamel rods with adjacent enamel rods. The clinical significance is that gnarled enamel can not undergo cleavage easily like regular enamel. They are more resistant to use of enamel, chisels enamel hatchets & enamel hoes.

**9. IS ENAMEL PERMEABLE?**

**A:** Though enamel is very hard and dense, it is permeable to some ions. Dentinal fluid is supposed to permeate through enamel to the outer surface. Similarly salivary ions are also supposed to penetrate from the outer surface through enamel to varying depths. The route of penetration could be through hypomineralized area of enamel, rod sheathes, enamel cracks and any other defective areas. the clinical significance of this is the ability of preventing caries by topical fluouride application. One way of preventing caries is by increasing the resistance of the tooth to acid dissolution. By repeatedly applying high concentration of fluoride, over the surface of a formed tooth, it is found that the fluoride was able to penetrate through the enamel for several microns and form fluorapatite, replacing soluble salts of calcium phosphate (hydroxyapatite) containing manganese & carbonate which are lost during acid demineralisation. Calcium fluorapatite is more resistant to acid attack. Fluoride is also antibacterial by interfering with bacterial enzymatic activity. Fluorides (from dentists direct topical application, from dentifrices (tooth pastes), from drinking water, from mouth rinses) are all able to penetrate enamel and protect the superficial enamel

**10. WILL THE PERMEABILITY OF ENAMEL REMAIN THE SAME THROUGHOUT THE LIFE SPAN?**

**A:** Permeability decreases with age because of changes in enamel matrix though some permeability may remain. Generally a younger enamel is more permeable.

**11. IS ENAMEL A LIVING TISSUE?**

**A:** No. Enamel doesn't have any living cells. The enamel forming cells, the ameloblasts, degenerate after forming the enamel and form a protective layer over the enamel called secondaryenamel cuticle. Enamel is insensitive. While cutting enamel, there is no sensitivity. Enamel cannot regenerate or repair itself after an injury & fracture. The remineralization of a demineralized area cannot be said to be an act of repair as no cellular activity is involved and it is purely a chemical process.

**12. WHAT IS MEANT BY PULP DENTINE COMPLEX?**

**A:** Dentine is a hard tissue. Pulp is a soft tissue. But both are specialized connective tissue derived from mesoderm. Pulp forms the dentine and dentine protects the pulp. The cells forming dentine (odontoblasts - some prefer to call these cells dentinoblasts) are present in pulp, though the cytoplasmic extension of odontoblasts (called Tomes fibres) are present in dentine. Pulp and dentine are interconnected. Changes occuring in dentine affects the pulp and it reacts to the changes. Hence many authors do not view the structures as different but as a single functional unit. They have named it pulp dentine complex.

**13. WHERE IS DENTINE PRESENT?**

**A:** Dentine is present both in the coronal (crown) and radicular (root) portion of teeth as the single largest portion of tooth structure. In the crown portion, the enamel covers the dentine and the root portion, the cementum covers the dentine. Sometimes in the neck of the tooth, a portion of dentine might not be covered neither by enamel nor cementum. Cementum or enamel, because of their thinness might be abraded away easily and clinically patient is likely to have hypersensitivity.

**14. WHEN DENTNE IS EXPOSED WHY THERE IS HYPERSENSITIVITY?**

**A:** Dentine consists of dentinal tubules and inter-tubular dentine. The dentinal tubules tranverse from the dentino enamel or dentino cemental junction to the pulp and they contain the cytoplasmic extension of odontoblasts and dentinal fluid (tissue fluid in dentine). The diameter of the dentinal tubules could 2 to 3 micrometers near the pulpal end but only 0.5 to 0.9 micrometers at the dentino-enamel junctions. Stimulation of dentine with an instrument, blowing hot or cold air over dentine, application of hot or cold substances, contact of sweet or sour substances initiate movement of fluid in the dentine either in outward or inward direction, pulling on or pushing the peripheral cells & the nerve tissue in pulp. This hydodyamic theory is the explanation of sensitivity of dentine.

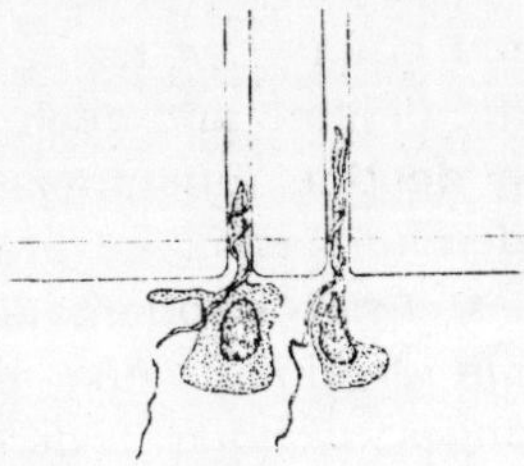

*Fig. 7.2 Dentinal tubules*

**15. WHY DOES A PATIENT HAVE MORE SENSITIVITY AT DENTINO ENAMEL JUNCTION?**

**A:** At the level of dentino enamel junction, the dentinal tubules undergo dicotomy(branches into two) and the cytoplasmic processes also divide into two. These increased number of cytoplasmic processes may be responsibile for the increased sensitivity. The clinical significance is that the cavity depth is never kept at the dentino enamel junction because of the possibility of increased hypersensitivity. In such situations the cavitydepth is taken further 0.5 milli meter into dentine where the number of dentinal tubules might be only half that present at dentinoenamel junction and so is less sensitive.

**16. WHAT IS PRIMARY DENTINE?**

**A:** Primary dentine is that portion of dentine formed by odontoblastis during the formative stage of the tooth. For the coronal dentine this will stop at about the eruption time of dentine but radicular dentine might be formed upto 3 years after eruption of tooth. The rate of formation of primary dentine is high.

**17. WHAT IS SECONDARY DENTINE?**

**A:** Unlike enamel formation, dentine formation occurs throughout the lifespan of an individual. After the formation of primary dentine, the odontoblasts continue to deposit dentine at a much reduced rate. There is no external stimulus for this deposit and occurs throughout the surface of dentine. The difference from primary dentine is the slight alteration in direction of dentinal tubules & slightly reduced number of tubules.

**18. WHAT IS TERTIARY DENTINE?**

**A:** Tertiary dentine is otherwice called reparative detine. This reparative dentine is formed in response to specific external stimulus of mild irritants which may be chemical, thermal or biological (bacterial) following dental diseases like attrition, abrasion, erosion, minor trauma, slowly progressing (chronic) caries cavity cutting procedures and some medicaments. When there is an irritation due to any of the above diseases, the pulp tries to protect itself by creating a dentine barrier between itself and the irritants.

**19. IN WHICH PART OF THE TOOTH IS REPARATIVE DENTINE FORMED?**

**A:** Reparative dentine is not formed throughout the tooth but only in the area of pulp closest to the area of irritation. It is a local phenomenon.

**20. WHICH CELLS FROM THE REPARATIVE DENTINE?**

**A:** If the irritation is mild, it stimulates the odontoblasts that form the primary and secondary dentine, and the odontoblasts continue to from the reparative dentine at a fast rate. If the irritation in that area is severe enough to kill the existing odontoblasts, new odontoblasts that are differentiated from the existing undifferentiated mesenchymal cells of the pulp, take their predecesor's place and start producing reparative dentine. However, it takes 2 to 3 weeks for the new odeontoblasts to differenciate from undifferentiated mesenchymal cells.

**21. WHAT IS THE RATE OF FORMATION OF REPARATIVE DENTINE?**

**A:** Initially the rate of formation of reparative dentine could be 1.5 to 3.5 micrometer per day. This rate decreases after 21 days, and ceases in 135 days.

**22. HOW MUCH TIME DOES IT TAKE TO FORM ABOUT 0.1 MILLIMETER OF REPARATIVE DENTINE?**

**A:** Assuming new odontoblasts are to be differentiated from undifferentiated mesenchymal cells (approx 20 days), it may be between 80 and 90 days.

**23. WHAT IS THE MICROSCOPICAL APPEARANCE OF REPARATIVE DENTINE?**

**A:** Reparative dentine is highly atubular. The minimal tubules existing are also not orderly or oriented in a particular direction. This makes the reparative dentine imprevious to the irritants.

**24. WHAT ARE DEAD TRACTS IN DENTINE?**

**A:** Sometimes, the irritants kill the odontoblasts and their cytoplasmic extentions leaving the dentinal tubules empty. These dentinal tubules appear empty when viewed as ground sections of teeth under transmitted light. The pulpal end of the dentinal tubules appear to be sealed with formation of reparative dentine. Dead tract formation may be a form of pulpal protection.

**25. WHAT IS SCLEROTIC DENTINE?**

**A:** In some cases of milder irritation, there is deposition of calcified material in the dentinal tubules and this calcification process might proceed from the dentino enamel junction towards the pulp. Such hypercalcified areas are harder, denser, less sensitive. This is another way of pulp protection. Clinically such a sclerotic dentine will appear hard, dark and shiny and is known as eburnated dentine. The clinical significance of eburnated dentine is that they are more resistant to caries attack and need not be removed from a cavity.

**26. WHAT IS THE CHEMICAL COMPOSTION OF DENTINE?**

**A:** Inorganic constituents form 75%, organic components form 20% and the remaining 5% is formed by water. The clinical siginificance of the composition is any dentine adhesive should be able to bond in a wet atmosphere. Many of the dentine adhesives are biploar molecules with the hydrophilic end combing with dentine and hydrophobic end uniting with the composite. Glass ionomer and polycarboxylate cements combine directly with the calcium of clean dentinal surface.

**27. HOW TO DIFFERENTIATE BETWEEN DENTINE AND ENAMEL DURING CAVITY CUTTING?**

**A:**

1. Dentine is yellower than enamel. Enamel is whiter than dentine.
2. Enamel is shiny and reflects light better but dentine is opaque and dull.
3. Enamel is harder than dentine and a sharp probe tends to get caught in dentine.
4. When an instrument is passed over enamel there will be a metallic sound (sharper and higher pitched) than in dentine.
5. When an instrument is passed over dentine, there will be hypersensitivity but over enamel there won't be any sensitivity.

**28. HOW TO REDUCE HYPERSENSITIVITY WHILE CUTTING DENTINE?**

**A :**

1 Using copious water spray over the revolving rotary instrument to dissipate the frictional heat.

2. Avoiding dehydration of dentine due to repeated drying with compressed air blasts.
3. Using sharp burs and instruments
4. Doing intermittant cutting

5. Applying lesser pressure

6. Reassuring the patient.

**29. HOW PERMEABLE IS THE DENTINE?**

**A:** Dentine is more permeable than enamel due to the presence of dentinal tubules. But coronal dentine is more permeable than radicular dentine. Through these communicating channels, bacterial toxins, enzymes, bacterial metabolites as well as microorganisms can penetrate. From a restoration, base or luting cements, chemicals like acids, unreacted monomers & mercury may penetrate and irritate the pulp. At the same time, medicaments can also leach out of a liner and penetrate through the tubules to give a beneficial effect. Common examples are Zinc Oxide Eugenol and Calcium hydroxide.

**30. WHAT IS A SMEAR LAYER?**

**A:** Whenever dentine is cut or abraded with a rotary instrument, the cut dentine surface will be covered by an amorphous layer of denatured collagen, hydroxyapatite and cutting debris. Such debris may cover dentinal tubules also forming dentinal plugs. Smear layer is relatively weak & might be sequestrated along the margins of restoration & smear layer will prevent the close adaptation of the restoration with the cavity margin. Smear plugs, however, by reducing penetrability of dentinal tubules is benefical. So during toilet of cavity, smear layer is removed trying to leave the smear plugs in position.

**31. HOW ARE DENTINE BONDING AGENTS BONDED TO DENTINE?**

**A:** The claim of manufactures about the chemical bonding of dentine bonding agents to dentine is not accepted by the scientists. Scientists feel the bonding is mainly micro mechanical. They feel use of acid conditioners in dentine tend to remove the smear layer and partially demineralize the inter tubular dentine. Scientists feel that the bonding agents applied later adapt to the etched areas, interglobular dentine and the exposed collagen fibers and form a hybrid layer of inter-diffusion zone. After the bonding agent polymerizes, the composite is applied over it. Many scientists feel the retention is mainly micromechanical in nature.

**32. IS THE DENTINE A LIVING TISSUE?**

**A:** Though dentine does not contain any living cells within it, cytoplasmic extensions of odontoblasts are definitely present in dentine. When cut, dentine is painful. Irritants in dentine do result in formation of reparative dentine. Dentine is permeated by dentinal fluid. These features are in support in calling dentine vital. But dentine is avascular. Cut dentine does not repair or regenerate. The reparative dentine formation does not occur at the site of injury but at a place away from it. These features are in favour of calling the dentine nonvital. In case the dentine pulp complex is viewed as a single unit, then dentine can easily be called as vital.

**33. WHAT IS MEANT BY THICKNESS OF REMAINING DENTINE AND WHAT IS ITS SIGNIFICANCE?**

**A:** After a cavity has been prepared, the thickness of the dentine separating the floor of the cavity from pulp tissue is important. This layer of dentine may be the only calcified protection the pulp has. If the thickness of remaining dentine is more than 2 millimeters, there is enough thermal insulation. Only cavity varnishes need be applied to seal the dentinal tubules. Application of dentine bonding agents will also effectively seal the dentine. If the remaining dentine thickness is between 1 and 2 millimeters, an effective thermal insulating base is necessary. If the remaining dentine thickness is just 0.5 millimeter or less than 1 millimeter, use of protective subbases are needed below the thermal insulating bases.

**34. HOW IS IT POSSIBLE TO ASSESS THE THICKNESS OF REMAINING DENTINE, CLINICALLY?**

Clinically it is very difficult to assess the thickness of remaining dentine below the pulpal floor or axial wall. At the maximum, it could only be an intelligent guess. But it is possible to calculate reasonably accurately the thickness of remaining dentine from an undistored radiograph of the tooth after cavity preparation is complete. From this radiograph, it is possible to measure the thickness of enamel from a proximal wall (say, mesial wall). It is also possible to measure the thickness of the remaining dentine from the radiograph. Clinically it is possible to directly measure the thickness of the enamel in the proximal wall (same wall whose thickness was measured in radiograph). By using the formula.

$$\text{Actual thickness of remaining dentine} = \frac{\text{Radiographic thickness of remaining dentine}}{\text{Radiographic thickness of enamel}} \times \text{Actual thickness of enamel}$$

(or)

$$\text{A.T.R.D.} = \frac{\text{R.T.R.D.}}{\text{R.T.E.}} \times \text{A.T.E.}$$

it is possible to approximately calculate the actual thickness of remaining dentine. A similar formula called Crossman's formula is used in Endodontics to calculate the working length of tooth.

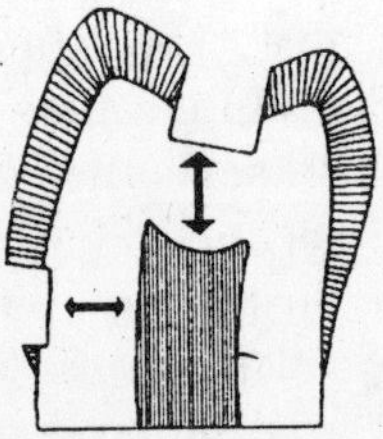

*Fig. 7.3. Remaining dentine thickness*

## 35. WHAT IS PULP TISSUE?

**A:** Pulp tissue is a special form of connective tissue consisting of cells, collagen fibres, blood vessels and nerve tissue.

It is the living portion of the tooth that provides vitality to the tooth.

**36. IS THE PULP NECESSARY FOR A TOOTH TO REMAIN IN THE MOUTH?**

**A:** No. Pulp is not necessary for a tooth to remain in the mouth. Pulp is not part of the attachment apparatus of the tooth. Many times a properly treated and restored pulpless tooth remains functional for many years in the mouth.

**37. WHAT ARE THE CELLULAR COMPONENETS OF PULP?**

**A:** Formative cells, defence cells and reserve cells form the cellular components of the pulp.

**38. WHAT ARE THE FORMATIVE CELLS OF THE PULP?**

**A:** Odontoblasts and fibroblasts are the formative cells of the pulp. Odontoblasts are the dentine forming cells and fibroblasts produce the collagen of the connective tissue odontoblasts are present in a single layer around the periphery of pulp and cytoplasmic extension from odontoblasts extend into the the dentinal tubules. Fibroblasts are present distributed throughout the pulp tissue. The clinical significance of the presence of odontoblasts is that if stimulated, the odontoblasts are capable of forming reparative dentine to wardoff the irritant.

**39. WHAT ARE DEFENCE CELLS OF PULP TISSUE?**

**A:** They are histiocytes and lymphocytes. The number of defence cells may be few in normal pulp, but will increase greatly in inflamed pulp. These are wandering cells derived from blood. They try to combat microorganisms & their toxin damaged tissue cells are removed by macrophages.

**40. WHAT ARE THE RESERVE CELLS?**

**A:** They are the undifferenciated mesenchymal cells present around the blood vessels. These cells are pluripotent and generally remain quiescent. When some odontoblasts undergo damage or destruction, these undifferenciated mesenchymal cells migrate to their place, differenciate into odontoblasts and take over the production of dentine. Some authors postulate that fibroblasts dedifferentiate into the primitine cells and then redifferentiate into odontoblasts.

**41. HOW IS THE VASCULARITY TO PULP?**

**A:** The blood vessels that enter through the apex and accessory canals are small. the largest is only an arteriole, but within the pulp tissue it forms a well connected network. The capillaries form a network just below the odontoblasts. The clinical significance of this is when there is a microscopical exposure of pulp not involving the sub odontoblastic capillarieis, the absence of bleeding may lull the operator to think that there is no pulp exposure. It must be remembered that pulp exposures are possible without heamorragic evidence. The blood vessels of pulp do not have any good anastamoses and the arterioles entering the pulp are end arteries. The clinical significance of this is that in case of trauma to the arteriole of the pulp there is no effective collateral circulation to maintain the vitality of pulp.

**42. HOW IS THE NERVE SUPPLY TO PULP?**

**A:** Myelinated and unmyelinated nerve fibres enter through the apical foramen. The unmyeliniated fibres are sympathetic fibres surrounding the blood vessels and they help control blood flow. The myelinated fibres are dental branches from inferior dental nerve or the branches from alveolar branches of maxillary division and these fibres are sensory. Pulp has only A δ (delta) fibres and C fibres that conduct superficial and deep pain sensation. The clinical significance of this is, be the stimulation thermal, touch, pressure, or electrical, the sensation felt in the tooth is only pain.

**43. IF THERE IS A PULPAL EXPOSURE, WILL THE PULP DIE?**

**A:** Not necessarily. Pulp is a tissue surrounded by rigid dentinal walls. It is usually said that if there is a pulpal inflammation and if there is an inflammatory oedema, the lack of space causes the increased intra pulpal pressure compress the blood vessels decreasing the blood circulation and possible strangulation of pulp. But such pulpal death need not occur in every pulpal inflammation. It depends on the extent of irritants, be it becterial, chemical, thermal, mechanical or electrical, the state of closure of the apex of tooth, the general health of the patient, the condition of dental pulp (whether it was subjected to innumerable insults in the past and is already degenerated) etc. There is a popular saying that "A frown can wither away a pulp but an axe cut might see it flourish". This does not mean a severe injury won't cause any harm but a mild trauma will result in irrepairable damage. The saying merely highlights the unpredictability of pupal behaviour. Dentists should take all possible precautions during cavity preparation to protect this delecate tissue.

**44. WHAT MEASURES ARE A DENTINST SUPPOSED TO TAKE DURING RESTORATIVE PROCEDURES FOR PULP PROTECTION?**

**A: 1. WHILE CAVITY CUTTING:**

a) Never cutting a tooth dry, to avoid excess generation of frictional heat.

b) Trying to do a conservative cavity - cutting less number of dentinal tubules and odontoblastic processes.

c) Avoiding repeated drying of dentine with hot air - to avoid dessication.

d) leaving enough thickness of healthy remaining dentine above pulp tissue.

e) Avoiding direct exposure of pulp

f) Avoiding leaving microorganisms in the cavity before filling - from residual caries is or saliva contamination.

g) using sharp instruments and cutting tools.

**(2) DURING RESTORATION**

a) Avoiding irritant restorations.

b) use of protective varnishes, liners, sub bases or bases, if an irritant restoration is to be given.

c) Avoiding or minimising microleakage or marginal leakage.

d) Minimising trauma during insertion of the restoration

e) Avoiding saliva contammination during restoring a tooth

f) Avoiding use of dissimilar metals in opposing teeth to prevent galvanism.

**45. WHICH RESTORATIVE MATERIAL CAUSES LEAST IRRITATION TO PULP?**

**A:** Zinc Oxide Eugenol causes least irritation to pulp. Calcium hydroxide also causes least irritation to pulp. This is the reason for using these two materials closest to pulp as sub bases.

**46. IS THE PERIODONTAL HEALTH RELATED TO THE RESTORATIONS?**

**A:** Yes. Faulty restorations can adversely affect the health of the periodontium. Care should be taken while restoring a tooth to ensure continued periodontal health. If one of periodontal tissue is affected, it can affect the other tissues of periodontium.

**47. WHERE IS CEMENTUM PRESENT?**

**A:** Cementum covers the root dentine. Its thickness is more near the apex and is only 20 micrometer to 50 micrometer thick near the neck of the tooth. Because of this thickness and its poor wear reistance, cementum gets abraded away very fast following gingival recession and the exposed dentine is highly sensitive.

**48. IS CEMENTUM A STRONG TISSUE?**

**A:** Among the hard dental tissues, cementum is the softest. The clinical significance of this is, in any gingival seat, cemetum should not form part of it. If cementum is present in the gingival seat, it should be scraped away.

**49. IS CEMENTUM A LIVING TISSUE?**

**A:** Cementum is avascular. There are no living cells within cementum. The formative cells of the cementum, the cementoblasts are present in the periodontium and they may cause cemental repair on the external aspect. If cementum is considered as part of the periodontium, then it could be considered vital. The situation is similar to dentine.

**50. HOW DOES PERIODONTAL LIGAMENT ATTACH THE TOOTH TO THE ALVEOLAR BONE?**

**A:** Periodontal fibres are inserted on one side to alveolar bone and on another side to cementum. There are gingival, transeptal, alveolar crestal, transverse, oblique, apical and inter radicular fibres. These fibres are alligned in different directions and are attached to alveolar bone, gingiva and cementum. There are blood vessels, nerves and lymphatics in periodontal ligaments. The fibres are collagen fibres and very strong. Collagen fibres of 1 millimeter thickness are capable of withstanding 10 to 40 kilogram load before breaking. It is this high tensile strength of collagen that makes it withstand the masticatory pressure.

**51. DOES A SINGLE FIBRE EXTEND FROM ALVEOLAR BONE TO THE CEMENTUM?**

**A:** The same fibre does not extend all the way from cemntum to bone. They are in three parts - the outer fibre attached to the bone runs towards the cementum, the inner fibre attached to the cementum, running towards bone and the intermediate fibre joining the outer and inner fibre. This middle fibres undergo modifications depending on function.

**52. ARE THE PERIODONTAL LIGAMENT FIBRES STRAIGHT?**

**A:** No. The fibres follow a slightly wavy course which straighten under load. The clinical significance of this is the ability to use separators without causing permanent damage to periodontium. Normal healthy teeth have physiological movement due to the wavy course of the fibres.

**53. WILL TOOTH SEPARATION CAUSE PERIODONTAL DAMAGE?**

**A:** When the tooth separation is done slowly and upto 0.2 and 0.5 millimeter, there won't be any periodontal damage. After separation, the seperator must be stabilized, other wise periodontal damage can occur.

**54. WILL WEDGE APPLICATION CAUSE PERIODONTAL DAMAGE?**

**A:** Not usually, only improper and prolonged wedging may cause damage to periodontal ligament.

**55. CAN RESTORATIONS DAMAGE PERIODONTAL LIGAMENT?**

**A:** If the restorations are above the occlusal level, there may be premature contacts leading to traumatic periodontitis of that tooth. During lateral movements of the mandible, if there are occlusal interferences, it will definitely cause periodontal damage.

**56. CAN PACKING OF A RESTORATIVE MATERIAL INTO THE TOOTH CAVITY LEAD TO PERIODONTAL DAMAGE?**

**A:** Application of excessive forces during condensations of direct filling gold may cause periodontal damage. Normal condensation forces do not cause any damage to periodontium.

**57. WHAT IS THE FUNCTION OF GINGIVA?**

**A:** One of the functions of gingiva is protection of the underlying periodontium. Gingiva consists of the free gingiva and attached gingiva. Free gingiva forms on the inner aspect of the gingival crevice or sulcus, with the outer surface of the tooth, and below the sulcus, the epituelical attachment. The epithelial althachament when intact, protects the periodontium from mechanical and bacterial attack. The epithelial attachment is 5 to 15 cell layer thick.

58. **HOW DAN GINGIVA BE INJURED IN RESTORATIVE PROCEDUES?**

A: Gingiva might be injured by faulty use of instruments and improperly built restorations.

59. **HOW FAULTY INSTRUMENTATION CAN INJURE GINGIVA?**

A: 1) Careless use of rotary instruments on the tooth area near the gingiva can traumatize and lacerate the gingiva.

2) Improper selection and application of the rubber dam clamp can injure the gingiva.

3) Slipshod placement of the separator jaws over the gingiva can injure it.

4) Using a matrix band without trimming the gingival excess may impinge on the inter dental gingiva.

5) Using uncontoured and improperly placed wedge can injure the inter dental papilla.

60. **HOW DO IMPROPERLY PREPARED RESTORATIONS AFFECT GINGIVAL HEALTH?**

A: 1) Failure to replace the preexisting contact points between teeth might result in food impaction between teeth resulting in loss of interdental col and further periodontal diseases.

2) Over contouring the restoration denies the normal massaging action, the masticated food gives the outer surface of gingiva for its strength. There might be plaque accumulation and poor gingival health.

3) Undercontouring a restoration can result in masticated food being thrust into the gingival sulcus leading to pocket formation.

4) Restorative overhangs due to non-placement of wedge can mechanically displace the gingiva. It will accumulate plaque and chemically irritate the gingiva.

5) Improperly finished restorations, because of rough surface accumulate plaque faster & be a cause of gingival irritation.

6) Irritants like unreacted acids from cements, unreacted monomers from composites can chemically irritate the gingiva.

**61. HOW DOES PESIDONTAL HEALTH INFLUENCE RESTORATIONS?**

**A:** Before starting any restorative treatment, the periodontal status of the tooth should assessed. The tooth should be free from periodontal diseases. If any periodontal disease exists, it should be corrected before restorative treatment is undertaken.

# CHAPTER : 8

# PRELIMINARY CONSIDERATIONS BEFORE CAVITY PREPARATION

**1. WHAT ARE THE PRELIMINARY CONDITIONS TO BE CONSIDERED BEFORE CAVITY PREPARATION?**

**A:** Arranging the patient's and operator's positions during the restorative treatment, pain and saliva control during the procedures, handling the instruments are some of the preliminary considerations before cavity preparation.

**2. ARE THESE PRELIMINARY CONSIDERATIONS NECESSARY DURING PRECLINICAL TRAINING ALSO?**

**A:** Some procedures like pain control and saliva control might not be valid in preclinical procedures but only in clinical situations. But proper seating of the dental surgeon, the posture he has to adapt during the various procedures, the way he should hold and use the various instruments are all necessary to reduce operator fatigue, increase the operator efficiency and prevent any injury to the patient. The preclinical student should also have a good knowledge of patient management, saliva and pain control though he will be encountering them only during the clinical years.

**3. WHY THE PATIENT'S POSTURE DURING DENTAL TREATMENT IS IMPORTANT?**

**A:** When a patient enters a dental clinic, he is usually apprehensive about the forthcoming treatment. Many patients associate pain and discomfort with dental procedures, especially cavity cutting. When they are sitting in the dental chair, usually they are tensed up. If patient's body is not well supported by the dental chair and the patient is sitting in an uncomfortable postion, the physical tension will only add upto his mental tension. On the other hand if the patient's sitting position is comfortable, physically the patient is relaxed. Many comfortable ergonomically designed body contoured dental chairs are currently available to provide comfort to the patient. A physically relaxed patient is more likely to relax mentally also.

**4. WHY IS THE DENTAL SURGEON'S POSTURE DURING TREATMENT IMPORTANT?**

**A:** In the olden days, dental surgeons used to stand by the side of dental chairs and performs the work for long hours. They also tend to bend laterally or forward to have better visibility and access in the back of the patient's month. Such uncomfortable operating postions for prolonged periods led the dental surgeon to suffer from various occupational diseases like varicose veins, low back ache, scoliosis, (lateral bend in the back bone) Kyphosis (forward bending of the backbone) etc. A dental surgeon's active professional life might span for a period of 30 years or more. If the dental surgeon adapts a good working posture, the chances of him maintaining good health is much higher. Operating stools are presently available where the dentist can sit and do the work. These stools, provide effective support for the dental surgeon's thigh and back.

**5. WHAT IS MEANT BY SITTING DENTISTRY?**

**A:** When the patient is conveniently seated in the dental chair, the dental surgeon does all the restorative procedures from a sitting position to relieve the stress on the legs and to support the operator's back.

**6. WHAT IS MEANT BY FOUR HANDED DENTISTRY?**

**A:** When a dental surgeon is helped by a qualified dental assistant while doing restorative work, it is known as four handed dentistry, because of the four hands (two operating and two helping hands) involved.

**7. HOW SHOULD THE PATIENT BE SEATED?**

**A:** The dental chair should give good support for the patient's head, back and legs. The neck rest cushion or the headrest is adjusted for the patient's back is at an angle of 45°. But even in supine postion, the head should not be at a lower postion than the leg except when the patient has fainted.

8. **HOW SHOULD THE OPERATOR BE SEATED?**

A: The operating stool's height should be adjusted so that when the dental surgeon is sitting on the chair, his legs should be touching the floor, his thighs parallel to floor and back ably supported by the back rest. The dental surgeon should sit erect with back and chest held upright.

9. **WHAT SHOULD BE THE LEVEL OF THE FIELD OF OPERATION TO THE DENTAL SURGEON?**

A: The dental assistant should be seated at a slightly higher level than the dental surgeon for having better visibility to anticipate the dentist's requirements and pass on the instruments. The assistant's feet should rest on the foot rest of assistant's chair. Assistant's back should be straight.

10. **WHERE WILL THE DENTAL SURGEON AND HIS ASSISTANT SIT IN RELATION TO THE PATIENT?**

A: If the dental surgeon is right handed, he will sit to the right of the patient and the dental assistant will sit to the left of the patient. If the dental surgeon is left handed, he will sit to the left of the patient and the dental assistant to the right of the patient. Though most of the dental equipment are made for the right handed operator, they can be altered for the left handed operator.

11. **WHAT WILL BE THE CONVENIENT POSITIONS FOR THE OPERATOR TO WORK IN VARIOUS PARTS OF THE MOUTH?**

A: If the field of operation is the centre of an imaginary clock face, the dental surgeon who is right handed sits usually between 7' O clock and 12'O clock postion (between 12'O clock and 5' O clock postions for the left handed dental surgeon) and the dental assistant sits between 2'O clock and 4' O clock postions if the dental surgeon is right handed (or between 8' O clock and 10' O clock postions if the dental surgeon is left handed). When a right handed operator is working on the mandibular teeth and maxillary anterior teeth the operator sits at 7'O clock postion. When the right handed operator work on the facial surfaces maxillary teeth and mandibular right posterior teeth he usaully work from 9'O clock postion. When the right handed operator works on lingual, incisal and occlusal surfaces of maxillary teeth and left mandibular teeth, the preferred postion is 11'O clock postion. the 12'O clock postion is used for working on lingual surfaces of mandibular anterior teeth.

**12. SHOULD A DENTAL SURGEON WORK ONLY FROM THESE FIXED POSTIONS?**

**A:** There is no rule which state the dental surgeon should work only from fixed postions. These positions are suggested as most comfortable for operating on some areas. If the operator finds another postion more comfortable, he can work from that position. But the stated postions are time tested and proven. For working on the upper teeth, usually indirect vision is used by using a mouth mirror. Many students find preparing the cavity under indirect vision a difficult task, but with practice it is possible to master the technique. Direct vision for maxillary teeth is also permitted when the operator sits at 7' O clock postion and thepatient's back is at an angle of $130^0$ to $140^0$ to the floor.

**13. HOW CAN A DENTAL STUDENT MASTER THE CAVITY CUTTING FOR UPPER TEETH UNDER INDIRECT VISION?**

**A:** Initially the student is advised to sit in front of a mirror with a pencil and a paper in which a tooth's occlusal out line is drawn. By looking into the mirror image, the student should draw the outline of the cavity on the occlusal surface drawn on paper. He should repeat this till he masters it on different occlusal outlines. When the drawing has become perfect, he can start cutting the cavity under indirect vision. To start with, the natural tooth should be viewed in the mirror for the caries involvement and groove pattern. With the mirror in position, the outline form should be imagined mentally. Later the probe should be passed repeatedly over the imagined outline. Repeated tracing of the imaginary outline from with a probe gives a good mental picture of the proposed outline. Now a handpiece and bur can be used to cut the cavity. By repeatedly preparing the cavity under indirect vision, it is possible for the dental student to master the technique.

**14. WHAT WILL BE PRESENT BETWEEN 12'O CLOCK POSTION AND 2'O CLOCK POSTION FOR A RIGHT HANDED OPERATOR?**

**A:** That will be the static zone where equipment and instruments are present. Any additional instrument or equipment needed can be taken from this place.

**15. WHAT WILL BE PRESENT BETWEEN 4' O CLOCK AND 7' O CLOCK POSTION FOR A RIGHT HANDED OPERATOR?**

**A:** This zone is called transfer zone. This is the area where the assistant passes to the dentist the required instruments.

**16. HOW DOES THE ASSISTANT PASS ON THE INSTRUMENT TO THE DENTIST?**

**A:** While passing the instrument, it should never be passed over the face of the patient lest it falls on the face and cause any injury. The instrument should be carefully passed over the chest of the patient. While passing single ended instrument, the assistant should hold the instrument in such a way that the blade of the instrument is facing towards the assistant and the handle of the instrument is facing the operator. If it is double ended instrument, it should be held in such a way the handle is perpendicular to the operator's hand. Care should be taken that sharp instruments do not tear the gloves.

**17. ARE GLOVES ALWAYS NECESSARY WHILE WORKING ON A PATIENT?**

**A:** Oral cavity contains numerous microorganisms. To avoid contamination from the oral cavity to Dental surgeon's hands, it is imperative that gloves are worn by the dental surgeon. It is doubly necessary when the dental surgeon has any minor abrasion/cuts in his fingers. This is to prevent cross infections. (i.e. to prevent infection from the patient to dental surgeon as well as from the dental surgeon to patient.)

**18. WHAT OTHER PRECAUTIONS DOES THE DENTAL SURGEON TAKE?**

**A:** The dental surgeon and his assistant should always wear protective, disposable masks to prevent air borne infection. It is also preferable for the operator to wear eye goggles to prevent any splatter of saliva, tooth chips, old restoration or a broken bur from the operating field to the operators eyes.

**19. HOW ARE PAIN AND SENSITIVITY CONTROLLED DURING CAVITY PREPARTION?**

**A:** Patient reassurance, use of sharp cutting tools, use of intermittant cutting, use of sufficient coolants during cutting with rotary instruments help **reduce** the pain and hyper-sensitivity experienced by the patient. But use of local anaesthesia help **eliminate** the pain.

**20. WHAT ARE THE BENEFITS OF LOCAL ANAESTHESIA?**

**A:** Apart from pain control, local anaesthesia also reduce bleeding if present from soft tissue - rare to occur in cavity cutting. Local anaesthetics also reduce reflex stimulation of saliva. The operator efficiency is also increased because of a calm cooperative patient.

**21. WHAT ARE THE DISADVANTAGES OF CONTAMINATION OF THE CAVITY BY MOISTURE?**

**A:**
1. Saliva contamination of cavity can cause bacterial contamination of cut dentine, which is more prone for penetration by bacteria into pulp.
2. Salivary contamination of cavity can interfere with the properties of the restorative materials. a) causing delyed expansion of zinc containing silver amalgam, b) Weak-

ening the cements c) Direct filling gold cannot cohere to each other in the presence of saliva. d) Saliva contamination will prevent penetration of bonding agent in acid etched areas. e) Saliva contaminations will prevent bonding of glass ionomer.

3. Salivary contamination can increase aerosol infection due to the spray from the hand piece.
4. Salivary contamination reduces the visibility.

**22. HOW CAN SALIVA BE CONTROLLED FROM THE OPERATIVE FIELD?**

**A:** Saliva can be controlled either by reducing the secretion, removing saliva from the oral cavity or by isolating the operative area from the mouth. These methods may be used in combination also.

**23. WHAT DRUGS ARE USED TO CONTROL SALIVARY FLOW?**

**A:**

1. Anti sialagogues, the drugs used to control the salivary flow are a) atropine sulphate 0.25 to 1 mg given orally 1 to 2 hours prior to the procedure. The drug's effect will last for approximately 4 hours but the side effects could be dilatation of pupils, tachycardia (faster heart rate), dry, hot skin (due to sweat gland inhibition) urinary retention. Atropine is contraindicated in mongoloids, nursing mothers and glaucoma cases. b) Bathine 50 mg given orally as a single dose and is effective for 4 to 6 hours. The side effects are similar to that with atropine, though rare for a single dose of bed time. It is contraindicated in glaucoma. c) Belladonna tincture 10 to 12 drops given orally will be effective for 2 ½ to 3 hours. The side effects and contraindications are similar to atropine.
2. Anaesthetics like lignocaine also causes a reduction in salivary secretion as the patient is more comfortable, less anxious and the oral tissues are less sensitive to oral stimulation (reflex stimulation of saliva is reduced) Touch of the operator's hands, instruments on the oral mucosa does not elicit increased salivary flow.

## 24. HOW IS SALIVA REMOVED FROM THE ORAL CAVITY?

**A:** Saliva can be removed from the mouth either continuously or intermittently. Continuous evacuation involves use of saliva ejectors or high volume evacuators. They are commonly known as low volume and high volume suction apparatus. They run on negative pressure that sucks the saliva and the coolant spray collected at the floor of the mouth. The ejector tips could be made of metal (reusable after sterilization) or plastic (disposable, single use pieces). Plastic ejector tips can be bent and shaped with fingers and the inner metal wire in the disposable tip help retain the bent shape. While using the ejectors, care should be taken that the ejector tip does not impinge, on the mobile tissue of the floor of the mouth as it could be sucked into the tip. High volume evacuators are more useful during surgical procedures.

## 25. WHAT IS A SVEDOPTOR?

**A:** Svedoptor is a combination of saliva ejector with cheek retractor and tongue depressor.

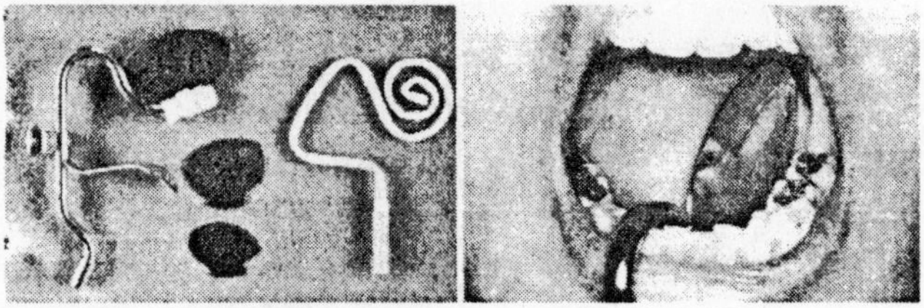

*Fig. 8.1 Svedoptor*

## 26. WHAT ARE THE INTERMITTENT METHODS OF SALIVA REMOVAL?

**A:** These methods involve placement of absorbent materials is some areas of the oral cavity to absorb saliva, and when saturated, are periodically removed and new ones replaced. The absorbent material could be cotton pieces, cotton rolls, cellophane wafers and sponges. Ready made cylinderical cotton rolls are available in different sizes. Cotton wisps from bigger rolls may also be twisted into rolls and used. Cellophane wafers are also available in different shapes. Gauze pieces and sponges may also be used as absorbent materials. These materials could be used when absolute dryness is not essential. The dental assistant can periodically change the cotton. Cotton roll isolation is not used during use of rotary instruments for two reasons. For one, the coolant spray saturate the cotton faster necessitating very frequent changes and another, if the cotton fibres get entangled to the revolving bur, there will be a messy splatter of saliva and other fluids over the operator, assistant and the patient.

**27. WHERE IN THE MOUTH ARE THESE ABSORBENT MATERIALS KEPT?**

**A:** They are kept in the buccal sulcus and labial sulcus of upper and lower teeth and the lingual sulcus. When kept in the upper buccal sulcus, the cotton roll absorbs the parotid secretions, as the stenson's duct opens opposite to the second permanent molar. In the lingual sulcus, the submandibular secretions and sublingual secretions from wharton's and Barthoin's ducts to staguate and the cotton rolls are placed subbingually to absorb them. While using cotton rolls for cement base placement, and condensing intra orally made restorations, air syringe or a chip blower can be used by the dental assistant to keep the area dry.

**28. WHAT ARE COTTON ROLL HOLDERS?**

**A:** Cotton roll holders are metallic devices with a bow and two arms to hold the cotton rolls in buccal and lingual sulci.

**29. HOW IS ISOLATION OF THE OPERATING AREA OBTAINED?**

**A:** Isolation of the operating field is achieved by Rubber dam.

**30. WHAT IS THE PRINCIPLE OF RUBBER DAM?**

**A:** The principle of rubber dam is creation of a barrier between work area and the mouth. It is the use of a rubber sheet to separate the tooth from the oral cavity. In the rubber sheet one or more holes are made (depending on the need) and the rubber sheet is pushed over the corresponding teeth, permitting them to project through the prepared holes. Because the hole made is always smaller than the circumference of the tooth, the elastic rubber closely hugs the tooth without any gap. the rubber sheet prevents saliva, blood and gingival fluids from coming into contact with the tooth preparation. Similarly, the coolant liquids from hand pieces are prevented by the sheet of rubber from entering the oral cavity.

**31. WHAT ARE THE ADVANTAGES OF USING A RUBBER DAM?**

**A:** 1. Provision of physical barrier to moisture which results in better properties of restorative materials and avoiding bacterial contamination of pulp.

2. Prevention of small objects (like inlays, jacket crowns, pins, rearmers and files) being swallowed or aspirated.

3. Prevention of cross infection through oral route

4. Prevention of bleaching liquids & endodontic irrigants irritating the mucosa.

5. Prevention of soft tissue interferences (tongue, lips and cheek).

6. Better visibility due to unobtrusive dark background.

7. Better access due to tissue retraction.

8. Protection of soft tissues from injuries.

9. Gingival retraction.

10. Clean aseptic field for endodontic therapy.

11. Avoiding frequent rinsing & unnecessary talking bypatient. (Less wastage of chairside time).

12. Prevention of closed mouth swallowing by patient

13. Isolation of teeth for thermal/electrical pulp testing

**32. WHAT ARE THE DISADVANTAGES OF RUBBER DAM?**

A: 1. Minor damage to marginal gingiva and cervical cementum by clamps.

2. If the clamps are applied to porcelain crowns, possibility of chipping of porcelain crowns.

3. Possibility of ingestion or inhalation of rubber dam clamp (long dental floss tied to the clamp can help in easy retrieval of ingested or inhaled clamp).

4. Possibility of allergy to rubber which can manifest either as contact allergy or angio neurotic oedema.

**33. WHAT ARE THE MATERIALS AND INSTRUMENTS USED IN PLACING A RUBBER DAM IN POSITION?**

**A:** Rubber dam sheets, rubber dam punch, rubber dam clamp forceps, rubber dam clamps, rubber dam frames, rubber dam harness and rubber dam napkins, are the materials and instruments used in rubber dam placement.

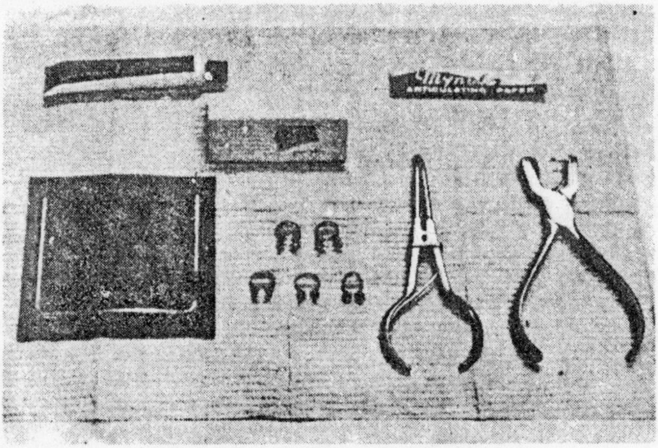

*Fig. 8.2 Rubber Dam kit*

**34. HOW ARE RUBBER DAM SUPPLIED?**

**A:** Rubber dam is made from natural latex rubber and is supplied either as continuous rolls of 12.5 cm or 15 cm width (5" or 6" width) or precut into 5" or 6" square. They are available in 5 colours and 5 thicknesses. Black and grey rubber dams give good colour contrast to the tooth. Green and blue colours give good background for colour photographs and translucent rubber dam helps in visualizing the radiographic film position while taking a radiograph. Out of the five thicknesses the thin (0.15mm/0.006") and medium (0.2mm/0.008") are easy to enter interdentally. The thicker varieties, heavy (0.25mm/0.01") extra heavy (0.3mm/0.012") and special extra heavy (0.35mm/0.014") have better tear resistance and better gingival retraction.

**35. WHAT IS THE SHELF LIFE OF RUBBER DAM SHEETS?**

**A:** The shelf life of rubber dam sheets is 9 months from date of manufacture, if stored at room temperature.

**36. WHAT IS A RUBBER DAM PUNCH?**

**A:** Rubber dam punch is an instrument used to produce clean cut holes in the rubber dam through which the tooth can be isolated.

**37. HOPW MANY PATTERNS OF RUBBER DAM PUNCHES ARE AVAILABLE?**

**A:** Two types, They are 1. Ainsworth pattern 2. Ivory pattern

**38. DESCRIBE A RUBBER DAM PUNCH?**

**A:** Rubber dam punch consist of a conical stylus (punch point) that will fit into different sized holes (diameter ranging from

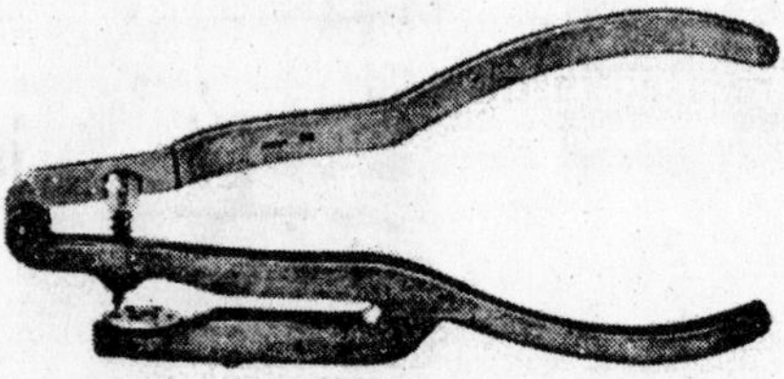

*Fig. 8.3. Rubber Dam punch*

0.5 mm to 2.5 mm) in an adjustable anvil. Different sized holes in the anvil are intended for making different sized holes in the rubber dam for various sizes of teeth. Smallest hole is for the lower incisors and largest for mandibular molars. The conical punch point (stylus) should correctly be aligned for obtaining a clean cut hole in the rubber dam. After selecting the appropriate sized hole, the anvil and stylus are correctly aligned and the selected and marked rubber dam is positioned in between the anvil & stylus and the hole punched.

**39. WHAT IS MEANT BY MARKING THE RUBBER DAM?**

**A:** Marking the rubber dam means identifying and marking the places the holes are to be made in the rubber dam as per the number of teeth to be isolated. The marking can be done by keeping the dam over a template which shows the normal positions of teeth in an average jaw or by keeping the rubber dam over the patient's teeth and marking the individual positions of the teeth to be isolated. The centre of incisal edge or an occlusal surface is marked & over the marked areas holes are punched.

**40. WHAT ARE RUBBER DAM CLAMPS?**

**A:** Rubber dam clamps or retainers are one of the means of holding the rubber dam in position. The rubber dam clamps consist of jaws that encircle the teeth and are connected by one or two bows. The jaw may have wings that facilitate placement of the clamp and rubber dam together on to the tooth.

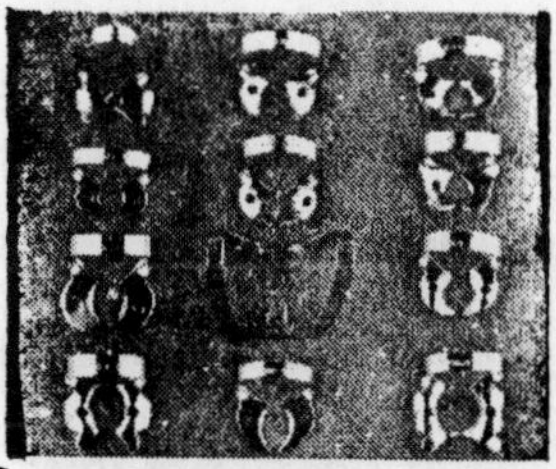

*Fig. 8.4 Rubber Dam Clamps*

**41. HOW ARE CLAMPS CLASSIFIED?**

A: 1. According to the number of bows, if could be a single

bowed or double bowed clamps. A double bowed clamp is used for anterior teeth and it is known as butterfly clamp.

2. According to the presence or absence of wings, they are classified into winged and wingless clamps. Wings are flanges on the outer edges of jaws. Winged clamp help in placing the rubber dam and clamp together on to the tooth.

3. According to the direction of jaws, they are classified into bland and retentive clamps. A bland clamp has flat jaws pointing directly towards each other and are designed to grasp the tooth at or above the gingival margin. The retentive clamp has downward (gingivally) directed jaws to grasp the tooth below the gingival margin. It is useful for partly erupted tooth where maximum bulk of tooth is sub gingival and for gingival retraction in class V cavities.

4. Accoridng to the material with which it is made, clamps can be divided into metallic and non metallic. Metallic clamps are stronger, thinner and more elastic' but radiopaque. Non metallic polycarbonate clamps are radiolucent. It is a benefit while taking radiographs for endodontic procedures. A radiopaque shadow of the clamp in an endodontic radiograph can mask the features.

**42. FROM WHAT METALS A RUBBER DAM CLAMP IS MADE?**

**A:** Retainers are made from tempered carbon steel, stainless steel or steel gold plated with diamond grit.

**43. WHAT ARE RUBBER DAM CLAMP FORCEPS?**

**A:** Rubber dam clamp forceps is also known as rubber dam clamp carrier. They are used to stretch the jaws of the clamp open in a controlled manner and carry the clamp during placement and removal. The beaks of the clamp forceps are placed in the holes present in the jaws of the clamp and slightly stretched. the sliding ring present between the forceps handles and hinge can be used to lock the forceps open and so hold the clamp under tension.

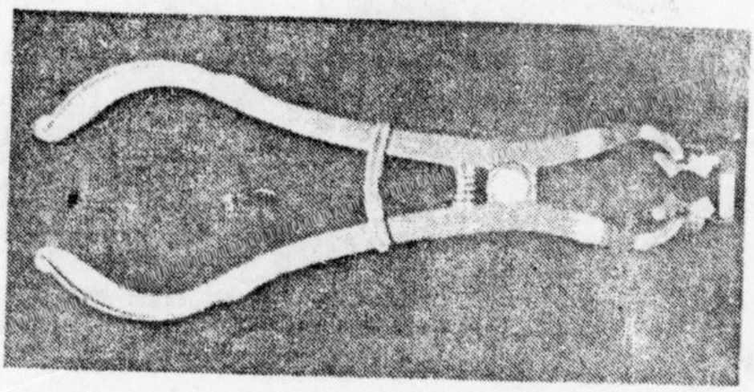

*Fig. 8.5 Rubber Dam Forceps*

**44. WHAT ARE RUBBER DAM FRAMES?**

**A:** Rubber dam frames are made of metal or plastic and are used to support the edges of rubber dam & retreact the soft tissues, improve access to isolated tooth. Plastic radiolucent frames need not be removed while taking a radiograph.

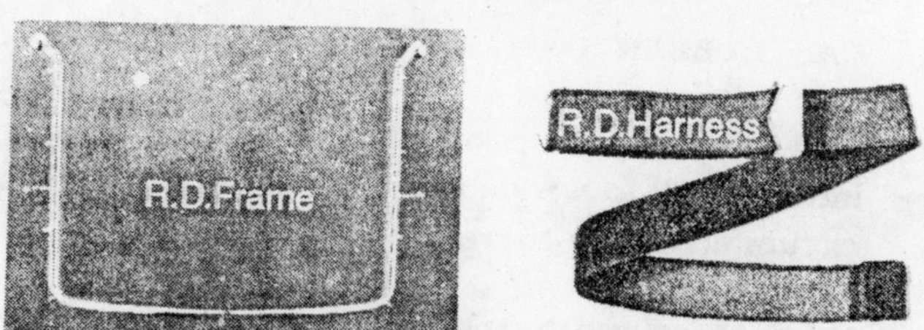


*Fig. 8.6 Rubber Dam Frames & Harness*

**45. WHAT IS A RUBBER DAM HARNESS?**

**A:** Rubber dam harness retracts only the sides of the rubber dam. The harness is attached to the vertical edges of then rubber sheet by metal clips from which elastics pass around the back of the head and apply traction to the edges of the rubber sheet. Ref. fig. 8.6.

**46. IN THERE ANY RUBBER DAM THAT DOESN'T REQUIRE A FRAME OR HARNESS?**

**A:** "Dry dam" does not require a frame or harness to hold the dam in position. It consists of a small sheet of rubber set into the centre of an absorbent paper sheet with light elastics on either side to pass over the ears. It is useful for quick isolation of anterior teeth. They are not suitable for bleaching or for isolating posterior teeth.

**47. WHAT ARE RUBBER DAM NAPKINS?**

**A:** Rubber dam napkins are precut sheets of absorbent material which can be placed between the rubber sheet and skin. They act like cushions kept over lips and prevent the stretched dam apply pressure over the lips. They also absorb saliva at the corner of mouth. Napkins also prevent the contact between skin and the rubber dam to prevent any possible allergy.

**48. CAN RUBBER DAM BE RETAINED WITHOUT CLAMPS?**

**A:** Wedges, wood sticks or pieces of rubber dam can be used interdentally to wedge the dam. Ligatures can also be used circumferentially to retain the dam.

**49. HOW IS RUBBER DAM PLACED ONTO A TOOTH?**

**A:** 1. Calculus removed from teeth to be isolated.

2) Contact points are tested with dental floss to know its tightness.

3) Suitable rubber dam clamp is selected, tested for four point contact on the tooth and a long dental floss is tied to the clamp as a safety measure and clamp placed.

4) Suitable rubber dam sheet is selected.

5) Marking done for the teeth to be isolated

6) Suitable punch hole selected in the anvil & hole punched on the marking.

7) Lubricant applied on the mouth side of the rubber dam.

8) Rubber dam stretched over the bow of the clamp.

9) Rubber dam stretched over buccal jaw and allowed to settle beneath the jaw.

10) Rubber dam stretched over the lingual jaw and released to settle beneath the jaw.

11) Rubber dam is passed through the contact. Alternatively, the rubber dam can be inserted first and clamp positioned later or the rubber dam and a winged clamp can be placed together and the streched rubber dam can be released from the wings.

**50. WHAT ARE SEPARATORS?**

**A:** Separators are instruments used to partly displace two neighbouring teeth in opposite directions to create a space in between.

**51. WHAT ARE THE PURPOSES OF SEPARATION OF TEETH?**

**A:** The purpose of separation of teeth are

1) examination
2) access for restoring
3) Proximal polishing
4) establishment of tight contact
5) Insertion of matrix band

**52. WHAT ARE THE TYPES OF SEPARATION?**

**A:** There are two types of separation. They are

1) slow separation and

2) rapid separation

**53. WHAT ARE THE SLOW SEPARATION METHODS?**

**A:** Slow sepation methods are

1) separating wires

2) oversize tempornies

3) orthodontic appliances

**54. WHEN ARE SLOW SEPARATORS USEFUL?**

**A:** Slow separation is achieved in days or weeks and they are useful in orthodontic treatment.

**55. ARE RAPID SEPARATORS USEFUL?**

**A:** Rapid separators are useful in conservative treatment procedures.

**56. WHAT ARE THE PRINCIPLES USED IN RAPID SEPARATION OF TEETH?**

**A:** The principles used in separation of teeth are wedge principle and traction principles.

**57. WHAT ARE THE METHODS OF ACHIEVING RAPID SEPARATION OF TEETH?**

**A:** In olden days, insertion of the operators nail between two adjacent teeth was done to achieve tooth separation. Nowadays with univeral usage of gloves by the dental surgeons, nail insertion is no longer done. However for brief separation, the flat end of a plastic instrument can be inserted between two teeth. Wedges made of wood, metal or plastic may also be used as a rapid separator.

**58. WHAT ARE MECHANICAL SEPARTORS?**

They are instruments designed for achieving teeth separa- on rapidly. These instruments work either under wedge principle or traction principle. They are Elliot's, True and Ferrier separators.

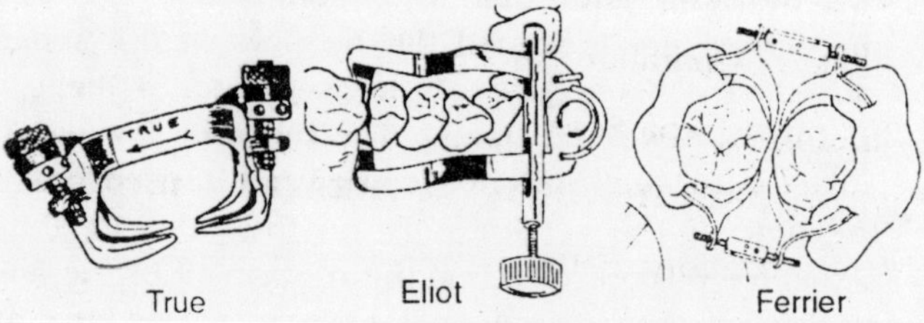


*Fig. 8.7 Different Separators*

**59. HOW DOES ELLIOT'S SEPARATOR WORK?**

**A:** Elliot's separator consists of a cental tube through which two jaws pass perpendicular to it and the jaws end in triangular wedge like projections facing each other. When the screw on one end of the central tube is tightened (turned clockwise) it compresses the jaws to bring the two wedges closer to each other. While in use, the two opposing wedges of the separator are positioned gingival to the contact area of the teeth to be separated, not impinging on the interdental papilla or interseptal rubber dam. Then the screw knob is slowly tightened (turned clockwise) and the two wedge ends move towards each other, wedging the teeth apart. Elliot's separator does not need stabilization and, is used for short peiords of separation. Elliot's separator works under wedge principle. It is a single bow separator.

**60. HOW DOES THE TRUE SEPARATOR WORK?**

**A:** True separator works under traction principle. Traction means pulling apart. In wedge principle, the force is in the insertion of the wedge which tend to push the teeth apart, whereas in traction principle, the teeth are pulled apart. The forces are more balanced when traction principle is used.

**61. DESCRIBE THE TRUE SEPARATOR?**

**A:** True separator consists of a bow with two fixed jaws that end in two wedges opposite to each other. Attached to the bow, are two screws, which, when adjusted, move the two movable jaws that are connected to it. Before use, the screws are loosened till the jaws of the separator are closed. The fixed jaw of the separator is kept over the tooth to be worked upon. The movable jaw will push the adjacent tooth. Softened compound is used now to cover the bow of the separator & on the sides to stabilize the separator without affecting the movement of the jaws. After stabilizing the separator, a wrench is used to move the movable jaws, first on the buccal side and next on the lingual side, alternatingly till the desired separation is achieved.

**62. WHY IS TRUE SEPARATOR KNOWN AS A NON INTERFERING SEPARATOR?**

**A:** Because the True separator can be adjusted even after stabilization (as stabilization does not interfere with the movement of the movable jaw), it is known as a non interfering separator.

**63. DESCRIBE THE FERRIER DOUBLE BOW SEPARATOR?**

**A:** It consists of two bows with jaws perpendicular to it with their tips ending at right angles to the jaws and facing each other. The two bows face each other so that the tips are nearer to each other. Two connecting rods that can rotate on screws unite the two bows. By adjusting the connecting rods with a wrench, the separator tips could be brought nearer or farther.

**64. HOW IS FERRIER SEPARATOR USED?**

**A:** The four tips are adjusted so that the tips hold a corner of proximal surfaces of adjacent teeth. The tips should be gingival to the contact area not impinging on the gingiva or rubber dam. Wrench is applied first to buccal for quarter turn and then to lingual connecting rods alternatingly every 30 seconds till the desired separation is achieved. Then the separator is stablized with softened impression compound to teeth.

**65. IN HOW MANY SIZES ARE FERRIER SEPARATOR AVAILABLE?**

**A:** Ferrier separators are available from size 1 to 6 & sizes 1 or 2 (smaller) are used for most anterior teeth.

**66. WHAT IS MEANT BY THE WORDS GRIP AND GRASP?**

**A:** Though the two words are used synonymously in English language, a subtle difference can be made between them to emphasise two important points for the dental student. The dental student should remember that while using any instrument (hand cutting or rotary instrument), if he permits the instrument to slip out of his hand, it can result in soft tissue injury. To avoid slippage, the student should have a firm grip (hold) on the instrument. This is for patient protection. While using the instrument, maximum mechanical advantage should be obtained to minimize the effort required. In addition, even mere holding a rotary, instrument for prolonged periods (during cavity preparation) could be tiring. Depending on the area of work in the oral cavity, how a instrument is held for operator's convenience and obtaining mechanical advantage can vary. How the instrument is held in different areas for maximum comfort of the operator can be called grasp. This is for better operator efficiency. While a firm grip is needed in all situations, the grasps may very depending on which part of the mouth is being worked upon.

**67. HOW CAN GRIP ON THE INSTRUMENTS BE IMPROVED UPON?**

**A:** A well fitting glove improves the grip. Serrations in the handle of the instrument improves the grip.

**68. WHAT ARE THE DIFFERENT GRASPS?**

**A:** There are three main grasps. They are a) the pen grasp b) inverted pen grasp and c) palm and thumb grasp.

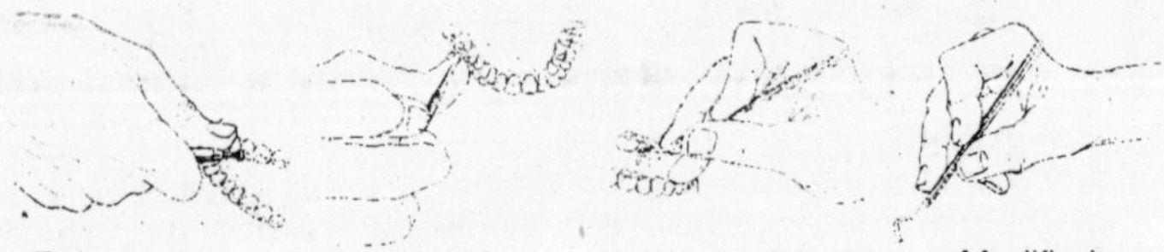


*Fig. 8.8 Different types of Grasps*

**69. WHAT IS A PEN GRASP?**

**A:** As the name implies, the instrument is held like a pen except that the instrument does not rest on the side of the first phalange but the pads of thumb, index finger and the middle fingers. The pad of the first phalange of the middle finger should be just above the shank on the top side of instrument to generate adequate pressure if needed. The ring and little fingers can act as rests.

**70. WHAT IS INVERTED PEN GRASP?**

**A:** In inverted pen grasp, the palm is rotated upwards with the pad of thumb and index fingers closer to each other but the middle finger is farther down the shank.

**71. WHAT IS PALM AND THUMB GRASP?**

**A:** In palm and thumb grasp, the handle of the instrument is held between the palm and four fingers firmly with the tip of the thumb acting like a rest. This position gives possibility of applying more pressure precisely.

**72. WHICH GRASP IS THE BEST?**

**A:** There is no such thing as a best grasp. Depending on the convenience of the operator, he can use any grasp he finds comfortable and stable.

**73. WHERE ARE PEN GRASPS USED?**

**A:** Pengrasps are used for lower teeth.

**74. WHERE ARE INVERTED PEN GRASPS USED?**

**A:** Usually inverted pen grasps are used for upper teeth.

**75. WHICH GRASPS ARE COMMONLY USED?**

**A:** Pen grasp and inverted pen grasp are commonly used.

**76. WHERE ARE PALM AND THUMB GRASPS USED?**

**A:** They are not used commonly. They can be used in both arches, but used more frequently in the maxillary arch. When more control and precision is needed this grasp can be used.

**77. WHAT IS A REST?**

**A:** While working with a rotary or hand instrument, it is absolutely necessary to rest one of the fingers of the hand holding the instrument over an adjacent tooth, gums or the external aspect of the jaw. This rest not only provides a place from which pressure can be applied but also protects the patient. If the patient accidentally turns his head while being treated, if there is no rest, the instrument might injure an adjoining tissue because of the unexpected mvement. If a rest is present, the hand, holding the instrūment is also likely to move along the direction of the head movement & there is less likelihood of tissue injury. The dental student should learn that he should never work on any patient without having a firm finger rest. Freehand usage of instruments (the working hand holding the instrument floating on air) should always be avoided. The rests should preferably be close to the area of work.

**78. WHAT IS A GUARD?**

**A:** While using any instrument, there is a possibility of slipping and accidents, occuring. To prevent injuries, guards are needed. Guards may be mouth mirrors, cheek retractors, tongue guards, lip retractors or even the operator's own finger of the other hand. The guards should be placed in the direction of movement of the instrument. The operator's finger is probably the most efficient guard as nobody wants to hurt himself.

**79. IS IT NOT THE DUTY OF THE PATIENT NOT TO SUDDENLY MOVE THE HEAD?**

**A:** An ideal patient should not do that. But many patients who come to the dentist are apprehensive, anxious and agitated. Many people are conditioned by their friends or relatives to expect pain during a visit to the dental surgeon. So every patient should be reassured to avoid unnecessary fear. Every dental procedure should be explained to the patient so that the patient knows what to expect. Patient management is a big art & a preclimical student should learn to be understanding, kind and compassionate when he comes to clinical side.

**80. WHAT IS MEANT BY LIP RETRACTOR?**

**A:** Lip retractors help in gently pushing the lips away from the field of operation. the lips fit into the concave portion of the retractor and it is very useful for class III, IV and V carifies in an anterior tooth.

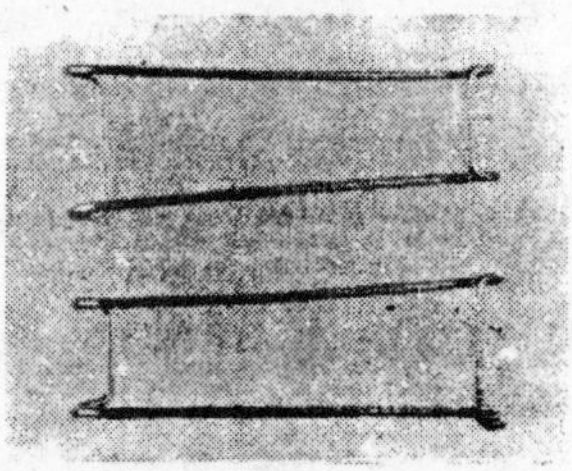

*Fig. 8.9. Lip retractors*

**81. WHAT IS A MOUTH PROP?**

**A:** Mouth prop is a device intended for keeping the mouth open. Some patients have difficulty in keeping the mouth

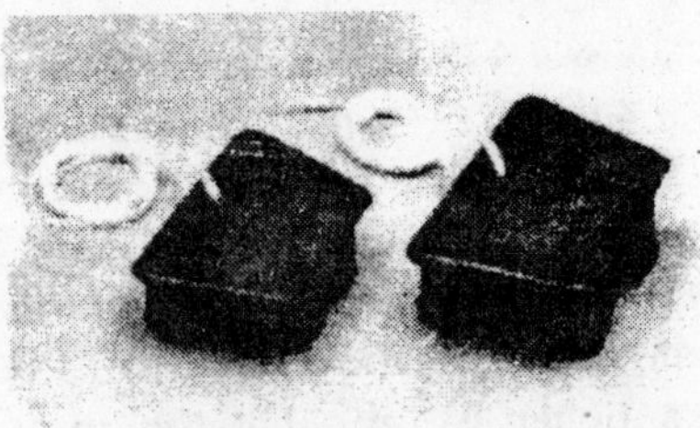

*Fig. 8.10. Mouth prop*

open They may require some devices called mouth props to keep their mouth open. Mouth prop may be made of metal or rubber, the later being move comfortable for the patient. They are usually triangular in shape with blunted corners. They have serrations on the sides touching the occlusal surface of teeth. The mouth prop is placed on the unoperated side with the narrower end placed posteriorly. It is placed as posteriorly as possible and patient is asked to bite on to it. If mouth prop is used, it should be removed intermittently for the patient to relax his. muscles during the dental procedure.

**82. WHAT IS THE ROLE OF STERILIZATION IN RELATION TO RESTORATION OF TEETH?**

**A:** Sterlization means removal of all microorganisms including viruses & spores. Disinfection means removal of most of the pathogenic organisms. While sterilization of instruments have always been emphasized in dentistry, the possibility of hepatitis B infection and HIV (AIDS) spread through the dental instruments has necessiated adaptation of universal precautions. Under universal precautions, every patient is presumed to to be a potential source of infection and after treating every patient, the instruments are thoroughly sterilized to prevent infecting the next patient. The four accepted mode of sterilization are 1. Steam under pressure (Autoclave) 2. Chemical vapour under pressure (chemiclave) 3. Dry heat sterilization (dryclave) 4. Ethylene oxide sterilization. Out of these four methods, antoclaving and dry heat sterilization are commonly used. Use of boiling water, immersion in antiseptics, wiping with alcohol etc can achieve only disinfection, not sterilization. While a preclinical student is not expected to sterilize each of his instruments before using on the phantom heads, he is difinitely expected to maintain high degree of basic cleanliness. Instruments should never be exchanged between students & all instruments used for restoring should be cleaned thoroughly of cements & other restoratives.

**83. DESCRIBE THE WORK AREA IN PRECLINICAL OPERATIVE DENTISTRY?**

**A:** Instead of a patient, there will be a phantom head. There are numerous types of phantom heads trying to simulate the natural situation existing in a patient to give the student are a prelude of the working conditions in a clinical environment. A phantom head has provisions for attaching an upper arch and a lower arch. A phantom head also has a rubber face mask to give the student an idea about the limited access in the oral cavity. The phantom head can be tilted in an up and down direction as well as in the sides to permit the student to adjust and keep it in a natural postion for good visibility and access. The height of the phantom head can also be increased or decreased depending on the need.

**84. WHAT SORT OF TEETH ARE USED FOR PRECLINICAL TRAINING?**

**A:** Most of the dental colleges use readymade acrylic teeth mounted on an acrylic base specially made for the preclinical student training. The acrylic base has a nut on the fitting surface that can be fastened to the screw in the phantom head. The individual teeth are attached to the base either with individual screws or a friction grip.

**85. WILL TRAINING IN ACRYLIC TEETH HELP IN THE CLINICAL SITUATION?**

**A:** The hardness and abrasion résistance of the natural enamel and dentine are much higher than the acrylic teeth. The acrylic teeth are much easier to cut than natural enamel and dentine. The students training in acrylic teeth definitely do not get the feel of cutting natural teeth & they may have difficulties in adjustment on coming to clinical side. To overcome this, some colleges advocate collection of intact teeth from cadavers or from dental clinics (intact teeth extracted for orthodontic, periodontal or prosthetic reasons) and mount the full set of teeth in acrylic bases with an embedded nut on the fitting surface and these prepared models are fixed to the phantom head & used. When a preclinical student works on these teeth, he gets the natural feel. However, currently, improved quality acrylic teeth are also available for preclinical training.

**86. WHAT ARE THE ADVANTAGES OF READY MADE COMMERCIALLY AVAILABLE MODELS HAVING ACRYLIC TEETH?**

**A:** 1. Because the acrylic teeth's sizes are all proportionate and standardized, occlusion will be good. Contacts between teeth and the occlusal level of teeth will be uniform.

2. If an error is made during cavity preparation,that tooth alone can be easily removed and replaced.

**87. WHAT ARE THE ADVANTAGES OF NATURAL TEETH?**

**A:** 1. preclinical students get the feeling of cutting enamel& dentine.

2. It is economical.

**88. WHAT ARE THE DISADVANDAGES OF NATURAL TEETH?**

**A:** 1. Because the natural teeth are obtained from various sources, occlusion can not be obtained.

2. Replacement of individual teeth will be difficult.

**89. WHAT CUTTING TOOLS ARE USED?**

**A:** In many dental colleges, airotors {high speed instrumentation} are used for gross cutting and cavity refining are done with air motor or micromotor instruments (slow speed instrumentation) the student should familiarize with the equipment used for cutting tooth.The air pressure needed for running the individual airotor units will be coming from a central compressor. The compressed air supplied should be clean and dry. Ussually compressed air is supplied through copper tubing rather than iron pipes because of the latter's susceptipility to corrosion. Particulate debris like dust and rust can interfere with the air motors or turbines and cause damage. The compressed air at high pressure is stored in a reservoir tank.

**90. HOW SHOULD THE RESRVOIR TANKS BE MAINTAINED?**

**A:** The compressed air in the reservoir tank cools inside the tank, releasing water vapour. The water accumulates in the tank and it should be periodically drained to prevent corrosion inside the tank and the distributing tubes.

**91. WHY THE COMPRESSOR AND THE RESERVVOIR TANK ARE NOT KEPT IN THE WORK AREA BUT AWAY FROM IT?**

**A:** Usually compressors are noisy. Only when they are kept at a distance the noise levels in the operatory will be less.

**92. WHERE DO THE COPPER TUBES CARRYING THE COMPRESSED AIR END?**

**A:** The copper tubes will come to individual units and will end in a pressure regulator in a control box.

**93. WHAT IS A CONTROL BOX?**

**A:** A control box is an assembly having distribution net work for air and water lines. It will be having a pressure regulator for air, distribution lines to, foot control, airotor or air motor outlets, airline to booster bottle, a changeover switch and a three way syringe.

**94. WHAT IS A PRESSURE REGULATOR? WHY IS IT NEEDED?**

**A:** The pressure needed to run an airturbine (airotor) hand piece is between 30 and 40 psi. This will usually be specified by the manufacturer. But the pressure in the reservoir tank must be high (between 80 and 120 psi). Such high pressures may be needed when a number of individual units may work simultaneously creating large demand, for shorter periods. These pressure regulators can be adjusted for each individual unit to permit air at a reduced pressure. Usually the pressure regultor would have been kept at the optimum position and unnecessary meddling with it by the student should be avoided.

**95. WHAT IS A FOOT CONTROL?**

A: Foot control is a device to control the rate of activation of a rotary instrument. In addition, it can also be a means of activiating any mechanism (eg. raising a dental chair) For airotor and air motor, the foot control will be operated by pressing over it and for micromotors and hanging laboratory motors it could be pushing the control lever to the right or left. By altering the pressure applied by the foot or the extent of pushing the control lever, the speed of rotation can be altered. The idea of using a foot control switch to operate the rotary cutting tool is to keep the hands free for holding the cutting tool in one hand and holding the retracting tool in another.

**96. WHAT ARE AIROTOR & AIR MOTOR OUTLETS?**

A: These outlets have couplings to which a airotor hand piece or an airmotor can be directly attached.

**97. WHAT IS A BOOSTER BOTTLE?**

A: Booster bottle is a small storage tank for keeping clean water to be used as a coolant. Compressed air forces the water to flow through the waterline to come through the water outlet in hand piece or the three way syringe. Many booster bottles have an air inlet and outlet knobs to permit entry and release of air from the bottle. There may also be a pressure guage to denote the air pressure inside the bottle.

**98. WHAT IS A CHANGE OVER SWITCH?**

A: It is a switch for selecting the airotor or air motor line for working. When one is working, the other may be inoperable.

**99. WHAT IS A THREE WAY SYRINGE? WHERE IS IT USED?**

A: A three way syringe is an instrument with a single nozzle and two control buttons. There is a airline and a water line entering the syringe. When the air button is pushed, compressed air comes out of the nozzle & it is used as a chip blower. When the water button is pushed, water jet comes out of the nozzle. when both buttons are simultaneously pressed air-water spray comes through the nozzle. Because of the triple action, the instrument is called a three way syringe. It is used to clean the debris from a cavity, wash an area of etching, to remove food particles from an area of mouth etc.

**100. HOW IS THE LIGHTING ARRANGEMENT IN THE WORK AREA?**

**A:** Apart from the overhead lights, each phantom head will have one operating focus light with flexible arms. It should be directed to the operating area but kept atleast at a distance of 18 inches.

**101. HOW ARE THE INSTRUMENTS ARRANGED IN THE WORK AREA?**

**A:** Clean set of instruments should be arranged in proper sequence on the operating tray. If a tray is not available, the instruments should be arranged on the work table over a clean towel. They should be arranged in the probable working order. After using every instrument, if should preferably be returned to its allotted place. Such work eithics improves the operator efficiency in the long run.

**102. HOW FAR IS STERILITY MAINTAINED IN PRECLINICAL AREA?**

**A:** Sterility may not be needed for preclimical work place, but absolute cleanliness is essential. The student should be dressed clean, and should always wear a clean coat. Nails should be pared, hair well groomed and should give a clean appearance.

**103. WHAT SHOULD BE THE DISTANCE BETWEEN THE STUDENT AND THE PHANTOM HEAD?**

**A:** It is preferable to train the dental student to keep some distance from the patient while doing the work. Leaning on the torso of phantom head or hugging the head etc. should be avoided, lest it continues into clinical area. Most of the patients do not like unsolicited body contact. Maintaining good working distance from the patient is important. Patients can very well distinguish between procedural necessities and unnecessary contacts. The face of the operator should not come too close to the face of the patient. Atleast one foot distance should be maintained preferably. It is always preferable to work with a dental assistant or have a patient's relative as a witness during the dental procedure. These precautions can help avoid law suits of personal nature.

# CHAPTER - 9

# DESCRIPTION OF CAVITY PREPARATION AND FEATURES IN THE PREPARED CAVITIES

**1. WHAT TYPES OF CAVITIES ARE PREPARED IN THE PRECLINICAL TRAINING?**

**A:** During preclinical training, cavities are prepared only in noncarious normal teeth. The student is presumed to assume that there are only minimal caries in all the involved teeth. In these cavities the outline will not be affected by extent of caries. The depth of the cavity can be kept at the minimum, cavity width can be at the minimum. In short, ideal cavities will be prepared by the student.

**2. HOW RELEVANT ARE THESE IDEAL CAVITIES IN RELATION TO THE CLINICAL SITUATION?**

**A:** In clinical situation, preparation of ideal cavities might not be too frequent. However, the idea of preclinical training is only to obtain hand control and precision. When a student knows what features are expected in a cavity, he must be able to incorporate those features in the cavity with precision. First the dental student should have a mental image of the cavity to be prepared (attained through theoretical knowledge) and he must be able to bring that cavity shape to the normal tooth with his instruments (attained with his skill). Some people have innate skill and precision. Most people develop such skills by repeating the procedure a number of times.

**3. WHAT ARE THE PRELIMINARY CONSIDERATIONS TO BE DONE BEFORE CAVITY CUTTING IN A CLINICAL SITUATION?**

**A:** While treating a patient, his caries index and oral hygine index should be assessed to decide the conservative or conventional outline. Patient's stress bearing area should be located so as not to end the margin of the restoration in that area. If it is a tooth coloured restoration, shade matching should be done. Any existing silicate, glass ionomer or composite restoration should be protected with cocoa butter or vaseline to prevent drying up. Preoperative radiograph will give an idea of closeness of the caries to pulp and the thickness of remaining dentine below the caries. If it is a proximal cavity, preoperative wedging achieves separation and insertion of a matrix band between the affected tooth and its neighbour help prevent damage from the revolving bur to the unaffected tooth. Local anaesthesia, if needed and if patient is not allergic, is administered. Isolation of the tooth is achieved by rubber dam, cotton rolls and saliva ejectors. For gross cutting, high speed instrumentation is advised and for finer cutting slow speed instrumentation is advised. Enamel penetration is done with diamond point and dentine cutting done with tungsten carbide bur with sufficient coolant spray.

**4. WHAT ARE THE PRELIMINARY CONSIDERATIONS TO BE DONE BY A PRECLINICAL STUDENT BEFORE CAVITY CUTTING?**

**A:**

1. Adjustment of the phantom head at the proper position (field of operation at elbow level of the operator) and adjustment of the operating stool for comfortable seating at the correct operating position depending on the tooth to be worked upon.
2. Checking the water level and air pressure in the booster bottle.
3. Checking the hand piece for the appropriate bur having been fixed firmly.
4. Activating the bur and checking the correct amount of coolant spray falling on the revolving bur.
5. Arranging the hand instruments in order.
6. Deciding about the outline of the cavity and having a clear mental picture of the extent of the cavity.

7. Airotor cutting for gross cavity preparation and air motor/ micro motor cutting for finer cavity preparation.

8. Enamel penetration with diamond points and dentine cutting with carbide burs.

**5. HOW IS THE BUR SELECTED FOR THE CUTTING PROCEDURE?**

**A:** For cutting enamel, preferably diamond points & for cutting dentine, preferably tungsten carbide are used. While using slow speed handpieces for the entire cavity cutting, a round bur was used for initial penetration through enamel, cavity extension was done either with an inverted cone bur or a straight fissure bur. Pressure was also needed while cutting with a slow speed handpiece bur. With the evolution of high speed instrumentation, initial penetration with a round bur may be superfluous and use of inverted cone bur is also limited to smoothening of pulpal floor & placing undercuts. In an amalgam cavity, a pear shaped bur is preferable because of the rounded tip to provide rounded line angles and the slight divergence of the bur head from the neck, which can provide the inverted truncated shape for the cavity in a buccolingual direction. If the cavity is for an inlay, a tapering fissure bur is chosen to provide pulpoocclusally divergent walls. If the overall size of the tooth is small, a smaller bur is chosen and if the overall size of the tooth is large, a large bur is chosen. A very small size round bur is useful in placement of retentive grooves. But the preclinical student should be aware that even with a small bur, it is possible to prepare a wide cavity if proper hand control is not exhibited. For airotor burs, no pressure should be exerted & light brushing strokes checked for smooth advocated.

**6. HOW IS THE DESIRED DEPTH OF CAVITY MAINTAINED?**

**A:** If the thickness of enamel is presumed to be 1.5 millimeter to 2 millimeters, the depth of penetration required may be 2 to 2.5 millimeter. In the bur, the length of the bur head could be 1 millimeter (for a short head bur) or 3 millimeter (for long head burs). With a scale, the 2 millimeter level should be measured and mentally noted. During cavity cutting this depth should be maintained throughout the preparation. Later, if the pulpal floor is found to be still in enamel, uniform deepening for additional 0.5 millimeter to 1 millimeter is done. Calculating upto what depth the bur head should go below the occlusal surface and maintaining it ensures having a uniform pulpal floor 0.5 millimeter below the dentino enamel junction.

**7. DESCRIBE THE PROCEDURE OF CUTTING A CLASS I CAVITY WITHOUT EXTENSION IN A LOWER FIRST MOLAR TOOTH?**

**A:** A pear shaped diamond point no. 008 or 010 is fixed to the airotor hand piece. A right handed operator sits at the 7'O clock or 9'O clock position for preparing the cavity. The rubber check is retracted with the mouth mirror held in the left hand of the operator and light is reflected onto the operating surface. The right hand holding the airotor hand piece in pen grip is postioned with proper finger rest on either of the premolars on the same side. The diamond point is kept perpendicular to the imaginary occlusal plane (plane touching all the cusp tips.) The diamond point should be rotating with sufficient coolant spray. Initial penetration is made in the central pit area as a punch cut for the calculated depth of 2 millimeters. A puch cut means direct downward penetration without any lateral tilting. This will result in a cylinderical cavity 2 millimeter deep and 0.8 or 1 millimeter diameter. The floor can be checked now to determine whether it is in dentine. If not, it may be deepended till it is in dentine (evaluated by colour, texture and sound by a passed probe). Once, pulpal floor is established, now the cavity can be extended to the predetermined conservative, or conventional outline For extending the cavity outline along the fissure the rotating bur is reinserted into the prepared punch cavity & extended along the central fissure at the same depth, cutting equally on both sides of the fissure and holding the bur perpendicular to the occlusal plane upto the marginal pit.

Care should be taken at the marginal pit area not to undermine the marginal ridge. The hand piece should be tilted slightly (the operating hand moving slightly away from the occlusal surface) so as to create a pulpoocclusally divergent proximal wall. The central fissure at the proximal (mesial or distal pit) is likely to bifurcate. A dovetail shape is prepared to include as much of the fissure as possible without weakening the marginal ridge. If the proximal pit or the marginal fissues are deep, enameloplasty can be done. If the cavity is a conventional one, the cavity should similarly be extended to the other marginal ridge. While extending the cavity, care should be taken to maintain the same depth. One common mistake a student does is to have more depth mesially and less depth distally, having a pulpal floor sloping mesially. If the cavity is a conservative one, the outline should stop at the central pit itself. From the central pit, the buccal & lingual fissues pass between the two buccal & two lingual cusps respectively. Dovetailing and enameloplasty may be needed in this without weakening the tooth structure. Had the cavity been cut without lateral movement of the bur, the thickness of the cavity will not be much more than the thickness of the bur. While the bur passed along the central groove, it would have created pulpo occlusallly converent walls of $8^0$ (the long bur taper). Now selective cutting should be done with the same sized carbide fissure burs to rounden the walls for creating smooth flowing curves & maintaining cuspal contour. Selective grinding is done on the sides of the cusps close to the central and proximal pit, to create the smooth curves. The cavity should again be floor walls and smooth floors. If the wall or floor is rough, gentle passing of the bur along the surface will ensure smootheness. An inverted cone bur, if used for smoothening, should be used without much downward pressure and preferably not touching the lateral walls for fear of creating sharp internal angles that can lead to stress concentration. Specific undercuts also need not be placed when buccal wall and lingual wall have pulpo-occlusal convergence.

8. **WHILE EXTENDING A CAVITY, WHY SHOULD A " BUR THICKNESS CAVITY" BE FIRST MADE AND THEN MODIFIED WITH SELECTIVE CUTTING? WHY NOT CREATE THE SMOOTH FLOWING CURVED WALLS SIMULATANEOUSLY?**

**A:** There are two aspects to be carefully monitored during cavity extension. One is maintenance of varying width (depending on branching of grooves, crossing of ridges, maintenance of cuspal contour). It may be very difficult to concentrate on all factors & prepare an ideal cavity. If there is a slight overcutting, it might spoil the entire cavity and there are no corrective measures for overcutting. While preparing a bur thickness initial cavity, the concentration is only on maintaining the ideal depth of the cavity and cutting equally on both sides of the groove while extending. No doubt this results in a smaller sized cavity which is not conducive for instrumentation. But a smaller cavity can easily be modified to a slightly larger size with suitable subtle alterations. So in the second stage, attention is paid to creating smooth and flowing walls maintaining cuspal contour. Such two stage procedure will be of immense use to the dental student, during the rotary instrumentation.

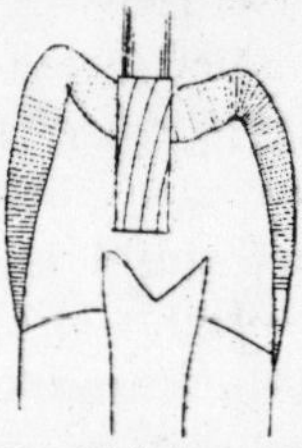

*Fig. 9.1. Bur thickness cavity*

9. **WHAT ABOUT RESISTANCE AND RETENTION FORMS?**

**A:** Creating a smooth pulpal floor parallel to intercuspal plane (an imaginary plane touching all the cusp tips), avoiding overcutting so as not to weaken the remaining tooth tissue, having sufficient depth and width of the cavity for providing sufficient thickness of restoration, ensure good resistance form. For retention, the buccolingual occlusal convergence itself would have been adequate. If it is felt additional retention is needed, with 005 round bur, retentive grooves can be prepared at the bucco pulpal line angle at the expenses of buccal wall and at the linguo pulpal line angle at the expense of lingual wall.

**10. WHAT ABOUT THE CONVENIENCE FORM?**

**A:** The student should try to insert the small plastic instrument and small amalgam condenser into all parts of the cavity to verify the convenience of base placement and condensation. If even the small instrument is not able to enter in some parts of the cavity, slight cavity widening is done at that place so that the instruments enter easily.

**11. HOW IS THE FINISHING OF ENAMEL MARGINS DONE?**

**A:** Removal of remaining caries does not arise in preclinical work as cavities are done in non carious teeth. For amalgam cvities a $90^0$ (butt joint) cavo surface margin is ideal for the strength of amalgam. The inverted truncated shape buccolingually, usually results in a $90^0$ cavosurface occlusally. To remove the unsupported enamel rods, straight enamel chisel enamel hatchet or enamel hoe can be used. If a straight enamel chisel is used, it can be used in a planing motion along the buccal and lingual cavosurface margin with the bevel of the chisel facing away from the cavity margin. With a firm ring finger resting on the premolar, the straight enamel chisel is held in pen grip, with the cutting edge in contact with the cavosurface margin. A protective guard in the form of a mouth mirror or operator's left thumb is placed distally to stop the instrument in case of slipping. With firm push stroke from mesial to distal along the buccal cavosurface margin, unsupported enamel rods are scraped off. Firm hand pressure is used to remove the unsupported enamel rods. After finishing the buccal cavosurface, the straight chisel is rotated along its long axis by $180^0$ and used on the lingual cavosurface margins. Instead of a straight enamel chisel, enamel hatchet could also be used on the buccal and lingual cavosurface margins. The enamel hatchet should be held on the buccal cavosurface with the bevel facing away from the cavity & downward push is given to remove the unsupported enamel rods. The motion is continued all along the buccal cavosurface margin. For lingual cavosurface margin, the other enamel hatchet (of the pair) is used. For mesial cavosurface margin, a distally beveled hoe is used in a downwardly directed stroke and for distal cavosurface margin, a mesially beveled hoe is used.

**12. IT IS PERMISSIBLE TO FINISH THE ENAMEL CAVOSURFACE MARGIN FOR AMALGAM CAVITY WITH A ROTARY INSTRUMENT?**

**A:** No. Usually there is a possibility of creating a bevel along the cavosurface margin if a rotary instrument is used leading to thin amalgam edge which may break at a later date. Use of hand instruments can not result in a bevel in enamel cavosurface.

**13. HOW IS TOILET OF CAVITY DONE?**

**A:** Usually blowing air from a chip syringe or a three way syringe is sufficient. If a block of debris is struck in any corner of the cavity, use of a probe can loosen it then it and could be blown off. Rarely dilute hydrogen peroxide can also be used to clean the cavity.

**14. WHAT ARE THE FEATURES EXPECTED IN A CLASS I CAVITY WITHOUT EXTENSION?**

**A:**
1. Outline (conservative or conventional) consisting of smooth flowing curves, including the pits and fissures of that area, with margins not in a stress bearing area.
2. Box like cavity with definite floors and walls. Walls should be pulpo occlusally straight. Mesial and distal walls should be either perpendicular to pulpal floor or pulpo occlusally slightly divergent. Buccal and lingual walls should be pulpo occlusally convergent. The internal line angles should be rounded.
3. Smooth flat pulpal floor parallel to inter cuspal plane 0.5 millimeter below the dentinoenamel junction.

4. Width of the cavity not more than 1/3 of the inter cuspal distance, but with enough convenience for instrumentation.
5. Butt joint cavosurface margin.
6. Undercuts, if needed at buccopulpal line angle and Linguo pulpal line angle at the expense of buccal and lingual walls.
7. No unsupported enamel rods at cavo surface margin.

**15. DESCRIBE THE PROCEDURE OF PREPARING A CLASS I CAVITY IN A LOWER FIRST PREMOLAR TOOTH?**

**A :** There are two factors that differenciate the lower first premolar from other teeth. One is that the lingual cusp is much smaller than the buccal cusp and the other is the inter cuspal plane for the lower first premolar is sloping lingually. Because of the differences, alterations are needed during class I cavity preparation in a lower first premalor tooth. The sizes of burs used should be the smallest available because of the smaller size of the tooth. 008 Pear shaped diamond point & carbide bur in an airotor hand piece could be used. A right handed operator sits at the 7'O clock or 9'O clock position with the patients' head slightly tilted towards the operator. The cavity is prepared under direct vision. The left hand holding the mouth mirror is usually kept lingual to the lower first premolar not only for illuminating the tooth with reflected light, but also to prevent tongue intrusion to the work area. Tongue retration assumes greater importance became of the lingual tilt of the crown and necessity of holding the cutting tool more lingually. The right hand holding the airotor hand piece in pen grip is positioned with a ring finger rest on the canine or lateral incisor on the same side. The diamond point is held perpendicular to the intercuspal plane (This mens marked tilting of the hand piece lingually) The diamond point should be rotating with sufficient speed with enough coolant air water spray. In the bur about 1.5 millimeter, thickness is measured, the initial penetration is made at the marginal pit for a depth of 1.5 millimeter, taking care not to thin out the marginal ridge. After satisfying that dentine is reached, the diamond point is changed to a tungsten carbide bur 008 and the cavity is extended to the other marginal ridge without altering the position of the hand piece. The lingually tilted hand piece creates a lingually sloping pulpal floor. While extending along the central groove, more tooth structure (about 2/3rd) is cut buccal to the central groove and less tooth structure (about 1/3rd) is cut lingual to the central groove. This excessive cutting buccal to groove is to preserve the small lingual cusp. Such preferential cutting should be done in situations where one cusp is small (eg. disto palatal cusp of a upper molar). The lingually sloping pulpal floor is also helpful in preventing exposure of the projecting buccal pulphorn. When the extension of cavity reaches the other marginal pit, care is taken not to undermine the other marginal ridge. Walls and floors are smoothened and straight enamel chisel or enamel hatchet and enamel hoes having small blades are used for finishing the enamel margins. Convenience form is tested with smallest plastic instrument and amalgam condenser, and minimum enlargement made, if needed. Toilet of cavity is made with thorough washing with airwater spray and drying the cavity.

**16. WHAT FEATURES ARE PRESENT IN A CLASS I CAVITY IN A LOWER FIRST PREMOLAR?**

**A:**

1. Outline form consists of smooth flowing curves and is 'U' shaped which is the usual groove pattern in a lower first premolar tooth. The outline to include all pits and fissures and cavity margin should not end in stress bearing areas.
2. Box like cavity with definite walls and floors. Walls should be straight pulpo occlusally. The internal line angles should be rounded. Mesial and distal walls are either perpendicular to the pulpal floor or slightly divergent pulpoocclusally.

3. Smooth flat pulpal floor, parallel to inter cuspal plane. The lingual slope of the pulpal floor will be perpendicular to the occlusal forces and help avoid possible exposure of the projecting buccals pulp horn. Pulpal floor to be located 0.5 millimeter below the dentino enamel junction.
4. Width of the cavity to be 1/4 of the intercuspal distance because of the small dimention of the lower first promolar.
5. Butt joint cavosurface margin.
6. Undercuts, if needed is placed at bucco pulpal line angle at the expence of buccal wall. Because of the small lingual cusp, lingual undercut is not given. Pulpo occlusally converging buccal and lingual walls give the necessary retention.
7. All unsupported enamel rods are removed from the cavosurface margin.

**17. DESCRIBE THE PROCEDURE OF CAVITY PREPARATION FOR A CLASS I CAVITY WITH BUCCAL EXTENSION, IN A LOWER MOLAR TOOTH?**

A: The right handed operator sits between 7'O clock and 9'O clock position for doing this cavity. An appropriate sized pear shaped diamond point is selected and fixed to the airotor hand piece. The phantom head is tilted slightly towards the operator. If the tooth to be operated is on the right side, the student sits at 7'O clock position and retracts the right cheek with a mouth mirror. If it is a left side tooth to be worked upon, the student sits at 9'O clock position and left arm is brought around the patient's head (without touching the patient's head) and retracts the left check with a mouth mirror. The mouth mirror should act as a guard when the buccal extension is done, as there is a chance of slippage of a rotary instrument and injuring the buccal mucosa. Initially, a class I cavity without extension is done in the tooth as described earlier. Specific underut is made on the linguopulpal line angle at the expense of the lingual wall because of the necessity of partial breaking of the buccal wall for the extension. After preparing the occlusalbox satisfactorily, the proposed buccal extensions should be mentally visualized. The inter cuspal distance between the mesio buccal & distobuccal cusps should be measured and the portion of tooth structure cut between them should be between 1/4 and 1/3 of the inter cuspal distance. The mesial and distal walls will flare out axio buccally, to conform to the direction of the enamel rods as well as to obtain a cavo surface margin of 90° for the amalgam. The mesial and distal walls of the buccal box should also have a gingivo occlusal convergence. The gingival seat should be in the middle third, at the level of the buccal pit, and not lower. With this mental picture, the extension of the occlusal box is continued buccally. The pear shaped diamond point or tungsten carbide bur is held perpendicular to the occlusal surface and bur thickness cavity is done, at the level of the pulpal floor, towards the buccal groove till the buccal enamel is reached without breaking it. Once this guiding cut is made, it is easy to prepare the mesial and distal walls of the buccal box by tilting the burs by 3° or 4° and are creating a pulpo occlusally convergent mesial and distal walls in the buccal box. Again care is taken not to break the buccal wall. Presently the axio buccal flare of the mesial and distal walls (for conforming to enamel rod direction and having a butt joint) is checked and adjusted. Now the buccal enamel wall is thinned further and the dentinoenamel junction is located in the buccal box. Now the cavity is deepened by keeping the bur on the dentino enamel junction at the mesial wall with the same taper kept earlier and the axial wall is kept 0.5 millimeter within the dentino enamel junction. The cervical extension of the gingival seat is upto the level of the buccal pit in the middle third of the buccal surface. The bur is extended distally and tilted to create the distal wall with the same gingivo occlusal convergence. While extending the cavity, the axial wall is made slightly convex, parallel to the buccal surface of the tooth. The gingival seat and axial walls are smoothened. Once the inner cavity details are satisfactorily prepared, the thin buccal enamel can be broken with hand instruments. The idea of keeping the buccal enamel wall intact till the final stages of finishing the cavity is as a safety measure against injuring the buccal mucosa. The enamel hatchet is used in a gingival direction along the mesial and distal cavosurface margins and the mesial gingival marginal trimmer is used along the gingival cavosurface margin of the buccal box. In the gingival cavo surface margins, if there are any unsupported enamel rods, they will be removed by the use of mesial gingival marginal trimmer. The axio pulpal line angle is rounded. The cavity walls and floors are checked for smoothness and retentive grooves are placed with 005 round burs in a slow speed hand piece at the mesio axial, disto axial and gingivo axial line angles of the buccal box at the expense of mesial, distal and gingival walls of the buccal box. The grooves are made in dentine from gingival seat to the level of pulpal floor. The cavity is washed and airdried to clear the debris.

**18. WHAT ARE THE FEATURES OF THE CLASS I CAVITY WITH BUCCAL EXTENSION IN A LOWER MOLAR TOOTH?**

**A:** 1) Outline form consisting of smooth flowing curves including all the pits and fissures of the cavity and cavity margin not in stress bearing areas. Intact mesial, lingual and distal walls with interrupted buccal wall that has an isthumus of 1/4 to 1/3 of the intercuspal distance as width extending to a buccal box which is having an inverted truncated shape gingivo occlusally but slightly diverging mesial & distal walls axio buccally.

2) Box like cavity with definite floors and walls. Pulpo occlusally the walls are straight. Mesial wall and distal walls of the occlusal box are either straight or slightly divergent to prevent weakening of marginal ridge. Lingual wall and part of the buccal wall of the occlusal box converge pulpo occlusally. The same mesial and distal walls of the buccal box diverge axio buccally.

3) Smooth, flat pulpal floor, parallel, to inter cuspal plane and flat smooth gingival seat parallel to the pulpal floor. The pulpal floor and axial walls should both be in dentine at a distance of 0.5 millimeter below the dentino enamel juncation The axial wall to be convex and parallel to the buccal surface.

4) Width of the cavity generally not more than 1/4 to 1/3 of intercuspal distance but with sufficient room for instrumentation.

5) No cavosurface bevel and butt joint at the cavosurface margin, except gingival cavosurface.

6) Specific undercut at the linguopulpal line angle and retentive grooves made in the buccal box. The retentive grooves at the mesio axial, disto axial and gingivo axial line angles of the buccal box at the expense of mesial, distal & gingival walls of the buccal box are an absolute necessity as they are the only means of retention for the restoration in the buccal box in a buccal direction. The axio buccal divergence of the mesial and distal walls necessitates the presence of these grooves.

7) Rounded axio pulpal line angle to avoid stress concentration.

8) Beveling of the gingival cavosurface margin.

**19. IF THERE IS CARIES IN THE OCCLUSAL SURFACE OF A MOLAR AND ON THE BUCAL PIT OF THE SAME TOOTH IS IT ALWAYS NECESSARY TO MAKE A CLASS I BUCCAL EXTENSION?**

**A:** No. If the caries involvement is minimal and the intervening tooth structure between the two buccal cusps is not weakened, it is advisable to prepare separate buccal and occlusal conservative cavities.

**20. DESCRIBE THE PROCEDURE OF A MESIO OCCLUSAL CLASS II CONSERVATIVE CAVITY PREPARATION FOR A LOWER MOLAR TOOTH?**

**A:** The right handed operator sits between 7'O clock and 9'O clock positions. The phantom head is adjusted so that the field of operation is at the level of the operator's elbow and the phantom head is slightly tilted towards the operator. The cavity is prepared under direct vision. Adjascent premolar is preotected with a metal band. The left hand holds the mouth mirror used for retraction of cheek as well as reflecting the light onto the operative area. A diamond pear shaped point 010 is fixed to the airotor hand piece and held in the pen grasp and the ring finger is rested on the premolar. The bur is held perpendicular to the intercuspal plane and the punch cut is made in the central pit to a depth of 0.5mm below the dentino enamel junction (approximately 2 to 2.5 millimeter from the outer enamel) At the central pit, dovetail can be made to partly include the buccally & lingually occlusal grooves. This distal wall created is vertical. Maintaining the same depth, a bur thickness cavity can be made upto mesial pit. Changing into a 010 tungsten carbide bur, the cavity is modified to produce cuspal contour of the mesio buccal & misiolingual cups. But before bringing the cavity outline upto the mesial margin, the extent of contact area with the second premolar should be verified. The margins of the cavity should be just outside the contact. The buccal and lingual extent of the contact area and the necessity of having a $90^0$ angle cavosurface (butt joint) decide the flare of the proximal walls. This invariably will result in axio mesial divergence of the buccal and lingual proximal walls. The buccal wall maintaining the cuspal contour of mesio buccal cusp should continue in a gentle sweeping curve into the buccal embrassure and the lingual wall maintaining the cuspal contour of the mesiolingual cusp should continue in a gentle sweeping curve into the lingual embrassure. While extending the occlusal box onto the proximal side, the proximal wall is thinned so that only the enamel wall alone remains. The pulpo occlusal convergence of the occlusal cavity is continued to the proximal box. Proximal ditch cut is made with the cutting bur held 0.5 millimeter in dentine and 0.2 or 0.3 millimeter in enamel to deepen the mesial box cervically upto the cervical extent of the contact area. The cutting bur is tilted to the extent of pulpo occlusal convergence to create the inverted truncated shape of the buccal and lingual walls. The axial wall is defined and made parallel to the proximal surface. Axio pulpal line angle is rounded. The thinned out mesial enamel is removed with enamel chisel, enamel hatchet, enamel hoe and the mesial GMT only. One common error most of the dental students make while breaking the contact is using a bur to break the buccal & lingual contact areas. This results in bringing the margins too far buccally or lingually than is necessary. The bur should be judiciously used only to thin out the enamel just outside the contact area as to easily remove it with hand cutting instrument. The contact should also be broken cervically. After breaking the contact, the gingival marginal trimmer should always be used to remove the unsupported cervically directed enamel rods that will be present in the gingival cavo-surface margin. In case of a broad contact area, if it is felt that the broad sweeping curve from the occlusal cavity may result in an acute margin for the amalgam, the curve may be reversed in direction to end in a butt joint cavosurface margin. The cavity walls and floor are smoothened. Retentive grooves are made with a 005 round bur held in a slow speed contra angle hand piece at the buccoaxial lineangle at the expense of wall, linguoaxio line angle at the expense of buccal wall, linguoaxial line angle at the expense of gingival seat. Hand cutting intruments are used to remove unsupported enamel rods from all the cavosurface margins. It is felt that the retention in the proximal box is insufficient, a retentive lock (reverse bevel) may be made in the gingivial seat. A 010 inverted cone bur can be fixed to a contra angle slow speed hand piece, and with distal tilt of the bur, an apical slope is created in the dentinal portion of the gingival seat. The cavity is cleaned with air water spray to remove the debris & dried.

21. **LIST THE FEATURES EXPECTED IN A CLASS II MESIO OCCLUSAL CONSERVATIVE CAVITY?**

**A:** 1. Occlusal outline is for access, occlusal dovetail for retention of the proximal restoration in a proximal direction, the outline is from central pit only (conservative cavity). Cavity margins not in stress bearing areas, cavity walls as smooth flowing curves, maintaining cuspal contour, diverging proximally to include the contact areas and to maintain butt joint.

2. Inverted truncated shape due to buccal & lingual walls converging occlusally both in occlusal & proximal boxes.

3. Pulpal floor and gingival seat, smooth and flat and parallel to intercuspal plane and present in dentine. Axial wall is parallel to proximal surface and in dentine.

4. The distal wall in central pit is perpendicular to the pulpal floor or slightly pulpoclusally divergent.

5. Supragingival gingival seat just below the contact area.

6. Proximal cavity margins are located just outside the buccal, lingual and cervical contact areas.

7. All internal line angles, of the cavity are to be rounded.

8. Retentive grooves in the proximal box, in the bucco axial line angle at the expense of buccal wall, linguo axial line angle at the expense of lingual wall and axio gingival line angle at the expense of gingival seat.

9. Bevel creation only at gingival cavosurface margin and axiopulpal line angle. Other cavo surface margins are at $90^0$ butt joint.

10. Width of the cavity 1/4 to 1/3 of intercuspal distance with enough convenience form for instrumentation.

22. **IS AMALGAM USED FOR A CLASS III CAVITY?**

**A:** Usually for an anterior tooth, a tooth coloured restoration is preferable. An amalgam restoration is avoided not only for its colour but also because of the discoluration of the tooth later due to corrosion products. However the stresses occurring on the distal surface of upper canines are more and could not be withstood buy the softer tooth coloured restoration. Moreover the distal surface of canine will not be that visible and a well polished amalgam done from a lingual access might be unobtrusive.

**23. WHICH APPROACH IS CHOSEN FOR A CLASS III CAVITY FOR AMALGAM IN DISTAL ASPECT OF UPPER CANINE?**

**A:** Unless caries has involved the distolabial aspect of the canine, the approach is only from the lingual aspect, for aesthetic reasons. The cavity is prepared under indirect vision.

**24. IS IT POSSIBLE TO DO A CLASS III CAVITY IN DISTAL ASPECT OF CANINE, CONFINED ONLY TO THE PROXIMAL SURFACE?**

**A:** If the first premolar is absent, it is possible to do a triangular cavity with intact labial, gingival and lingual walls. Such cavity may also be feasible, if sufficient space exists between canine and premolar or desired tooth separtion is obtained. If the access is not adequate, it may be necessary to sacrifice the lingual wall to obtain good access to all parts of the cavity. Trying to make a class III cavity by having a gingival turn or incisal turn (removing part of the lingual wall gingivally or incisally) might put constraints on the operator by limiting his vision and access.

**25. DESCRIBE THE PROCEDURE OF PREPARING A CLASS III CAVITY FOR SILVER AMALGAM?**

**A:** A right handed operator sits at the 1'O clock position. The phantom head is tilted slightly away from the operator (i.e to the left side). The cavity is done in indirect vision. A metal band is inserted in between the canine and first premolar as a protection agianst inadvertent cutting of the premolar while preparing a cavity on the distal side of the canine. It is preferable to use a small round diamond point for initiation of the cavity over a smooth surface. A 006 round diamond point is fixed to the hand piece. The mouth mirror is held in the left hand encircling the phantom head (without touching it). The handpiece is held in an inverted pen grasp with ring finger resting on the premolars and the diamond point is held with its long axis perpendicular to the lingual surface in the distal marginal ridge. The diamond point should be rotating before penetrating the enamel. While inserting the bur from the lingual surface, it is advisible to cut the tooth just mesial to the distal surface to have thin plate of distal enamel intact, if possible, which will help protect the neighbouring tooth from being cut. That distal plate of enamel can be removed at the final stage of cavity preparation. While cutting the tooth, the bur should cut into the proximal surface cutting 0.5 millimeter only into dentine. Though the penetration into dentine is only 0.5 millimeter below the dentino enamel junction, the extent of cervical cutting will be less than in the middle third due to variation in thickness of enamel. In other words, the width of gingival seat will be less (due to less enamel thickness) than the width of incisal wall (due to more enamel thickness). After penetrating through the enamel from the lingual surface, the round diamond point is changed to a pear shaped point of appropriate. size (008 or 010) and the point is passed occluso cervically to prepare an inverted truncated shape (that is, the gingival seat and the incisal wall converge labio lingually) to provide retention in the lingual direction. While preparing such inverted truncated shape from the lingual side, the bur should be angulated and moved gingivally and incisally upto the extent of the contact point (for tooth coloured restorations, complete breaking of contact area is not done as the restorative materials are weaker than the natural tooth structure). While defining the gingival seat and incisal wall mesidodistaly, they should diverge axio distally to correspond to the direction of enamel rods. The labial extent of the cavity should be upto the labial embrassure. Axial wall is made usually flat for better access, but if sufficient access exits, it can be slightly convex linguolabially. Incisal extension is also made conservatively to preserve the distoincisal corner to have a canopy of tooth structure for better retention and aesthetics. Retentive grooves are made at the axio gingival line angle at the expense of gingival seat and at the inciso-axial line angle with the 005 round bur. If it is felt that the lack of lingual wall has reduced the retention, a lingual dovetail can be prepared for additional retention. The lingual dovetail is made just coronal to the cingulam and should not cross the midline. The cavity is extended just into the dentine. A straight fissure bur with rounded tip can be used for doing the dovetail extension. thined distal enamel is removed with chisels. Intact enamel wall labially may remain in the cavity but unsuported enamel rods are removed with a Wedlstadt chisel. Air water spray is used for removing debris and air syringe is used to remove visible moisture.

**26. WHAT ARE THE FEATURES IN A CLASS III CAVITY FOR AMALGAM?**

**A:**

1. Outline from is triangular in shape if a direct access is available. If it is not available and a lingual approach is taken, the cavity is slot like when viewed from the palatal side. Cavity margins may be just outside the contact area gingivally and incisally. The labial extension is just into the labial embrassure.
2. Box like cavity with incisal and gingival walls converging towards each other lingually in an inverted truncated shape, but the incisal wall and gingival wall will diverge slightly axio distally.
3. Axial wall is flat or slightly convex, 0.5 millimeter below the dentinoenamel junction of the proximal side.
4. Butt joint of the cavosurface margin.
5. Wider incisal wall & narrower gingival seat due to variation in the thickness of the enamel.
6. Retentive grooves at axiogingival line angle at the expense of gingival seat and inciso axial line angle at the expense of incisal wall for retention in the proximal side.

7. Lingual dovetail, restricted to the mid point of palatal surface.

**27. IS AMALGAM USED IN A CLASS IV CAVITY?**

**A:** In olden days class IV cavity for the distal aspect of canine used to be filled with amalgam. Presently amalgam is not used. It is preferable to use a cast metal for such situation or reinforced porecelain could be used.

**28. IS AMALGAM USED IN CLASS V CAVITIES?**

**A:** In olden days it was very frequently used. With the development of tooth coloured restorations, glass ionomer and composite resin have replaced amalgam. However, amalgam in also used by some dental surgeons as a class V restoration due to their durability and cost effectiveness.

**29. DESCRIBE THE CAVITY PREPARATION PROCEDURE FOR A CLASS V CAVITY FOR AMALGAM?**

**A:** Care should be taken not to injure the gingival during cavity preparation. Gingival retraction may be beneficial in clinical cases. On buccal surfaces of many teeth, class V cavities could be done under direct vision. On palatal or lingual surfaces, many times indirect vision may have to be resorted to. The cavity out line is usually kidney shaped or bean shaped. Cavity is usually confined to the gingival one third of the buccal or lingual surface of any tooth. The gingival seat is usually kept supragingivally. The mesial and distal walls should not cross the axial angles. Usually the cavity is limited to the extent of the lesion and usually no extension for prevention is needed. The phantom head is adjusted by the student to operating level. The head it tilted towards the dental student so that the tooth (say upper canine) is under direct vision. Either an inverted cone bur 008 or a tapering fissue bur 008 is used for cutting the cavity. The enamel is penetrated by keeping the edge of the rotating bur tip at the smooth surface of the tooth rather than the flat end of the bur which may crawl over the smooth surface. After entry into the tooth, the walls are maintained perpendicular to the external tooth surface till 0.5 millimeter below the dentino enamel junction is reached. Because of the variations in thickness of enamel in the cervical 1/3 of the tooth and the neck of the tooth, the width of occlusal wall could be 1.5 to 2 millimeters but the width of gingival seat could only be 0.75 millimeter. The upper limit of the cavity (occlusal wall) is upto the height of contour of the tooth and the lower limit (gingival seat) in prepared just above the free gingiva. The gingival margin of the cavity is parallel to the gingiva and the occlusal surface is also concave and parallel to the free gingiva. The proximal walls are kept within the buccal surface without crossing the axial angles. The axial wall is smoothened with 010 tungsten carbide bur. Retentive grooves are prepared, with 006 round bur at the occlusoaxial line angle at the expense of occlusal wall and gingivoaxial line angle at the expense of gingivial seat. Instead of these two grooves, four retentive coves could be made at the four point angles for retention. A mesial GMT could be used to remove the unsupported enamel rods from the gingival cavosurface margins and chisels and hatchets may be used in other cavosurface margins to remove the unsupported enamel rods. Instead of kidney shape, the outline can also be trapezoidal with rounded corner for amalgam restorations. The finished cavity in cleaned with air water spray and air dried.

**30. WHAT ARE THE FEATURES OF A CLASS V AMALGAM CAVITY?**

**A:**

1. The cavity outline could be bean shaped or trapezoidal with rounded corners. The lower limit of the cavity is preferably supragingival, the upper limit of the cavity just at the height of contour of the tooth. The mesial and distal walls should be within the axial angles.
2. Axial wall in dentine 0.5 millimeter below the dentino enamel junction. Axial wall is curved.
3. Occlusal, mesial, distal & gingival walls are perpendicular to the external surface and walls are diverging axio buccally.

4. Retentive grooves in occluso axial line angle at the expense of occlusal wall and gingivoaxial line angle at the expense of gingival seat, or retentive coves at the four point angles.

5. Variations in width of gingival seat and occlusal wall is due to differences is the thickness of enamel.

**31. WHAT MATERIALS ARE USED FOR PREPARING INLAYS?**

**A:** Noble metal alloys, base metal alloys, castable ceramics, feldspathic porcelain, heat cured composite and CAD / CAM porcelain are some of the materials used for making inlays. Out of these materials, the first three inlays are prepared by the lost wax process. However the equipment needed for castable ceramics are different and costly. Fabrication of feldspathic porcelain & heat cure composite inlays are not by lost wax process but by addition and processing. CAD/CAM porcelain inlay is chariside fabrication of the inlay from a prefired porcelain block.

**32. WHAT ARE THE DIFFERENCES BETWEEN AN AMALGAM AND INLAY CAVITY?**

**A:** 1. In an amalgam cavity, buccal and lingual walls have pulpo occlusal converganee for retention but mesial and distal walls are either perpendicular or have slight pulpo occlusal divergence for better resistance of marginal ridges.

In an inlay cavity, all the walls will have slight pulpo occlusal divergence (or in any one direction) to facilitate removal of the wax pattern for processing or insertion of the finished casting into the cavity. Such divergence of walls is called taper and it could be 5 to $8^0$ for each opposing wall. Shorter the wall, lesser will be the taper.

2. In an amalgam cavity undercuts are made with the specific purpose of locking the restoration.

In an inlay cavity, no undercuts are prepared as they could prevent removal of the hardened wax pattern, or can distort a soft pattern resulting in loss of shape and an ill fitting restoration.

3. In an amalgam cavity, cavosurface bevel is given only at the gingival cavosurface margin and not other cavosurface margins. The reason is the lack of edge strength for amalgam which might fracture in function.

   In an inlay cavity for noble metal alloys, cavosurface bevels are created all along the margins for creating thin areas of alloys that could be burnished and adapted closely along the margins to reduce the extent of exposure of the luting cements to oral fluids and thereby reduce microleakage. But bevels are not made for base metal alloys and porecelain restoration.

4. For amalgam restorations, box type cavity preparation are done. Every restoration involving proximal side must have a gingival seat, for good resistance form.

   Inlay cavities involving proximal surfaces may be a box preparation or slice preparation. In slice preparations, minimal slicing of the proximal side in made to remove the minimal decay present and no gingival seat is prepared. This will be a conservative tooth reduction procedure and the absence of gingival seat does not reduce the resistance form of the tooth. For a single tooth restoration, slice preparation is not usually adviced as the thin wax pattern of the slice portion is likely to distort or fracture easily. Slice preparation is usually done when multiple teeth have adjacent minimal proximal caries. In such cases, occlusal boxes with proximal slices are made, impression taken, cast poured and wax pattern prepared in indirect technique and jointed inlays (a long single casting) prepared. It is known as Willets' inlay.

5. For increasing the retention of a restoration, tiny pins are fixed to the prepared cavity. Part of the pin will be buried in the dentine and part of it will be projecting into the cavity. When the cavity is packed with a plastic (soft) restorative material (like amalgam, composite or glass ionomer) the material surrounds the pin and hardens. The hardened material is locked to the pin

which is fixed in dentine, thereby increasing retention. For amalgam cavities such pins are placed in different angulation (each not placed parallel to other). Such non parallel pin placement enhances retention.

For increasing the retention of inlays, pins could be used. But such pins should always be part of the casting. These pins could be cast in the same material used for the inlay or could be a wrought pin made from a stronger alloy and embedded in the pattern.

But whatever is the type of pins used, the pin holes made for the pins should be parallel to each other, and to the direction of withdrawl of the pattern to facilitate removal of the pattern with (either wrought alloy pin or plastic pin) or insertion of the finished casting with wrought or cast pins. Parallel pin placement technique should be used for inlays if pins are to be used for additional retention.

6. For amalgam cavities, non parallelism of walls in the form of pulpo occlusal convergence of buccal and lingual walls enhances retention.

   For inlay cavities, if all the walls are parallel to each other, the amount retention is very high. However, if there is minimum taper of the walls, retention is not compromised much. With more taper (pulpo occlusal divergence) there could be more number of paths of insertion. With parallel walls, there could only be one path of insertion. In a cavity where the outer portion of walls diverge and the inner portion of the cavity walls are parallel, there might be a single path of insertion in the inner portion. The longer such single path of insertion, better will be the retention. Preparing exactly parallel walls is difficult and that is why taper is permitted. If however, it is possible to have parallelism of walls atleast in some part of the cavity, it will increase retention, as it can have longer single path of insertion.

7. Silver amalgam is not as strong as a cast alloy restoration. When the masticatory load is very high, cuspal coverage with silver amalgam might not succeed. Compared to inlay cavities, generally amalgam cavities are smaller.

A cast onlay restoration being a strong restoration can withstand masticatory load better. Generally an inlay/ onlay cavity can be large as the stronger restoration can protect weaker tooth structure. In short the differences in cavities for amalgam and inlay could be stated as 1. having pulpo occlusally convergent walls for amalgam & having pulpo occlusally divergent walls for inlays (intra coronal taper) 2. Necessity of undercuts for amalgam and absence of undercuts for inlays. 3. Only gingival cavosurfaces bevel for amalgam and having bevels in all cavosurface margins for inlay 4. Only box preparation for amalgam, having box or slice preparation for inlay 5. Non parallel pin technique for amalgam and parallel pin technique for inlays. 6. Non parallelism for amalgam but near parallelism for inlays 7. Usually a smaller sized cavity for amalgam compared to inlay.

**33. DESCRIBE THE PROCEDURE OF CLASS I INLAY CAVITY PREPARATION IN AN UPPER MOLAR TOOTH?**

**A:** A right handed dental student sits at the 11'O clock position in relation to the phantom head and the cavity is done under indirect vision. The phantom head is adjusted so that, the upper molar is at the level of the student's elbow. The phantom head is tilted back so that the student need not bend, to see the image in the mouth mirror. The student's left hand should hold the mouth mirror. The left hand should encircle the patient's head and ring finger of the right hand must be rested on a tooth or extraorally. A diamond point may be used for enamel penetration but only a plane cut tungsten carbide, tapering fissure bur be used for cutting the cavity as a smooth preparation surface is needed. Even cross cut tapering fissure tungsten carbide bur is not used as it might leave a rough surface. It is advisable for the student to fix the bur in the hand piece, and without activating the bur, the hand piece is held perpendicular to the intercuspal plane and the bur is moved along the grooves four or five times to familarize with the hand movement during the actual cutting. If it is a class I cavity, usually an inlay may not be indicated, unless the opposite tooth also has a similar inlay. If an amalgam restoration is given in the upper tooth when an inlay is present in the lower tooth, the dissimilar metals might undergo galvanic corrosion. To avoid it similar alloys should be used. For preparing a convertional class I cavity in an upper molar two conservative cavities are prepared initially on either side of the oblique ridge, and later they are joined together. The rotating tapering fissure diamond point with copious water spray is held perpendicular to the mesial pit and another punch cut is made in the distal pit for a depth of 2 millimeters. If the dentine is not reached, further deepening is done by 0.5 millimeter. Once dentine is reached, diamond point is removed and same size plane cut tungsten carbide tapering fissure bur is fixed to the hand piece. The rotating tungsten carbide bur is reinserted into the prepared punch cut at the mesial pit and moved buccolingually for 2 millimeters to create the dove tail. The bur is passed along the mesial groove which turns buccally to pass between the two buccal cusps. The bur, while extending along the mesial occlusal groove is held vertically at a depth of 2 to 2.5 millimeter & tooth tissue cut equally on both sides of the groove. The bur is stopped 2.5 millimeter from the buccal margin of the occlusal surface. This bur thickness cavity may judiciously be enlarged so as not to cut more than 1/3 of the oblique ridge. No undercuts should be incorporated in the cavity either. Similarly another c shaped cavity be made from the distal pit. It must be remembered that the distopalatal cusp is a small one & should not be weakened. The distal cavity is a smaller one stopping 2.5 millimeter from the lingual margin of the occlusal surface. Slight distal dovetailing is done. Cavity floors are smoothened and checked for undercuts. Once the two cavities are satisfactorily prepared, they should be joined together by cutting accorss the oblique ridge by not more than 1/4 to 1/3 of the intercuspal distance between the mesipalatal and distobuccal cusp. The cavity walls are smoothened and rounded. Had the bur been held perpendicular, the taper of the bur head (2 to $4^0$) will be transferred to the cavity walls and for a shallow cavity $2^0$ taper will be adequate. The pulpal floor Is smoothened. No cavosurface bevel is done for this inlay cavity as only a laboratory low fusing base alloy will be used as casting and it can not be burnished. Hand cutting instruments can be used to remove the unsupported enamel rods from the cavosurface margins. To find out whether there are any undercuts in the cavity, the mouth mirror must be held and the image visualized. If it is possible to see all the internal line angles and point angles atleast from any one angle, that will be the line of insertion and the cavity does not have any undercuts. Air water spray is used to clean the cavity and then air drived.

**34. WHAT ARE THE FEATURE SEEN IN A C1.I INLAY CAVITY?**

**A:**

1. Outline form consisting of smooth flowing curved walls, maintaining cuspal contour, with minimal cutting of crossing oblique ridge. The external outline form is larger than the internal outline form. All the walls have a pulpo occlusal divergence. Cavity includes all pits & fissures.

2. Absence of undercuts in the cavity.

3. Flat smooth pulpal floor 0.5 millimeter below the dentino enamel junction.

4. Cavity width not more than one third of the intercuspal distance.

5. Though inlay cavities are supposed to have cavosurface bevels of $135^0$ to $150^0$, for the preclinical training, if only base metal alloys are to be used for casting, no bevel should be given. If noble metal alloys are to

be used for preclinical training, bevels in the cavo surface margin are made.

**35. DESCRIBE THE PROCEDURE OF PREPARING A MESIOOCCLUSAL CLASS II INLAY CAVITY IN AN UPPER MOLAR TOOTH?**

**A:** The phantom head is adjusted, so that the field of operation is at the level of the operator's elbow. The right handed dental student sits at 11'O clock postion and prepares the cavity under indirect vision. The left hand of the operator encircles the phantom head (without touching it) and holds the mouth mirror. The ring finger of the left hand should be rested on a tooth or extra orally. A diamond point may be used for enamel penetration but a plane cut tapering fissue tungsten carbide bur with rounded corner & flat ends is used for cavity preparion. The tooth adjacent to the tooth to be worked upon (premolar) is protected with a metal matrix band. the diamond point is fixed to the hand piece and held perpendicular to the occlusal surface of the upper molar. The right hand of the dental student holds the hand piece in inverted pen grasps and the ring finger is used as a rest. The punch cut is made in the mesial pit to a depth of 2 millimeter to 2.5 millimeter to establish the pulpal floor in dentine. The diamond point should be rotating with sufficient water spray during insertion and removal. The diamond point should be rotating with sufficient water spray during insertion and removal. The diamond point is removed and tungsten carbide bur of the same size is replaced in the handpiece. Maintaining the same depth and the long axis of the bur kept perpendicular to the intercuspal plane, the cavity is extended along the mesial occlusal groove, cutting equally on both sides of the groove and stopping 2.5 millimeter short of the buccal margin of the occlusal surface. If it is a conservative cavity, oblique ridge should not be involved in the prepared cavity. The cavity is widened so as to have pulpo occlusally straight walls that diverege occlusally. Mesially the cavity is extended at the same depth with sufficient proximal flare to locate the margins of the cavitv in easily cleansable areas, just outside the contact area. The mesial enamel wall in the contact area can be thinned, but not broken till later, to protect the neighbouring tooth till rotary instrumentation is over. The buccal and lingual proximal walls should be in smooth flowing curves that diverge axiomesially to end at the cavosurface at 90°. The bur held at the dentino enamel junction at the mesial end of the pulpal floor, the cavity is deepened cervically upto the gingival extent of the contact area, creating a convex axial wall parallel to mesial surface. The buccal and lingual walls of the proximal box should have a gingivo occlusal taper. (Gingivo occlusal divergence). The gingival seat is established supra gingivally. Shallow grooves are made at the bucco axial and palato axial line angles from the gingival seat upto the level of pulpal floor. The grooves are made with a thinner tapering fissure bur so that the groove is narrower at gingival end & broader at pulpal end. These locking grooves are guidance grooves for correct seating of inlay. The thinned proximal enamel can now be broken and the jagged walls are smoothened with enamel chisels, enamel hatchets, enamel hoes and gingival marginal trimmers. The axio pulpal line angle is rounded or bevelled to have a thicker wax pattern at that location and to prevent air entrapment in the wax pattern at the sharp angle, during investing. If the student is going to use noble alloy for casting, he should create cavosurface bevels, with flame shaped fine grit diamond point, to create cavosurface bevels between 135° to 150°. This will create 30° to 45° inlay margins that are easy to burnish. Inlay margins that have less than 30° angulations are too weak and margins more than 45° are too thick to burnish. All the walls and floors are checked for smoothness and cavity is cleansed with air water spray, and dried with air syringe.

**36. DESCRIBE THE FEATURES PRESENT IN A CLASS II INLAY CAVITY?**

**A:** 1. Occlusal outline, in the form of smooth flowing curves to maintain cuspal contour, to include all the pits and grooves. Proximal outline is just outside the contact area buccally, lingually and gingivally.

2. Pulpo occlusally and gingivo occlusally, straight walls that diverge slightly.
3. Pulpal floor is flat, smooth and parallel to the intercuspal plane.
4. Width of the cavity between 1/4 and 1/3 of intercuspal distance but with sufficient convenience form for instrumentation.
5. Presence of definite but not sharp line and point angles.
6. Cavosurface bevel of 135° of 150° if noble alloy casting is to be made.
7. Pulpo occlusally and gingivo occlusally divergent walls..
8. No undercuts in cavity.
9. Axial wall parallel to proximal surface and flat supragingival gingival seat.

**37. DESCRIBE THE PROCEDURE OF CAVITY PREPARATION FOR CLASS III INLAY?**

**A:** A class III metallic inlay is preferred for distal surface of canine. The dental student sits at 11'O clock position and the cavity is prepared under indirect vision. The phantom head is adjusted so that the field of operation is at elbow level. The proximal cavity is reached from the lingual aspect. The prepared cavity could be a slot cavity with tapered retention grooves, slot type cavity with enhanced gingival & incisal retentive grooves or a slot type cavity with lingual dovetail. In any of the three types cavities, the line of insertion and withdrawal is lingual. A 009 tapering fissure diamond and tapering fissure tungsten carbide bur are used for gross cavity preparation. The initial cavity penetration is done with the diamond at the lingual marginal ridge of the enamel, penetrating towards the labial surface along the proximal dentino enamel junction. Intact thin enamel wall distally is preserved till the last stages of cavity prepartion, to protect the neighbouring premolar. The incisal and gingival walls diverge both labiolingually as well as axio mesially. The labial enamel wall is preserved and retention grooves are placed in gingivo axial line angle at the expense of gingival wall and inciso axial line angle at the expense of incisal wall, with a 005 round bur in a slow speed hand piece. Axial wall is flat. If these grooves are considered inadequate for retention, and more tooth substance are available, more enhanced cervico axial & inciso axial grooves are made cutting more deeply. Otherwise a lingual extension like a dove tail is made on the lingual side. After the proximal cavity is prepared, a tapering fissue bur is used to prepare the lingual deovetail at a depth of 1.5 to 2 millimeter. A short cavosurface bevel is prepared all along the cavosurface margins.

**38. DESCRIBE THE FEATURES IN A CLASS III INLAY CAVITY?**

**A:**

1. Slot like outline from with access from lingual side having an intact labial enamel wall.
2. Thicker carvical wall and a narrower incisal wall which diverge from the labial to lingual side providng the line of withdrawal.
3. Axio distal divergence of the gingival and incisal wall to correspond to the direction of enamel rods.
4. Orientation grooves that also help in providing retention are made at gingivo axial and inciso axial line angles.
5. Cavosurface bevel prepared to facilitate burnishing.
6. Lingual dove tail to enhance retention.
7. Smooth, flat axial wall.

**39. IS CLASS IV CAVITY PREPARED FOR INLAYS?**

**A:** Anterior inlays are prepared from cast metal as well as porcelain material. The anterior teeth are smaller teeth and incisal edges are stress bearing areas. Incisal restoration should be strong.

**40. DESCRIBE THE PROCEDURE OF MAKING A CLASS IV INLAY CAVITY IN AN UPPER INCISOR?**

**A:** The line of withdrawl for a class IV cavity can be lingual, provided the lingual wall is absent in both proximal and incisal boxes. As incisal withdrawal may also be possible if the lingual wall is absent in the coronal two thirds of the proximal box. Because of the shape of the anterior teeth, presence of a lingual wall will only interfere with the withdrawal of the pattern in an incisal or lingual direction. Proximal incisal withdrawal may not be feasibile if the neighbouring tooth is present. The dental student adjusts the phantom head in such as way as to have the field of operation at the level of the elbow. The dental student sits between 11'O clock & 12'O clock position and prepares the cavity under indirect vision. A tapering fissure diamond point 008 and a tungsten carbide bur 008 are used for preparing the proximal cavity and smaller burs are used for preparing the incisal cavities.The lingual access necessitates removal of lingual wall. The initial penetration is adjascent to the marginal ridge to establish the gingival seat and an intact labial enamel wall and a flat axial wall in dentine. Incisal preparation will be narrow necessitating use of smaller burs. As far as possible, incisal plate of enamel should be preserved for asthetics. The pulpal floor should be established in dentine. If retentive pinholes are made in pulpal floor and gingival seat, they should be oriented along the line of withdrawal, namely incisal. If noble metal alloy casting is to be done, cavosurface bevel is done an all margins to facilitate burnishing. The cavity walls are smoothened, washed with air water spray and air dried.

**41. WHAT ARE THE FEATURES IN CLASS IV INLAY CAVITY?**

**A:**

1. Outline form involving proximal and incisal surface of an anterior tooth. Usually lingual wall of the proximal box will be absent to facilitate incisal withdrawal of the pattern (especially when retentive pin is given). If a pin is not given, a highly divergent lingual wall may permit proximolingual withdrawl of the pattern.

2. Flat & smooth intact labial enamel wall and gingival seat.
3. Flat axial wall 0.5 millimeter below dentino enamel junction.
4. Intact labial enamel wall in the incisal box.
5. Pulpal floor in incisal box in dentine.

**42. WHAT MATERIALS ARE USED FOR CLASS V INLAY CAVITIES?**

**A:** Noble alloy castings are stronger. But in a class V cavity, if aesthetics is the primary concern, poercelain inlays or laboratory cured composite inlays are used. Temporary inlays could be made with tooth coloured acrylic resins.

**43. DESCRIBE THE PROCEDURE OF A CLASS V INLAY CAVITY PREPARATION?**

**A:** The dental student, if right handed, sits between 7'O clock and 9'O clock position and prepares the cavity under direct vision. The phantom head is adjusted so that the field of operation is at elbow level. The left hand holding the mouth mirror, retracts the lip. The right hand holds the airotor hand piece and bur in pen grip with finger rest in the canine tip or an adjacent tooth. A tapering fissure diamond 010 and tapering fissue plane cut tungsten carbide 010 bur are used for cavity preparation. To initiate the cavity, the diamond is used in the middle of the gingival third of the cavity. After penetrating to dentine, the tungsten carbide tapering fissure bur can be used to extend the cavity in a trapezoidal outline, with narrower arm cervically and the broader arm coronally. Maintaining the minimal depth of 0.5 millimeter below the dentine enamel junction, the cavity is extended by holding the bur perpendicular to the outer enamel surface. Because of the convexity of the labial surface, hand position holding the hand piece is subtly altered as the cavity is extended. It must be remembered that the thickness of enamel cervically is less than in the middle third so that the width of the incisal wall is more than the width of the cervical wall. By holding the bur perpendicular to the outer enamel surface all the walls are made diverging from the axial wall. The line angles are rounded. The axial wall is gently couvex and parallel to the outer surface. Because of the lesser depth of the cavity, it it is felt that the retention might not be adequate, two parallel pin channels for 1 to 1.5 millimeter could be made with 006 twist drill, on axial wall near mesial & distal walls. A cavo surface bevel is placed with a fine grit diamond point. The cavity is washed with air water spray and dried with air. Cavosurface bevels are not indicated for porcelain and laboratory processed composite inlays as these materials do not have enough strength in thin sections.

**44. WHAT ARE THE FEATURES PRESENT IN A CLASS V INLAY CAVITY?**

A: 1. Outline form is trapezoidal with rounded corners and the mesial, incisal, distal and cervical walls diverging axio buccally, to correspond with the direction of enamel rods.

2. Axial wall in dentine 0.5 millimeter below the dentino enamel junction and slightly convex mesio distally and inciso cervically.

3. No undercuts in any part of cavity.

4. Smooth walls

5. If necessary, parallel pin channels in dentine (axial wall) near the mesial and distal walls.

6. Cavosurface bevel for noble alloy cast restorations. No bevels for porcelain or composite restoration.

**45. WHAT ARE THE DIFFERENCES IN CAVITY PREPARATION FOR GOLD INLAY AND PORCELAIN INLAY?**

A: 1. BEVEL : a) No cavo surface bevel done for porcelain inlay, butt joint cavosurface margin for porcelain.

b) For gold inlays, $30^0$ to $45^0$ cavosurface bevel prepared.

2) TAPER : a) For porcelain inlays, greater taper $6^0$ to $8^0$ per each wall is needed as very little pressure is to be applied forty in.

b) For gold inlays, $2^0$ to $5^0$ taper per each wall is made.

3) INTERNAL LINE ANGLES AND POINT ANGLES:

a) For porcelain inlays, these angles shouid be well rounded to prevent stress concentration

b) For gold inlays, the internal angles could be definite but not well rounded.

4) PINS : a) For porcelain, no pins are to be used

b) For gold castings, parallel pins could be used.

**46. HOW ARE CAVITIES PREPARED FOR DIRECT GOLD RESTORATIONS?**

A: The cavities for direct gold restorations are similar to that for smaller amalgam cavities. The differences are

1) Internal line angles and point angles are sharp to prevent slipping of compacted gold foil.

2) Undercuts, and retentive starting and finishing pits are common to lock the compacted gold.

3) Bevels are made in cavo surface margins for burnishing of gold.

**47. WHAT TYPES OF CAVITIES ARE DONE FOR COMPOSITE RESINS?**

**A:** Conventional cavities like that for an amalgam used to be done earlier on. These cavities were box like prepartions with regular retentive features done for conventional composite resin restorations prepared without using acid etch technique. Such cavities are presently done only for root caries cavities that are prepared without any bevels but with a butt joint. The second type of composite resin restorations done presently are prepared while replacing on existing old restoration with an acid etched composite restoration. The old restoration is removed and bevels are created at appropriate areas of enamel, which are acid etched and then restored with composite.

The third type of cavity for composite restoration is the one done commonly for a new lesion. In all the lesions, acid conditioning of enamel and dentine are done and dentive bonding agents are applied. These cavities do not have any cavity wall configuration and there is no specific pulpal floor depth. Caries removal & any other defects are the only concerns. Even undermined enamel could be supported be bonded composite. For small lesions, minimal preparation of the tooth is adequate. For larger lesions, other retention modes may also be done in addition to acid etch technique.

**48. HOW IS THE TOOTH PREPARED IN ACID ETCHING TECHNIQUE?**

**A:** After removing the carious lesion, if dentine is exposed, dentine is protected with calcium hydroxide or glass ionomer cement. A bevel is created over cleaned enamel. The bevel in the enamel is created for a composite restoration for three reasons.

1. Having a larger surface area of enamel for etching.
2. Having the ends of the rods rather than the sides of the rods exposed to acid applied.
3. For better aesthetic result, because the line of demarcation between restoration and tooth is masked. There is a merging of the restoration with the tooth.

Tooth is dried & isolated. Acid jel containing 37% phorphoric acid is applied over the enamel for 15 to 60 seconds. The area is washed with copious water. The area is dried with oil free compressed air. The etched area will appear frosty. This is the stage when no contamination with saliva should occur. The enamel bonding agent should be applied in the etched area now.

Initially, when acid etching technique was introduced, instructions were given that only enamel should be etched and dentine should not be etched for fear of pulpal damage. But presently, many acid conditioners are supplied by different manufacturers for application over dentine, for conditioning the dentire, before application of the bonding agent. Manufacturer's instructions should be strictly followed while using any of the bonding systems.

**49. HOW IS THE TOOTH PREPARED FOR GLASS IONOMER CEMENTS?**

**A:** If the tooth is carious, caries is removed completely. The outline will be dictated by the lesion. Ragged enamel ends should be smoothened. If the tooth is non carious, the tooth is polished with fluoride free prophylaxis paste. Then the tooth is washed with copious water. Tooth is dried and isolated. In very deep lerions with remaining dentive thickness of 0.5 millimeter, calcium hydroxide base may have to be given for pulpal protection. 10% polyacrylic acid is applied over the tooth for 20 seconds followed by rinsing and drying with dry clean air.

**50. HOW IS A DEEP CARIOUS TOOTH PREPARED FOR AN INDIRECT PULP CAPPING?**

**A:** This is a clinical situation encountered by every dental surgeon. The dental student can not get an extracted tooth with deep caries without exposure, because such a tooth would not have been extracted at all! He can only get an extracted tooth with carious exposure. For training purpose the student is asked to ignore the exposure and excavate the caries from areas other than the exposure. The exposed area is supposed to be the deepest part of the lesion, to be treated by indirect pulp capping. All the soft caries from the freshly extracted tooth should be excavted with a spoon excavator used from periphery to the centre. Excepting the area of exposure, caries is removed from all other areas until hard dentine is encountered. This exercise is intended to make the dental student experience the feel of removing soft carious dentine with an excavator.

# CHAPTER 10

# MANIPULATION OF RESTORATIVE MATERIALS AND RESTORATION PROCEDURES

**1. WHY IS MANIPULATION OF A MATERIAL IMPORTANT?**

**A:** For obtaining the best properties of materials, it is necessary to follow the manufacturer's instructions regarding proportioning, dispensing, mixing, transfering the material to the prepared cavity, packing, shaping and polishing. Many materials are technique sensitive and require rigorous implementation of manufacturer's instructions. Even a material like silver amalgam which is not technique sensitive exhibits the best properties when manipulated correctly. Contamination during mixing should be avoided. While deliberate contamination will not occur, inadvertent contamination is a distinct possibility if the mixing surface or instruments still have remnants of earlier mixes. The dental surgeon should ensure absolute cleanliness of any reusable mixing instruments and equipment like cement spatula, plastic instruments, condensers, glass slabs, mortar and pestle and reusable capsules of mechanical amalgamators.

**2. WHY IS CAVITY ISOLATION IMPORTANT DURING PLACEMENT OF MATERIALS?**

**A:** Rubber dam isolation is needed while restoring with gold foil. It is also the best method of isolation of moisture. Direct filling gold will never cohere to the previously condensed gold if there is slightest contamination with moisture. After acid etching, if there is saliva contamination, it will lead to poor bonding. Adhesion of glass ionomer to tooth surface will be greatly affected due to contamination of saliva over tooth surface before placement of restoration. Moisture contamination of zinc containing silver amalgam alloy will result in delayed expansion. Contamination of moisture generally weakens the restorative, luting and base cements and dissolve them. When rubber dam isolation is not feasible, atleast cotton roll isolation should be done.

**3. WHAT ARE MATRICES?**

**A:** Matrix is a device used in some cavities for restoring the contour of the restoration.

**4. WHY A MATRIX IS NOT NEEDED FOR ALL RESTORATIONS?**

**A:** When the cavity has all the walls, it is possible to condense the material into the cavity easily and shape it. If one or more walls are missing, it may not be possible to fill the cavity and shape it easily to its natural contour. Moreover if a material has ample working time (eg. command set of a light activated material) it is possible to build up the contour patiently, without fear of hardening of the material, and shaping is completed. Most of the restorative materials are chemically activated and have fixed setting time and prolonged shaping (contouring) procedures might result in breaking the chemical bonds already formed. In such cases, it is preferable to use a precontoured matrix for shaping the restorations.

**5. WHAT ARE THE OBJECTIVES OF A MATRIX?**

**A:**

1. First objective is providing contour or the shape of the restoration.
2. Second objective is preventing intrusion of gingival tissue and rubber dam into the prepared cavity margin by retracting them away.
3. Third objective is assuring dryness and preventing contamination of the restoration.
4. Fourth objective is to have something against which the restoration could be condensed.
5. Fifth objective is to confine the restoration within the cavity.
6. Sixth objective is to maintain the shape of the restorative material while hardening.

7. Seventh objective is protection of the restoration from premature exposure of the cement to air or water before setting (eg: glass ionomer, silicate).

**6. IN A CLASS I CAVITY WITHOUT EXTENSIONS IN A POSTERIOR TOOTH, IS A MATRIX NEEDED TO PREVENT OCCLUSAL EXCESS?**

A: In a Class I cavity without extensions in a posterior tooth, no occlusal matrix is necessary as any occlusal excess of the restoration can easily be detected and corrected by requesting the patient to close his jaws in centric and eccentric postions and detecting occlusal prematurities. But on other surfaces, alterations of contour are not that easily and quickly identifiable, especially when it is minimal. it may take some time before the periodontal signs and symptoms point to the damage inflicted. Moreover gross occlusal excess during restoration will not occur because of better visibility. Due to poor visibility, proximal excess is frequently missed leading to disastrous results.

**7. WHAT ARE THE REQUIREMENTS OF A MATRIX?**

A: The matrix should be sufficiently rigid to retain the contour given to it so that it could be transferred to the restoration. The matrix should not react or adhere to the restoration. The removal of the matrix should be easy. The matrix should be contoured easily.

**8. WHAT MATERIALS ARE USED AS MATRICES?**

A: Stainless steel, cellulose acetate (cellophane) and cellulose nitrate (celluloid) and polymer materials are used as matrices.

**9. HOW ARE MATRICES SUPPLIED?**

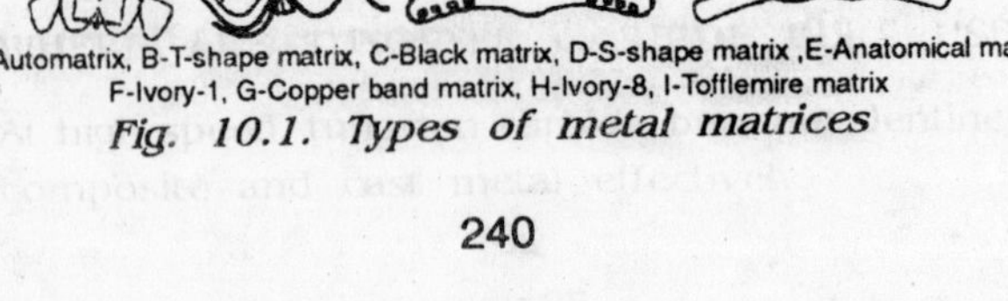


A-Automatrix, B-T-shape matrix, C-Black matrix, D-S-shape matrix ,E-Anatomical matrix F-Ivory-1, G-Copper band matrix, H-Ivory-8, I-Tofflemire matrix

*Fig. 10.1. Types of metal matrices*

**A:** Matrices are commonly supplied as strips of different dimensions. Matrices are also supplied as crown forms, split crown form, hollow cylinders, curved bands with one or more cervical extensions etc.

**10. WHAT IS THE THICKNESS OF MATRIX BANDS?**

**A:** Metal matrix bands are thinner. They may be 0.001" (0.025 millimeter) or 0.002" (0.05 millimeter) thick. The width of the matrix bands may be 1/4", 3/8", 5/16" or 1/8". Depending on the height of the restoration, suitable matrix band is selected. Crown forms and split crown forms are thicker than polyester strip matrices.

**11. WHAT ARE MATRIX RETAINERS?**

**A:** Matrix retainers are gadgets used to retain the matrix bands in position. Some matrices do not need any special mechanical devices to hold them in postion. Some matrices could be held by simple retainers like wire, silk thread, dental floss & impression compound. Some matrices need special mechanical retainers.

**12. WHICH MATRICES DO NOT REQUIRE A RETAINER?**

**A:** Self retaining matrices are 1. Copper band matrix 2. T Band matrix 3. Auto matrix 4. Celluloid crown forms 5. Aluminium crown forms 6. Soldered orthodontic (stainless steel) bands.

**13. NAME SOME OF THE MECHANICAL MATRIX RETAINERS?**

**A:** a. Ivory number 1. b. Ivory number 8. c. Ivory number 9. d. Tofflemire retainers e. Steel siquevland self adjusting retainer f. Bonnalie retainer g. Nygard retainer h. Howe's retainer i. Hick's retainer.

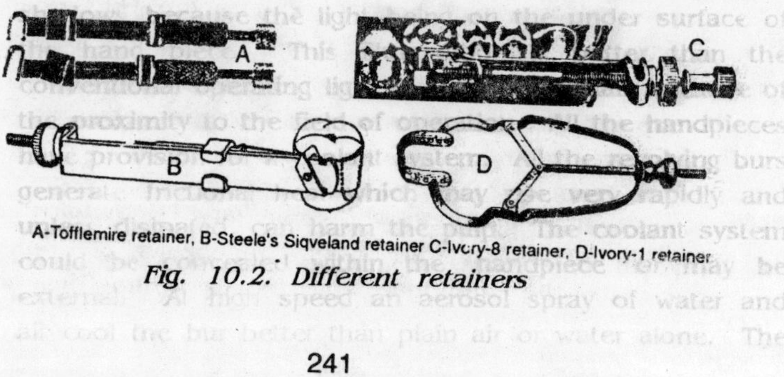


A-Tofflemire retainer, B-Steele's Siqveland retainer C-Ivory-8 retainer, D-Ivory-1 retainer

*Fig. 10.2. Different retainers*

**14. HOW ARE MATRICES CONTOURED?**

**A:** Matrices are contoured with contouring pliers. Matrices could also be contoured by the spherical or egg shaped burnishers with matrix held over compressible paper pads.

**15. ARE MATRICES REUSABLE?**

**A:** Because of the necessity of contouring of every matrix band for every restoration, it is wiser to discard the old matrices & use a new matrix for each restoration.

**16. DESCRIBE DIFFERENT METAL MATRICES?**

**A:** Matrices come as flat straight continuous strips or rolls. Required length could be cut and used. Matrix bands for individual retainers are also marketed. Matrix bands are also supplied with a convex outer border and a concave inner border. The inner border may have two convex projections in the mid portion. When this band is bent to form a loop, the upper convex border will correspond to the larger occlusal surface and the concave inner border will correspond to the smaller cervical surface of the tooth. Most of these matrix bands could be used in different retainers excepting Ivory No.1 retainer.

**17. WHAT IS UNIQUE ABOUT IVORY NO.1 RETAINER?**

**A:** Ivory No.1 retainer needs bands with perforations in the arms of the band. Ivory No.1 retainer and band could be used either in mesioocclusal or disto occlusal cavities but not for mesiooccluso distal (MOD) cavities as this band is only a partial converage (unilateral) band and not a circumferential band. This band can not be used for class I buccal or lingual extension either, Ivory No.1 retainer and band are easier to place than cicumfrential bands. With this retainer in positon, occlusion can not be checked.

**18. WHAT IS THE PURPOSE OF MILTIPLE HOLES IN THE IVORY NO.1 MATRIX BAND?**

**A:** The circumferences of teeth vary. Depending on the cicumference of the tooth, the beaks of the retainer engages the appropriate hole. Usually symmetrical holes are engaged so that the band engaging the proximal portion is properly centred.

**19. DESCRIBE THE MATRIX BAND USED FOR IVORY NO.1 RETAINER?**

**A:** This stainless steel band has a convex occlusal border and a concave cervical border with a central convex portion to project into the proximal gingival portion and 3 or 4 holes on the extending arms of the band.

**20. DESCRIBE THE IVORY NO.1 RETAINER?**

**A:** Ivory No.1 Matrix retainer consists of a compressible 'U' shaped metallic arm that continue at a lower plane as two prongs with beaks. A central screw passes through the metallic arm. The tip of the screw is connected by a hinge joint to two ends of the 'U' shaped metal arms. when the locking nut on the central screw is turned clockwise (tightened), it pulls the central screw out of the metallic arm and because of the pull of the laterally directed plates, the two prongs of the retainer are brought towards each other. When the nut is turned anticlockwise (loosened) it pushes the central screw into the metallic arm and because of the push of the laterally directed plates the two prongs of the retainer are pushed away from each other.

**21. WHY THE 'U' SHAPED METALLIC ARM OF THE IVORY NO.1 RETAINER CONTINUES AS TWO PRONGS AT A LOWER PLANE?**

**A:** The continuation of the metallic arm as two prongs at a lower level is to have clearance for the anterior teeth as the beaks holding the matrix band engage the gingival embrassure of the tooth worked upon. If the metallic arm and the two prongs are at the same level, it will interfere with positioning the retainer properly, and the metallic arm and nut will be at an ackward angle, interfering with restoration procedures. While applying the Ivory No.1 retainer, it should be correctly positioned so that the metallic arm and the nut are just clearing the occlusal surfaces of the anterior teeth. If the retainer is positioned upside down it will grossly interfere with condensation &

carving procedures. This problem does not occur while using the other retainers as most of them are placed buccally and few lingually.

**22. HOW IS IVORY NO. 1 RETAINER WITH BAND APPLIED TO THE TOOTH?**

**A:** First the circumference of the tooth is noted and an Ivory No. 1 matrix band of suitable length, width and thickness is selected and tried on the tooth. If there are any gingival impingement, the band is relieved in that area by cutting with a short sharp crown scissors. The band is contoured with contouring pliers. The correctly contoured matrix band is repositioned on the tooth and the holes in to which the beaks of the retainer should enter should coincide with the gingival embrassure of the intact proximal surface. For a mesio occlusal cavity, the beaks should engage the distal gingival embrassure and for a disto occlusal cavity, the beaks should engage the mesial gingival embrassure. After deciding which perforations of the band the beaks should engage, the band is removed and kept aside. The retainer is loosened so that the beaks of the prongs just clear the contact area of the intact proximal surface. Now the band is inserted at the selected holes. Before fixing the retainer and band onto the tooth, any gingivial excess is trimmed and the correct positioning of occlusal and gingival margins are checked. After ascertaining the correct positioning of the band, it is slowly inserted in the proximal side of the working area. Once the band is in position, the nut of the retainer is tightened so that the beaks enter the gingival embrassure of the intact proximal surface. The wedging effecting of the two beaks tighten the band and holds it in position.

**23. IS IVORY NO. 1 RETAINER STABLE?**

**A:** IVORY NO. 1 retainer is not very stable. Its only advantage is that it can be used when circumferential banding is difficult because of unduly tight contacts.

**24. IS THE WEDGING EFFECT OF THE RETAINER BENEFICIAL?**

**A:** No. The wedging effect of the beaks of the retainer occur at the (non working) intact proximal side which tend to push the tooth worked upon towards its other neighbouring tooth.(working side). If condensation of the restoration is done in this postion and after removal of the retainer, when the tooth regains its original postion, there will not be a tight contact with its neighbouring tooth. So the wedging effect of the beaks of the retainer are not beneficial. To ensure tight contact of the restoration with its neighbouring tooth, good wedging is necessary on the working side to overcome the wedging effect of the retainer.

**25. DOES ANY OTHER RETAINER HAVE SIMILAR WEDGING EFFECT?**

**A:** No other retainer has such adverse wedging effect.

**26. WHAT ARE THE DISADVANTAGES OF IVORY NO.1 RETAINER?**

**A:** 1. 1. Ivory No.1 retainer cannot be used for MOD cavities. 2. Ivory No.1 retainer cannot be used for class I buccal and lingual extensions. 3. Ivory No.1 retainer has adverse wedging effect. 4. Ivory No.1 retainer is not very stable. 5. Ivory No.1 retainer can not be used if the neighboring tooth on the intact (non working) proximal side of the tooth worked upon is abent. (eg. If M.O. cavity for tooth No.46 is done & 47 is absent, Ivory No.1 retainer can't be used).

**27. DESCRIBE ABOUT CIRCUMFERENTIAL BANDS AND THE RETAINERS USED TO HOLD THEM?**

**A:** Circumferential bands, when held with their ends together, form a loop. The ends of the matrix band pass through a slot in the fixed arm into a movable vice and tightly held by a long band locking screw to form a large loop that can encircle the crown of the tooth. The diameter of the loop is reduced by turning the large vice moving knob clockwise. For increasing the diameter of the loop, the vice moving knob is turned anti clockwise. This is the basic principle of circumferential matrix bands and the various matrix bands designed for them. Minor variations in band entry slots, locking vice designs, present of a mobile self adjusting metal slide result in various types of matrix retainers. Straight matrix retainers are used on the buccal side and contra angle matrix retainers are used on the lingual side. When the retainers are present on the buccal side, the advantage is, with proper occlusal trimming of the matrix band, it is possible to check the occlusion even before removing the matrix band.

**27. DESCRIBE THE IVORY NUMBER 8 RETAINER?**

**A:** The Ivory No.8 retainer has a slot in its fixed arm. The movable vice also has a slot which is in approximation with that in the fixed arm, when the vice is adjusted to the maximum movable position. With the two slots coinciding, the looped band is inserted first through the fixed arm, into the movable vice and the band locking crew is rotated clockwise to lock the band and prevent it from slipping. Activation of the vice moving knob clockwise results in reduction in size of the loop diameter. Adjustment of the vice moving knob could be minimal if the loop diameter is made just larger than the size of tooth, before locking it to the movable vice.

**28. HOW IS IVORY NO.8 RETAINER POSITIONED AROUND THE TOOTH?**

**A:** The retainer is adjusted till the movable vice slot is approximated to the fixed arm. The band is selected, the two ends of the band held together and inserted through the slot in the fixed arm and the approximated slot in the movable vice till the loop size is just larger than the tooth diameter. The band is locked in this postion by turning the band locking screw. The band is slipped around the tooth with the retainer remaining on the buccal side and parallel to the buccal surfaces of the teeth projecting anteriorly. Instead, if the retainer is kept buccally but perpendicular to the buccal surfaces of teeth and projecting laterally, the occlusoapical contour of the band will be altered.

**29. WHAT IS A UNIVERSAL MATRIX RETAINER?**

A: Tofflemire's matrix retainer is called the universal matrix retainer because of the diversity of situations where it will be of use.

**30. DESCRIBE THE TOFFLEMIRE RETAINER?**

A: Straight Tofflemire retainer is positioned on the buccal surface & contra angle Tofflemire is postioned on the lingual surface. The retainer consists of a fixed arm on which three guide channels are present for postioning the matrix band from the right, left or straight direction depending on the tooth to be worked upon. The movable locking vice has an angular slit through which the band ends should pass and the long band locking screw holds the band in the vice. The vice moving knob permits shortening of the loop diameter by moving the locking vice.

**31. HOW IS THE TOFFLEMIRE MATRIX RETAINER APPLIED OVER THE TOOTH?**

A: Appropriate tofflemire retainer is chosen (depending on buccal or lingual placement). If available, precontoured matrix band supplied by the manufacturer is selected or contouring of the band done with contouring pliers or an egg shaped burnisher tip with band held over a pliable paper pad. The band ends are held together to form a loop and the band is placed in the appropriate guide channels (right, left or straight depending on the tooth to be worked upon) and passed through the angular slit in the vice and locked in postion. Care is taken to enter the occlusal side of the band to pass though the guide channel & locking vice first. This will facilitate the placement of the retainer with guide channels & vice, gingivally directed and this help in easy removal of the retainer from the matrix band once the restoration is finished. The vice moving knob help in moving the vice and reducing the size of the loop.

The band is slipped over the tooth with due care to prevent gingival impingment and the guide channel & locking vice facing gingivally. The vice moving knob is activated to tighten the band. Care is taken to place the retainer parallel to the buccal surfaces of the teeth in that quadrant and not perpendicular to them to prevent alterations in the occluso gingtival contour of the band.

**32. DESCRIBE THE DOUBLE MATRICING TECHNIQUE?**

**A:** While restoring a buccal extension or lingual extension cavity, it it difficult to reproduce the occluso cervical contour of the buccal or lingual surface. The convexity of the occlusal one third is not easily achieved with a single matrix band. It is advisable to insert a second matrix band of suitable length to cover the buccal surface, between the single band already applied and the surface of the tooth and softened compound applied between the bands to stabilize them. This is the double matrix technique.

**33. IS IT EASY TO APPLY THE RETAINER AND BAND IN THE PRECLINICAL WORKING MODELS?**

**A:** Commercially available acrylic preclinical work models have detachable teeth. In these models, it is possible to place the bands and retainers easily. In custom made acrylic models holding fixed natural teeth the unyielding acrylic prevents the correct positioning of the retainers & bands. But a student must be able to show how the band & retainer is kept correctly.

**34. WHAT IS A RETAINERLESS MATRIX?**

**A:** Though matrices like Black's matrices, copper band matrix, soldered stainless steel matrix, anotomical matrix, 'T' Band matrix, crown forms etc. do not need a mechanical retainer for holding them in postion, the term retaineless matrix usually denotes an automatrix. It is also called Roll in band matrix. It comes in 3 widths (3/16", 1/4" and 5/16") and two thickenesses (0.0015" & 0.002") This matrix is a single use matrix (not reusable). The principle of this matrix is that one end of the matrix is held by an auto lock and the other ended is rolled over itself. The cirumference of the band could be increased or decreased. The rolled over coil can be further rolled with a hand held mechanical device to decrease the circumference of the matrix (for tightening the band around the tooth). For enlarging the circumference, the lock release hole is used to release the rolled band through the auto lock. After restoration is completed, the autolock is cut off and the band is removed. The advantage of this matrix is that no retainer is necessary to hold it in place & hence better visibility, less chariside time than adapting a copper band matrix and the feasibility to place the auto lock loop either buccally or lingually. The disadvantages are cost and the difficulty of contouring the bands.

**35. WHAT S BLACK'S MATRIX?**

**A:** Black's matrices are strips of metallic bands held by a wire or floss wrapped around it. The bands are trimmed to avoid gingival impingement and the corners are tucked over the encircled floss or wire to hold them in position. No other retainer in used.

**36: WHAT ARE COPPER BAND MATRICES?**

**A:** Hollow cylinders of seamless copper bands are available in differnt sizes. Suitable size of the copper band is selected by trying on the tooth. Gingival contouring is done by cutting with a short curved scissors or trimming with rotary stones.

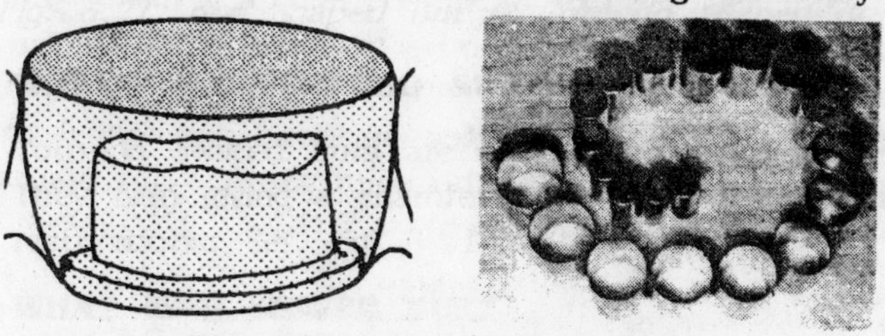

*Fig. 10.3. Copper Band Matrix*

Rough edges are smoothened out. Occlusal reduction of the band is also done if necessary so that the band is only 1 millimeter above the occlusal level. After restoration hardens, the excess is trimmed off, permitting closure of mouth. The band can also be thinned out from inside near contact areas without perforating it for tighter contacts. For contouring the copper band matrix, it is heated red hot and quenched in cold water, so that it is in a soft annealed condition permitting easier contouring. For removal of copper band matrix after restoration hardens, the band is cut with a disk or bur and removed.

**37. WHAT IS A SOLDERED STAINLESS STEEL MATRIX?**

**A:** A stainless steel orthodontic band of sufficient width is selected and cut longer than the size of the circumference of the tooth and soldered at the correct site. The band can be annealed like the copper band. The gingival and occlusal margins are suitably altered for a correct fit. Contouring pliers are used to contour the band. The gingival end of the band could be pinched with a flat bladed plier to form a tuck so that the band is tight.

**38. WHAT IS ANATOMICAL MATRIX?**

**A:** It is a custom made matrix with well contoured and closely adapted margins made in segments and held in position by wedges, and well adapted impression compound buccally & lingually joined by a staple wire.

**39. WHAT IS 'T' BAND MATRIX?**

**A:** They are commercially available matrices, shaped like a T with two short arms and one long arm. They may be mae of stainless steel or brass. The short arms of the band are bent one over the other to form a loop. The long arm is passed circumferentially around the tooth, passed through the loop to tighten the band and folded back to prevent opening up of the short arms. This matrix also does not need a retainer.

**40. WHAT ARE CROWN FORMS?**

**A:** Crown forms are matrices shaped like the crown of a tooth. They have the external morphology of crowns of different teeth in various sizes. They are hollow within. Sectional crown forms are also available and the split crown forms help in restoring a single proximal cavity. They are made of cellulose nitrate (celluloid) or aluminium. They are disposable materials.

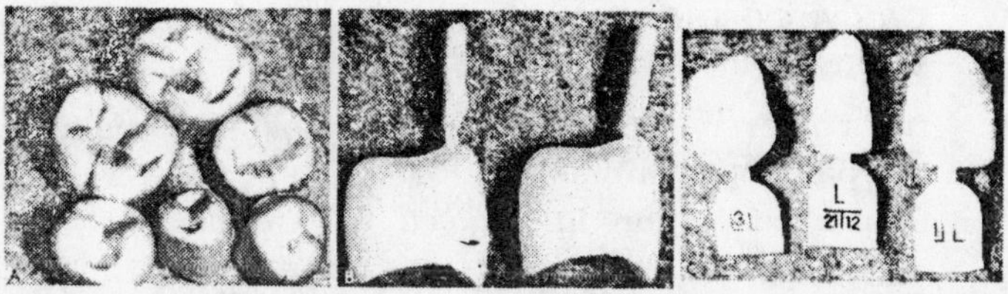

*Fig. 10.4. Crown Forms*

**41. WHAT IS A WINDOW MATRIX?**

**A:** It is a metal matrix in which a window is cut, through which restorative material is condensed in the cavity. It is used for class V cavities.

**42. WHAT ARE WEDGES?**

**A:** Wedges are devices used interndentally to ensure close adaptation of the matrix band with the gingival seat of the prepared proximal cavity. They may be made of wood, metal or plastic.

**43. WHAT ARE THE FUNCTIONS OF A WEDGE?**

**A:**
1. Close adaptation of the matrix band to the tooth margin of the cavity to prevent cervical overhangs of restoration.
2. To separate the teeth during the proximal restoration, so that it can compensate for the thickness of the matrix band and ensure tight contact area.
3. Protect the interdental gingiva and interdental rubber dam during instrumentation.
4. Prevent the interdental gingiva and inter dental rubber dam from pushing the matrix band away.
5. Stabilize the matrix band
6. Maintain gingival embrassure space
7. Define the gingival extent of contact area.

**44. WHAT IS SHAPE OF THE WEDGE?**

**A:** Wedges could be round in cross section or triangular in cross section.

**45. CAN A COMMERCIALLY AVAILABLE WEDGE BE USED AS SUCH?**

**A:** No. For every case, the wedge should be modified to suit the particular embrassure. Trimming of the wedge ensure proper adaptation in a given embrassure.

**46. WHAT IS THE ADVANTAGE OF WOODEN WEDGE?**

**A:** 1. Wooden wedges are easy to trim and adjust

2. Wooden wedges are cheaper

3. Wooden wedges absorb moisture & swell ensuring retention of the band.

**47. WHAT IS THE ADVANTAGE OF PLASTIC WEDGES?**

**A:** 1. Plastic wedges can be plastically moulded and bent to correspond to the shape of interdental col.

2. Transparent plastic wedges, can transmit light through and is of use while using light activated restoration.

**48. WHAT IS THE ADVANTAGE OF A METALLIC WEDGE?**

**A:** 1. Rigid metallic (Silver) wedges separate teeth easily.

**49. WHAT IS A CAVITY VARNISH?**

A: Cavity varnishes are solutions of natural or synthetic resins in volatile liquids like chloroform, alchohol or acetone. The resins could be copal resin, cowrie resin or rosin. They are intended to be applied on all exposed dentinal portions, of the tooth with the aim of blocking the dentinal tubules. After application over a surface of exposed dentine the volatile solvent evaporates, leaving a thin film of resin over the dentine surface which may not be continuous due to evaporation of the solvent.

**50. HOW SHOULD CAVITY VARNISHES BE APPLIED?**

**A:** Cavity varnish can be applied with a cotton pledget, small piece of sponge or a brush. A small cotton pledget held in a tweezer, is soaked in the varnish and taken to the cavity, pressed against dentine and varnish is squeezed out to spread over dentine. The pallet is resoaked and applied in another part of the cavity till the varnish covers all walls and floor. Usually three coatings are needed to have minimal porosity.

**51. WHAT IS THE FILM THICKNESS OF VARNISHES?**

**A:** The film thickness is 5 to 10 micrometers.

**52. WHAT ARE THE ADVANTAGES OF CAVITY VARNISHES?**

**A:** 1. It reduces post operative sensitivity

2. It protects pulp by sealing the dental tubules

**53. IS CAVITY VARNISH AN INSULATING MATERIAL?**

**A :** Cavity varnish is too thin to offer thermal insulation.

**54. WHAT ARE CAVITY LINERS?**

**A:** Cavity liners are aqueous or resinous suspensions of therapeutic agents like calcium hydroxide or zinc oxide. They are applied on dentine only. Calcium hydroxide has acid neutrallizing effect and is also bactericidal. Liners provide dentine protection.

**55. HOW ARE CAVITY LINERS APPLIED?**

**A:** Liners can be applied with a small cotton pledget, sponge or a brush and the application is similar to varnish application.

**56. WHAT IS THE THICKNESS OF CAVITY LINERS?**

**A:** The liner thickness is 20 to 25 micrometers and liners also do not have thermal insulating property.

**57. WHY THE VARNISHES AND LINERS ARE NOT APPLIED UPTO THE CAROSURFACE MARGIN?**

**A:** Liners and varnishes are soluble in oral fluids. If they are applied upto the cavosurface margin, after they are dissoloved, it will result in increased marginal leakage.

**58. WHAT IS A SUBBASE?**

**A:** A sub base is given in the deepest portion of a cavity for specific therapeutic effect.

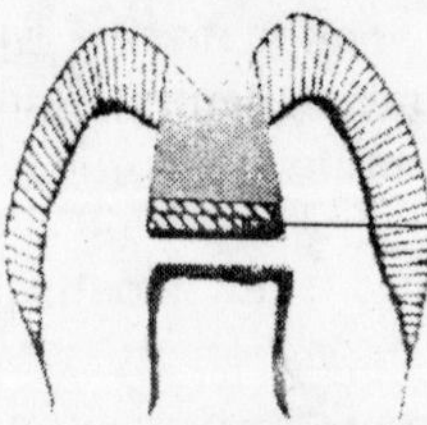


*Fig. 10.5. Sub base*

**59. WHAT MATERIALS ARE USED AS SUB BASES?**

**A:** Materials pulpally compatible are used as sub bases. Calcium hydroxide, zinc oxide eugenol, zinc poly carboxylate and glass ionomer may be used as sub bases. Out of these, calcium hydroxide and zinc oxide engenol are more commonly used.

**60. WHAT IS THE ACTION OF CALCIUM HYDROXIDE AND ZINC OXIDE EUGENOL AS SUB BASES?**

**A:** Calcium hydroxide changes of the area to alkalinity. It is also bactericidal. Calcium hydroxide is also capable of inducing reparative dentine formation. Zinc oxide eugenol has a sedative effect on a slightly inflamed pulp.

**61. WHAT IS THE DIFFERENCE BETWEEN A LINER AND SUB BASE?**

**A:** Liner is thin. Sub base is thick. Liner is applied in all the exposed dentine. Subbase is applied only on deepst part of the dentine. Liner is a liquid. Sub base can be a settable paste, powder or non setting paste.

**62. HOW IS A SUBBASE PLACED?**

**A:** If the subbase is a powder, it can be mixed with distilled water, anaesthetic solution or normal saline to make a paste and applied on the area. There is no chemical reaction involved, the mixing is done with a thick spatula and the mix is carried into the cavity with the flat end of the plastic instrument. If only dry powder is to be placed without a vehicle, it can be carried in an amalgam carrier & ejected into the cavity. If the subbase are two pastes (base and catalyst) and are chemically setting, equal amounts are taken, mixed as per manufactuer's instructions and mixed cement is carried into the deep cavity area and placed with a plastic instrument. If the subbase material is a light activated material, the material is placed in the cavity, manipulated into position and activated with light. If the subbase material is dual cured, the powder and liquid are mixed with a cement spatula on a paper pad and the mix is carried to the cavity, placed in postion and then activated with light for quicker setting.

**63. WHAT IS A BASE?**

**A:** Base is a material placed below a restoration on the dentinal surface for pulp protection.

**64. WHAT ARE THE FUNCTIONS OF A BASE?**

**A:** 1. To provide thermal insulation 2. To prevent chemicals from restorations leaching into the pulp through dentinal tubules 3. To prevent bacterial penetration into the pulp through marginal leakage 4. To provide mechanical support for the restoration and distribute local stresses to dentine 5. To block out undercuts, if present, in an inlay cavity 6. If zinc oxide eugenol is used as a base, it will have obtundent action. 7. If calcium hydroxide is used as a base, it can have anticariogenic effect due to its alkalinity. 8. If calcium hydroxide is used as a base, it may induce formation of reparative dentine.

**65. HOW ARE BASES MANIPULATED AND PLACED IN CAVITY?**

**A:** Most of the bases are supplied as powder and liquid while few are supplied as two pastes and some are light activated. While proportioning and mixing, manufacturer's directions be strictly followed for maximum efficacy. Either a clean glass slab or a clean mixing pad is used to mix the different components with a clean metallic or plastic spatula to the appropriate consistency and carried to the cavity in a plastic instrument and applied. (Details of mixing and placement of individual bases and sub bases are given under each cement).

**66. HOW IS ZINC OXIDE EUGENOL CEMENT USED IN CONSERVATIVE DENTISTRY?**

**A:** Zinc oxide Eugenol cement is available as unmodified zinc oxide eugenol cement, quick setting zinc oxide eugenol cement, reinforced zinc oxide eugenol cement, root canal sealant etc. Zinc oxide eugenol cement could be used as a temporary restoration, base and a temporary luting cement. A reinforced zinc oxide eugenol cement is preferred for temporary restorations and bases. Unmodified zinc oxide eugenol is preferred as a temporary luting cemnt though it can also be used as a base or restoration.

**67. WHAT CARE IS NECESSARY WHILE MIXING UNMODIFIED ZINC OXIDE EUGENOL?**

**A:** Unmodified zinc oxide eugenol is a slow setting material. If it is not handled properly, it can leave messy marks on the work table, instruments and hands of the operator. Eugenol can react with many organic materials leaving markings that are very difficult to clean. But properly handled, it will not mess up the area. For restorative pupose a very thick putty consistency is required. For luting purposes, a creamy consistency is favoured.

**68. HOW IS ZINC OXIDE EUGENOL MIXED?**

**A:** Either a paper mixing pad or a glass slab can be used for mixing. As the mixing reaction is not exothermic, there is no necessity to cool the pad or slab. A stiff bladed stainless steel cement spatula is used. Stiff blade is needed for the heavy spatulation that ensures maximum incorporation of powder into the mix. Cleaning up is easy if disposable paper pad is used. Manufacturer's recommendations regarding proportioning is, powder liquid raio of 6:1 by weight for restorative consistency and 4:1 by weight for luting consistency. The proportioning of powder and liquid is done as per the manufacturer's directions. Volumetric dispensers, if supplied by the manufacturer, could be used. Bulk of powder is mixed into the dispensed liquid and the mix is thoroughly spatulated and then a series of smaller increments are added till the mix is creamy for luting consistency and putty like for restoration. The mixing time could be more, as unmodified zinc oxide eugenol is very slow to set (upto 24 hours). The thick putty consistency zinc oxide eugenol cement is taken in the flat end of a plastic instrument, inserted into the cavity by wiping against the wall. It is condensed with a wet cotton pledget, as the presence of moisture hastens the setting reaction. Further additions of cement & condensation with wet cotton pledget ensures complete filling of the cavity. Some operators, after wiping their fingers with vaseline, roll the putty zinc oxide eugenol into a ball, place it with the tine of proble & carry it into the cavity. Some operators, for strengthening the unmodified zinc oxide eugenol cement, add wisps of cotton firbres in the eugenol before mixing with zinc oxide. Such cotton incorporated unmodified zinc oxide eugenol is found to last longer clinically. When zinc oxide eugenol is mixed to a creamy consistency for luting purposes, the cement from the spatula is directly transferred to the fitting surfaces of the restoration and the restoration is firmly seated on the cavity. The cement exuding from the sides are immediately wiped off.

**69. HOW ARE QUICK SETTING AND REINFORCED ZINC OXIDE EUGENOL CEMENTS MIXED?**

A: The apparatus used for mixing, proportioning, mixing technique, transfer to the cavity and condensation procedures are similar to that for unmodified zinc oxide eugenol materials. But quick setting and reinforced zinc oxide eugenol materials have a setting time of 3 to 10 minutes. Hence the mixing time for the modified zinc oxide engenol is 60 to 90 seconds.

**70. HOW IS ZINC OXIDE EUGENOL USED A BASE?**

A: Unmodified zinc oxide eugenol is not directly used in base thickness as its setting time is long and any material condensed over it, easily displaces it. However, when hardened temporary zinc oxide eugenol restoration is replaced by a permanent restoration, a portion of the hardened temporary restoration might be permitted to remain over the pulpal floor and/or axial wall as a base. When reinforced zinc oxide eugenol is used as a base, it is mixed to a putty consistency and is placed over pulpal floor and / or axial wall and condensed with a wet cotton pledget. Excess zinc oxide eugenol sticking to other walls are chipped off them with a sharp probe.

71. **WHAT IS MEANT BY PACKING FACTOR?**

A: While mixing unmodified zinc oxide and eugenol, it is possible to add much more powder before the material becomes a thick putty. This results in a material which has least amount of marginal leakage among nonadhesive cements. The ability to incorporate maximum quantity of powder into the liquid before setting is called packing factor.

72. **HOW ARE ZINC PHOSPHATE CEMENTS SUPPLIED TO DENTAL PROFESSIONALS?**

A: Zinc phosphate cements are usually supplied a powder and liquid. Sometimes they are also supplied as water settable (anhydrous) cements.

73. **WHAT ARE THE USES OF ZINC PHOSPHATE CEMENTS?**

A: Zinc phosphate cements are used for luting purpose. They are also used for base purpose. Base cements are also infrequently used as a temporary restoration.

74. **ARE THERE SEPARATE CEMENTS OF ZINC PHOSPHATE FOR USE AS BASE AND LUTING MATERIALS?**

A: Yes. Manufacturer advices using type I cement for luting purpose and type II cement for base purpose. The chief difference is in the particle size of the powder. The average particle size of a type I cement is 25 micrometer and that of type II cement, 40 micrometer.

75. **CAN A TYPE II CEMENT BE USED FOR LUTING PURPOSE?**

A: It is not advisable to interchange the materials as the film thickness achieved can be more than 40 micrometer.

76. **WHAT APPARATUS IS USED FOR MIXING ZINC PHOSPHATE CEMENT?**

A: A thick glass slab of atleast 6" x 3" size and a long narrow bladed stiff stainless steel spatula are used for mixing the cement. For slowing down of th setting reaction, it is preferable to cool the glass slab. A cool paper pad does not retain the chillness for a long period like a thick glass slab. The larger mixing area of the glass slab and cooling the glass slab help in dissipating the exothermic heat generated while mixing the zinc phosphate powder & liquid.

77. **HOW ARE THE POWDER AND LIQUID DISPENSED FOR MIXING ZINC PHOSPHATE CEMENT?**

A: Manufacturers provide scoops and droppers for volumetric dispensing of powder and liquid. As per the manufacturer's instructions, two scoops of powder are dispensed onto the centre of the glass slab and divided into six equal parts. The bottle of liquid is swirled before dispensing and with the orifice of the dropper held parallel to the glass slab, six or seven drops of liquid are dispensed by the side of the powder. The liquid should be dispensed just before mixing to avoid any evaporation of water from the liquid. The lid of the liquid bottle should be tightly closed before and after dispensing to avoid water loss or gain.

78. **IS IT ALRIGHT TO DISPENSE LESSER QUANTITY OF POWDER AND LIQUID FOR A SMALLER MIX?**

A: Manufacturers advice that it is undesirable to have one or two drop mixes as it might be too less for proper mixing and evaluating for correcting consistency.

79. **HOW ARE THE POWDER AND LIQUID MIXED?**

A: Initially one part of the dispensed powder is carried into the liquid and mixed in a wide area (atleast over half the glass slab) to allow dissipation of evolved beat: No areas of powder liquid stagnation should occur. After 15 seconds, the second increment is added and mixed for another 15 seconds, such additions are made till the desired consistency is achieved.

80. **WHAT IS THE DESIRED CONSISTENCY FOR ZINC PHOSPHATE CEMENT?**

A: The mixing procedure is the same for Type I and Type II cements. A putty (mouldable solid) consistency is desriable for base puspose. For luting purpose, when the creamy mixed mass is gathered together and the flat side of the spatula is laid on to it and lifted up, the cement should string up for 1 to 1½ inches before breaking and this is the correct consistency.

**81. HOW IS THE MIXED CEMENT USED?**

**A:** 1. The creamy luting cement is collected over the end of the spatula and applied evenly on the fitting surfaces of the extraorally made restoration and firmly seated over the prepared tooth surface and held under pressure to squeeze out the excess cement along the margins which are immediately removed.

2. The mixed base cement is collected over the flat end of the cement spatula. The ends of a stainless steel plastic instrument is dipped in alcohol or in dry powder of the cement to prevent adherence of the putty cement to the instrument. The flat end of the plastic instrument is ued to carry sufficient quantity of the cement on to the cavity and placed in the centre of the cavity. It could be the centre of the pulpal floor or axial wall for a simple class I, III, V or M.O.D. Cavity or axio pulpal line angle for class I with buccal or lingal extensions, class II, class III with lingal dovetail or class IV restoration. The purpose of keeping the base in the centre is it is easier to draw it to all corners of the cavity. The cylinderical end of the plastic instrument is now used to gently tease the putty material over the pulpal floor and/or axial wall as the case may be. Care should be taken that even thickness of material remain all around. Periodical dipping of the plastic instrument tip into dry powder or alcohol, and dragging motion of the instrument ensures even spread of the base. Excess cement on the side walls are carefully removed. If any undercuts were made earlier for extra retention and if the base has entered there, they are removed. Under cut areas should be filled by the restorative material to fulfill their purpose.

**82. IF THE QUANTITY OF CEMENT TAKEN IS INADEQUATE TO COVER THE ENTIRE PULPAL FLOOR AND/OR AXIAL WALL, CAN SUBSEQUENT ADDITIONS BE MADE?**

A: Patch work while giving a base is inadvisable. It will lessen the strength of the base. The inadequate base should be completely removed. A fresh mix is made & suitable quantity is used for covering the entire pulpal floor and/or axial wall with a single base.

**83. WHAT IS FROZEN SLAB METHOD?**

A: Zinc phosphate cement can be mixed in this method also. When multiple cementation of inlays or crowns are to be made, this method is advantageous as it provides larger working time but shorter setting time. The mixed cement remains in creamy state for a greater time but has a snap set. In this method, glass slab is cooled in a refrigerator between minus $10^0$ & $6^0$ No attempt is made on the slab and mix is made on the slab. It is possible to add 50 to 75% more powder than by the conventional method. Strength and solubility of the mix are not altered significantly in this method. Because of the low temperature, the working time is incrased but the setting time is decreased.

**84. HOW IS THE ANHYDROUS ZINC PHOSPHATE CEMENT MIXED AND USED?**

A: In an anhydrous cement, the liquid component is freeze dried and added to the powder. This powder, when mixed with distilled water, results in initial reconstitution of the acid and subsequent reaction with the powder. The proportioning and mixing are as per the manufacturer's directions and manipulation is similar to the conventional zinc phosphate cement. The lid of the powder bottle should tightly be sealed to avoid absorption of water vapour from the atmosphere.

**85. ARE THERE ANY ADVANTAGES IN A ANHYDROUS CEMENT?**

A: There are no advantages in an anyhydrous cement compared to a powder liquid version except it is a novelty.

**86. IS CALCIUM HYDROXIDE USED AS A BASE?**

A: As such calcium hydroxide is a weak material. It is generally used as a sub base. However, reinforced calcium hydroxide with polymers dissolved in salicylic acid esters have enough strength to provide mechanical support to the restorations and such settable calcium hydroxides can be used as base below silver amalgam and composite resins.

**87. HOW IS QUICK SETTING CALCIUM HYDROXIDE USED AS A BASE?**

A: The settable calcium hydroxide is supplied as two pastes. The base paste is white in colour and the catalyst paste is light brown in colour. The mixing is done in a disposable paperpad or a glass slab with a stainless steel spatula. Equal quantities of the two pastes are dispensed on the paper pad and mixed to a uniform consistency without individual streaks of colour. The mixed cement which is fluid in nature, is taken in a ball ended instrument and applied to the cavity. Material flows into the different parts of the cavity and on contact with dentine, sets fast. Chemically settable calcium hydroxide cannot be manipulated like other cements. Presently light activated calcium hydroxide is also available and they can be manipulated to the desired extent and only when the blue light is shown, does it set.

**88. HOW IS POLY CARBOXYLATE CEMENT SUPPLIED ?**

A: 1. Powder and liquid 2. Anhydrous cement 3. Premeasured disposable capsules.

Type I is used for luting & type II is used as base.

**89. WHAT APPARATUS ARE USED FOR MIXING POLYCARBOXYLATE CEMENT?**

A: Encapsulated polycarboxylate is mixed in a capsulator (mechanical mixer for premeasured capsulated material.) Powder & liquid as well as anhydrous cements can be mixed either on a glass slab or a paper pad with either a plastic disposable spatula or a stainless steel spatula.

**90. HOW ARE THE POWDER AND LIQUID PROPORTIONED?**

**A:** Manufacturer's directions should strictly be followed. The powder liquid ratio could be 2:1 or 1:1 by weight. Volumentric dispensers might be provided by the manufacturers. Powder is dispensed first and divided into two halves. Liquid is dispensed just before mixing to prevent evaporation and further thickening. The mixing time is kept short so that the working time is long. The mixing should be done between 30 and 60 seconds so that 2½ to 6 minutes of working time remains. The mixed cement might appear thick but when pressure is applied it flows. Attempts at reducing the quantity of powder mixed (lowering the powder/liquid ratio) will only weaken the cement strength. Clean tooth surface and clean fitting surface of the extraorally made restoration is necessary. Half the powder is incorporated into the liquid at once and after 15 seconds, the other half is incorporated and mixing is completed within 30 to 60 seconds. The mix which should appear glossy and creamy. When drawn up spatula, it should flow under its own weight. The creamy mix is applied on the fitting surface of the extraorally made restoration and seated with firm pressure to ensure good flow and a small film thickness. If zinc polycarboxylate is used as a base, Type II cement is mixed in the above way and a plastic instrument dipped in alcohol (to prevent sticking of the cement) is used to carry the cement to the pulpal floor & manipulated into position. If the surface of the mix appears dull, it means the setting reaction has progressed too far to have sufficient number of unreacted carboxyl groups for combining with calcium of dentine. Excess cement from the side walls of the cavity should be removed and used steel instruments be immediately cleaned.

**91. HOW ARE GLASS IONOMER CEMENTS SUPPLIED?**

**A:**
1. Powder and liquid
2. Anhydrous cement (water settable cement) where the liquid is freeze dried and added to powder.

3. Preportioned capsules with nozzles. (To be mixed in a mechanical mixer (capsulator) and applied with applicator guns).
4. Light activated glass ionomer.

Type I glass ionomer is the luting cement.

Type II glass ionomer is the restorative cement.

Type III glass ionomer is the liner.

**92. WHAT ARE THE DIFFERENCES BETWEEN THE VARIOUS TYPES OF GLASS IONOMER CEMENTS?**

**A:** Type I powder has smaller particle size and Type II powder has larger particle size while type III glass ionomer has better handling properties, greater flow & faster set.

**93. HOW ARE GLASS IONOMER MIXED?**

**A:** For luting purpose, Powder & liquid system :

1. Use of paper pad or glass slab.
2. Plastic spatula is used. Steel spatula may be abraded by ceramic powder particles & abraded material might contaminate the cement.
3. Proportioning done as per manufacturer's instructions powder liquid ratio is 1.5 : 1. Anhydrous type ratio is 3:4:1 Usually manufacturer supplies volumetric dispensers - scoops & droppers. Usually 2 scoops of powder are taken for 1 drop of liquid. Bottle to be held horizontal & slowly pressed to form the drop and then transferred to the pad.
4. One half of the powder is transferred to the liquid and mixed. The powder is mixed, collected & folded back and other half is incorporated & mixed, till creamy consistency is obtained. Mixed for 30 to 60 seconds.
5. Mixed cement is applied to the fitting surface of the extraorally made restoration and restoration seated on the isolated and cleaned tooth preparation.

6. Excess cement extruding out of the margin is removed.

For liner cement:

1. Mixed as above

2. Placed in the cavity with a ball ended instrument to permit the liner to flow and cover the pulpal floor and / or axial wall.

If liner is light activated material,

1. The powder and liquid are mixed to the proper consistency and placed in the pulpal floor and/or axial wall.

2. Visible light is shown for the required time to cure the material.

**94. WHAT ARE THE USES OF REIN CEMENTS IN DENTISTRY?**

**A:** Acrylic resin cements were once used as restorative materials. Their low strength, high co-efficient of thermal expansion, excessive wear and water sorption has prevented their use at present as a restorative material. Presently composite resin cements are used as a luting cement for extra orally made restorations, especially for minimal extension metallic bridges, veneers and composite bridges.

**95. HOW ARE RESIN CEMENTS SUPPLIED?**

**A:** Resin cements are supplied as chemically cured resins or dual cured cements. Exclusive light activated resin cements are not used for luting purpose, due to the difficulty of light reaching the cement through the extraorally made restoration.

**96. HOW ARE RESIN CEMENTS MANIPULATED?**

**A:** 1. Tooth is completely isolated

2. Acid etching done on the tooth as per manufacturer's direction. Bonding agent applied on etched area & cured.

3. Restoration's fitting surface is microroughened either by etching, sand blasting or silanated.

4. Equal quantity of base and catalyst paste of resin cement is taken in a paper pad and mixed with a plastic spatula till there are no individual streaks of colour.

5. Mixed resin cement is applied onto the tooth and the restoration seated over the tooth surface with firm pressure. If dual activated, light curing done.

6. Excess cement is removed around the margin.

**97. WHAT IS THE ADVANTAGE OF RESIN CEMENT?**

**A:** Resin cements are insoluble in oral fluids.

**98. WHAT ARE THE DISADVANTAGES OF RESIN CEMENTS?**

**A :** 1. Possible pulpal irritation from unreacted oligomer.

2. Polymerisation shinkage

**99. WHAT ARE THE RESTORATIONS DIRECTLY MADE IN THE ORAL CAVITY?**

**A:** Silver amalgam, composite resin, glass ionomer, gold foil and silicate cements are some of the restorations directly made in the oral cavity.

**100. HOW ARE SILVER ALLOYS AND MERCURY SUPPLIED?**

**A:** Silver alloy is supplied in powder form in bulk or as pellets for easy dispensing. Mercury is supplied in separate bottle. Silver alloy and mercury are also supplied in separate compartments in a premeasured (preproportioned) disposable capsules.

**101. HOW ARE POWDER AND LIQUID SEPARATED IN A PREMEASURED AMALGAM CAPSULE?**

**A:** In some capsules, amalgam alloy powder and mercury are kept separated by a plastic diaphragm. Before trituration, such capsules are to be activated (pressed along its long axis to displace the diaphragm and permit the alloy and mercury to come together) by special gadgets like Amal press or with fingers. The diaphragm will act like a pestle during mechanical titration. In some capsules, the mercury is present in a paper pouch along with alloy powder, without any diaphragm. These capsules do not require any activation and during titration, the friable paper pouch gets torn and mercury comes in contact with the alloy powder. After mixing, the plastic disphragm pestle and remnants of the paper pouch, if present, should be removed, before filling.

**102. HOW ARE ALLOY AND MERCURY DISPENSED FOR MIXING?**

**A:** Following manufacturer's instructions is the correct way for best results. The proportion might vary depending upon the type of alloy, trituration method and place of usage. The proportioning should preferably be done by weight though volumetric dispensing is also permitted.

**103. HOW DOES THE PROPORTIONING VARY DEPENDING ON THE TYPE OF ALLOY?**

**A:** Generally more mercury is needed for lathe cut alloy and less mercury is needed for spherical alloy.

**104. HOW DOES THE METHOD OF TRITURATION ALTER THE POWDER LIQUID RATIO?**

**A:** Hand (mortar & pestle) trituration needs more mercury Mechanical trituration requires less mercury.

**105. HOW DOES ALLOY MERCURY RATIO DEPEND UPON THE PLACE OF AMALGAM USAGE?**

**A:** Amalgam used around pins, in retentive channels and internal retentive boxes need more plastic amalgam and high mercury mixes are used.

**106. WHAT ARE REUSABLE CAPSULES?**

**A:** Reusable capsules are empty capsules into which alloy and mercury are dispensed and triturated by the operator. As the name implies, these capsules are not disposable and reutilized a number of times.

**107. HOW MANY TYPES OF REUSABLE CAPSULES ARE THERE?**

**A:** There are two types. One is two piece capsule which is opened and the proportioned alloy and mercury are placed inside and triturated. This capsule may or may not have a pestle. Another reusable capsule is a single piece one, whose open end is screwed on to the feeder channel of the hopper feed amalgamators with build in volumetric dispensers. Whichever reusable capsule is used, periodical checkups for cleanliness and leakages are necessary for better mercury hygiene.

**108. WHAT IS THE PROPORTION OF SILVER ALLOY & MERCURY?**

**A:** For high mercury techniques, lathe cut alloy and hand trituration, the proportioning is 6:5 by weight. For minimal mercury Eame's technique, with mechanical amalgamator is 1:1 by weight. For low mercury techniques with spherical particles and mechanical trituration, the alloy mercury ratio is 5:6 by weight.

**109. DESCRIBE THE METHOD OF PROPORTIONING?**

**A:** Pellets (tablets) of alloy powder are easy to dispense. Such pallets are first pulverized in a reusable capsule in a mechanical mixer before mercury is added. Volumetric dispensers for alloy powders are also available but they may not be accurate because of type of particle and its size. Volumetric mercury dispensers should atleast be half full with mercury and held vertically while dispensing, for correct measurement.

**110. WHAT ARE THE ADVANTAGES OF PREMEASURED DISPOSABLE CAPSULES?**

**A:** Preproportioned disposable amalgam capsules have the advantages of reliability, convenience and safety (avoiding mercury spillage during proportioning and trituration)

**111. WHAT ARE THE DISADVANTAGES OF PREPROPORTONED DISPOSABLE AMALGAM CAPSULES?**

**A:** The disadvantages of premeasured disposable amalgam capsules are higher cost and the inability to alter the mercury alloy ratio depending on the need.

**112. WHAT ARE THE TRITURATION METHODS AND WHICH IS BETTER?**

**A:** Hand trituration and mechanical trituration are the two ways of mixing alloy and mercury. Mechanical mixing is definitely superior because of safety (no mercury exposure to the surroundings and no skin contact with the operator) reliability (repeatable mixes due to no operator variables).

**113. IF MECHANICAL AMALGAMATION IS SUPERIOR, WHY IS HAND TRITURATION DONE?**

**A:** Mechanical amalgamators and capsulators are electrically operated. In case of electrical failures or in areas of no electrical supply, hand trituration is done. Due care is taken not to touch mercury or the mix during trituration (no touch technique) and to squeeze out the excess mercury out of the mix after trituration.

**114. WHAT APPARATUS ARE USED FOR HAND TRITURATION?**

**A:** A glass or ceramic mortar and pestle are used for mixing alloy and mercury. The pestle should fit closely with the mortar (the concavity of the mortar & convexity of the pestle should coincide). The vertical shape of the bowl & of the mortar be parabolic with a raised centre so that the mix always remain under the pestle. The pestle and mortar must be made of fine grained silicon carbide particles of 12 micrometer average size. If the new glass mortar and pestle are not coming in close contact with each other while mixing, it is advisable to repeatedly grind dry sand in the mortar and pestle till the surfaces of mortar and pestle abrade sufficiently to have a close fit.

**115. HOW ARE THE ALLOY AND MERCURY MIXED IN A MORTAR & PESTLE?**

**A:** Silver alloy and mercury are proportioned in 6:5 by weight into the mortar. The mortar is kept in a firm surface like a table top and held by the left hand. The right hand holds the pestle with two pounds pressure (800 to 900 gms) and firmly rotated clockwise with the alloy and mercury kept below the pestle, till a well cohered, homogeneous smooth, warm mix that separtes easily from the mortar & pestle is obtained. Once trituration is started, no further alloy or mercury is added. The correctly triturated amalgam mix is scrapped easily with a cement spatula onto a gauze piece or chamois leather for squeezing out the excess mercury with gloved hands. Once the excess mercury is squeezed out, the mix is ready for packing into the cavity. The fresh mix should be condensed into the cavity before three minutes. If more than three minutes has lapsed, the mix is discarded and fresh mix made.

**116. WHAT IS MULLING AND PALMING?**

**A:** In olden days, after mixing the alloy in a mortar and pestle, the collected amalgam used to be kept in the palm of the operator and squeezed with the thumb of the other hand to homogenize the material. Such procedures used to be done with bare hands. Nowadays if mulling or palming is to be done for homogenizing the mix, it is done with gloved hand to avoid absorption of mercury through skin as well as to prevent moisture (sweat) contamination of the mix that can cause delayed expansion of a zinc containing alloy. For mechanically triturated mixes also, to prevent layering, mulling is done by removing the pestle after mixing and reactivating the amalgamator for a few seconds. Mulling results in obtaining a homogeneous cohesive mix.

**117. HOW WILL UNDERTRITURATED MIX LOOK LIKE?**

**A:** Undertriturated mix will look grainy with beads of remaining mercury and free alloy particles.

**118. HOW WILL OVERTRITURATED AMALGAM LOOK LIKE?**

**A:** It will be a hot mix tending to stick to the mortar and pestle or capsule.

**119. HOW IS MECHANICAL MIXING OF AMALGAM DONE?**

**A:** When hopper feed amalgamator is used with reusable capsule:

1) a) reusable capsule checked for correct fixing and timer set as per manufacturer's instructions

b) The proportioning knob is turned to $180^0$ and back for a single mix proportioning. Knob turned twice for double mix proportioning.

c) Unit switched on to agitate the capsule (either in to and fro oscillation or full rotation) for the required time.

d) After the reusable capsule stops, it is unscrewed and the mixed amalgam should be condensed before three minutes.

2) When an amalgamator with holder attachment for a two piece reusable capsule is used:

a) The reusable capsule is opened, inner side cleaned of any old amalgam remnants.

b) Pestle of the capsule, if present is cleaned.

c) Proper proportion of alloy & mercury put in the capsule and closed.

d) An adhesive tape wrapped around the capsule to prevent mercury leakage.

e) Capsule kept in the arms of the holder attachment and amalgamator switched on.

f) To and fro movement of the capsule holder or complete rotation for the specified time allowed.

g) After the holder attchment stops, adhesive tape removed, capsule opened & pestle removed.

h) Capsule closed, tape refixed and amalgamator switched on for few fixed seconds for mulling.

i) Capsule reopened and mixed amalgam to be condensed before 3 minutes

3) When premeasured disposable capsules are used:

a) Capsule is activated, if necessary.

b) Capsule kept between the arms of the holder and capsulator (amalgamator with holder for mixing capsules) is switched on for the fixed time.

c) After capsulator stops, capsule is removed, diaphragm or remnants of paper pouch removed and the mixed amalgam is ready for condensation.

d) Mixed amalgam is to be packed within 3 minutes

**120. HOW IS MIXED AMALGAM CARRIED INTO THE CAVITY?**

**A:** Amalgam should never be carried into the cavity with bare fingers (to avoid absorption of mercury through skin and moisture contamination of mix). Amalgam is carried to the cavity with an amalgam carrier.

**121. HOW IS AMALGAM CARRIER LOADED?**

**A:** The mixed amalgam is collected in a dappen glass and amalgam carrier tip is repeatedly inserted into the mix in a pecking action till no more material can enter the tip. The carrier is taken into the matriced (if necessary) and lined (base applied) cavity to the deepest portion and a small portion of amalgam ejected.

**122. HOW IS AMALGAM CONDENSED INTO THE CAVITY?**

**A:** Condensation of amalgam can be done either with hand condensers or mechanical condensers. Different hand condensers are chosen for different parts of the cavity. In a prepared cavity, varnish liner or base is given as per requirement and matrix and wedges are applied where needed. The first place to condense amalgam will be into the retentive grooves and under cuts. In these areas even the smallest condenser tip available may be big. A straight probe with its sharp tip cut off might be the best instrument suited for condensing amalgam into the grooves and under cuts. Once the inner retentive areas are packed a small increment of amalgam is kept in the deepest portion of cavity and amalgam is condensed with a small condenser with sufficient pressure to eliminate voids and to adapt amalgam to the walls. Condensation is started at centre and slowly stepped towards the cavity wall. Condenser is forced into the amalgam mass under hand pressure. Force applied depends on the type of alloy particles. On completion of condensation of one increment, the surface must be shiny with mercury to diffuse through the next increment and unites it for homogenecity. Next increment is added & condensation continued till the cavity is over filled.

**123. WHAT IS THE NORMAL CONDENSATION PRESSURE FOR AMALGAM?**

**A:** The normal hand condensation pressure for amalgam restoration is 3 to 4 pounds.

**124. WHAT WILL HAPPEN IF TOO SMALL OR TOO LARGE A CONDENSER TO USED FOR CONDENSING THE AMALGAM?**

**A:** Too small a condenser will not effectively condense the amalgam, but will be packing holes through it. Too large a condenser will be transmitting lesser pressure per unit area because of the larger surface area and close packing of amalgam might not occur.

**125. WHY SHOULD THE CAVITY BE OVER FILLED AND THEN CARVED?**

**A:** Condensation brings out the excess mercury from the amalgam increment to the surface. Sequential increments are bound together by the upward movement of excess mercury. Hence the top most layer of the filling will be rich in mercury that will be weak. If the cavity is filled to excess and then carved to correct shape, the mercury rich surface layer could be removed during carving.

**126. HOW ARE MECHANICAL CONDENSATION DONE?**

**A:** Hand held instruments with detachable tips are available. Such mechanical condensers deliver either impact type of force or rapid vibration. Suitable tips are selected and amalgam is compacted in small increments and cavity is filled to excess. Care is taken that blows do not fall at the cavosurface enamel. Mechanical condensation is less fatiguing to the operator.

**127. WHAT ARE THE OBJECTIVES OF CONDENSATION?**

**A:**
1. Close adaptation of restoration to all the cavity walls.
2. Compacting amalgam alloy to form a dense restoration
3. Removing excess mercury from the mix by bringing it to the top
4. Lesser voids and air entrapment in restoration.

**128. WHAT IS BURNISHING?**

A: In noble alloy cast restoration, the term burnishing denotes closer marginal adaptation of the malleable and ductile alloys by using rotary and hand burnishers. The burnishing energy applied at the thin metal margins of the cast restorations over the cavosurface bevel results in reshaping the restoration margin thinner and closely adapted and protecting the luting cement. In amalgam restorations, the term burnishing refers to better marginal adaptation at the cavosurface margins and smoothening of the filling. No cavo surface bevel is created for the amalgam cavity and silver amalgam is not a malleable and ductile alloy either. In amalgam restoration, precarve burnishing and post carve burnishing are done.

**129. WHAT IS PRECARVE BURNISHING?**

**A:** Pre carve burnishing is done to ensure better marginal adaptation. A large burnisher is ued and it is firmly drawn from centre of amalgam to the cuspal slopes. Pre carve burnishing is a type of condensation only.

**130. WHAT IS THE CARVING PROCEDURE?**

**A:** Reshaping the condensed restoration to the tooth form is carving procedure.

**131. WHEN IS AN AMALGAM RESTORATION READY FOR CARVING?**

**A:** When amalgam has initially set and offers some resistance to carving, the restoration is ready for carving. A metallic scraping sound will also be heard during carving.

**132. WHAT INSTRUMENTS ARE USED FOR CARVING?**

**A:** Either a Hollenbach's carver, Wards 'C' carver or Frahm's (diamond) carver could be used for carving. Some operators prefer to use a sharp discoid or cleoid instrument.

**133. HOW IS CARVING DONE?**

**A:** First occlusal embrassure is created. Marginal ridge is next curved by keeping its level compatible to the neighbouring tooth. While carving the ridges and grooves, the carver should rest partly over unprepared tooth surface and partly in amalgam to ensure continuation of the cuspal incline. Edge of the blade should be kept perpendicular to the margin and moved parallel to the margin. Deep occlusal grooves are not to be carved lest it weakens the restoration. After carving, the outline of amalgam margin should show the location of the prepared cavo surface margin of the cavity.

**134. WHAT IS POST CARVE BURNISHING?**

**A:** The purpose of post carve burnishing is to ensure a smooth surface of the restoration. Light rubbing of the carved amalgam surface with a burnisher results in a smooth surface.

**135. WHAT BURNISHERS ARE USED FOR BURNISHING?**

**A:** Depending on the occlusal morphollgy either a ball (spherical) ended burnisher, cone (anatomical) burnisher or egg shaped burnisher is used.

136. **HOW IS THE MATRIX BAND REMOVED?**

**A:** After carving and burnishing is completed, the wedge is removed. The matrix retainer is loosened and removed without removing the matrix band. The matrix band is pushed against the neighbouring tooth and removed occlusobuccaly or occluso lingually with pressure applied against the adjacent tooth. The band is not removed directly occlusally to prevent occlusal displacement of the proximal restoration.

137. **HOW IS THE OCCLUSION CHECKED?**

**A:** In a patient's mouth, patient is asked to bite in centric and eccentric positions with an articulating paper kept in between the upper and lower teeth to find out any premature contact. The contacts should be evenly distributed and occiusal prematurities are removed. In case of preclinical training, if acrylic models are used, occlussion should be checked with opposing teeth. When natural teeth are used, because of their diverse origin, proper occlusion might not be there.

138. **WHAT IS MEANT BY MERCURY HYGIENE?**

**A:** It denotes the precautions taken by the dentist while preparing, inserting, condensing, polishing and removal of amalgam restorations.

139. **IS SILVER AMALGAM A HAZARDUOUS RESTORATION?**

**A:** All the dental associations of the world categorically state silver amalgam restorations do not pose any threat to the patient's health, except for a very minor proportion who are allergic to mercury. However, every dental text book cautions the dental surgeon and the dental student to take utmost care while handling elemental mercury. Mercury vapour is toxic and it has cumulative effect. Mercury can vapourize in room temparature and mercury vapour is odourless, colourless and tasteless. But if the dental personnel take enough precautions, the hazards of inhaling elemental mercury vapour for prolonged periods can be avoided.

**140. WHAT PRECAUTIONS ARE TO BE TAKEN WHILE HANDLING MERCURY?**

**A:**
1. Mercury should be stored in unbreakable, tightly closed containers to avoid accidental breakage & spillage.
2. All operations involving mercury shoud be done under closed areas (eg. Amalgamator). Use no touch technique.
3. If spillage occurs, it should be covered with sulphur powder immediately to prevent evaportion and should be collected with tin foil (tin reacts with mercury faster)
4. Capsules used for mechanical trituration should not leak.
5. Avoid skin contact with mercury to prevent cutaneous absorption.
6. All waste amalgam should be collected and stored under water, oil or used fixer solution to prevent evaporation of mercury.
7. Dental surgery work area should be well ventillated.
8. Carpets in work area to be avoided as spillages are difficult to clean.
9. Avoid using mercury containing solutions.
10. Heating amalgam by dry polishing, or sterilizing instruments (carrier, condensers) having amalgam remnants sticking to it should be avoided.
11. While removing amalgam enough coolant spray and efficient suction should be used.
12. Ultrasonic condensation of amalgam should be avoided
13. Biological samples (hair, nails & urine) of dental personnel should be periodically monitored for excretory level of mercury.
14. Ambient air levels of mercury in dental clinic be checked periodically.
15. Subordinates and students should be educated about proper handling of mercury.

**141. WHAT RESTORATION IS BEST SUITED FOR A VITAL TOOTH WITH FRACTURE OF INCISAL EDGE INVOLVING DENTINE?**

**A:** A composite restoration is best suited for such class IV restoration.

**142. DESCRIBE THE PROCEDURE OF RESTORING A CLASS IV DEFECT INVOLVING DENTINE WITH COMPOSITE RESIN?**

**A:**

1. Shade matching of tooth done in natural light, preferably wet tooth.

2. Selection of crown form matrix of appropriate size, if chemically activated composite resin is to be used. Preparation of lingual support with impression compound & mylar strip if light activated composite is to be applied.

3. Isolation from moisture - rubber dam/cotton rolls (in patient's mouth).

4. Protection of existing composite, glass ionomer or silicate restoration with varnish or cocoa butter to prevent drying (in patient's mouth)

5. No anaesthesia as no cavity cutting is to be done (in patient's mouth)

6. Removal of friable & ragged enamel edges, if present.

7. Cleaning the enamel surface to remove surface pellicle, plaque and food debris. Cleaned with fluoride free prophlaxis paste and bristle brush held in a slow speed conventional hand piece.

8. Washing with water to remove the prophylaxis paste.

9. Bevel created in enamel for 1 millimeter width on labial and lingual surface with a diamond point held at an angie to the incisal edge. Bevel creation is for (a) having more surface area for etching b) exposing ends of enamel for etching rather than sides of enamel c) blending the restoration with enamel better so that the line of demarcation is not clearly seen.

10. Dentine protection, if necessary, with calcium hydroxide or glass ionomer. If the effective thickenss of dentine is less than 0.5 millimeter, glass ionomer is avoided. Copal varnish is not used for dentine protection as it will interfere with retention, by preventing dentine conditioning, if used. Zinc oxide eugenol should not be used for dentine proection as eugenol will interfere with polymerisation of composite. If dentine is conditioned with acid, dentine bonding agent can be applied.

11. Acid etching of enamel done with 30 to 50% phosphoric acid. 37% phosphoric acid is commonly used. Acid gel is preferred to liquid acid because of controlled flow and limited area of etching. Etching is done for 15 seconds. Previously etching was done for 60 seconds. More etching time needed for fluorosed teeth & deciduous teeth (having prismless enamel). Acid gel applied with disposable brush or sponge.

12. The etched area is washed with oil free water for fifteen seconds.

13. The etched area is dried for 20 seconds with compressed air and tooth re-isolated (in patient's mouth). The etching has resulted in selective demineralisation of enamel leading to formation of micropores in enamel Clinically, etched area appears white and frosty.

14. Bonding agent, if chemically activated, comes in two bottles. A drop of each is mixed in a dappen glass, mixed and applied on the etched area with a new disposable brush. The brush is applied with gentle dabbing. No rubbing is done that can crush the delicate organic enamel matrix. The resin should flow by capillary attraction. If bonding agent is light activated, it will be a single liquid and it is taken in a new disposable brush and gently dabbed in the etched area. The blue curing light is shown for 20 seconds or as per the manufacturer's instructions to cure the bonding agent.

15. Dentine bonding agent applied to conditioned dentine if acid conditioning of dentine was done earlier. Presently single bonding agents are available that can be applied to both enamel and dentine.

16. If chemically activated composite is used, the crown form selected is vented (hole created in a corner) to permit excess composite material to flow out. The chemically activated composite is supplied as two paste system and equal quantities of base and catalyst pastes are dispensed by a double ended plastic disposable spatula, onto a paper pad, taking care to use separate ends of the spatula to dispense base and catalyst pastes. The two pastes are thoroughly mixed to a homogeneous colour without any air bubble incorporation. No individual streaks of colour should be seen. The mixed composite is loaded on to the crown form, the matrix is seated into position, holding with pressure & without movement forcing the excess composite to flow through the vent. Crown form is removed and gross excess is removed with a tungsten carbide bur.

17. If light activated composite used, the low fusing compound lingual support & mylar strip is positioned and composite resin is taken with a plastic or anodized aluminium plastic instrument and applied in small increments over the fractured site and manipulated into position. After shaping the restoration, blue curing light is shown from the labial side. Additions are made in increments of not more than 1.5 millimeter thickness and cured with light till the restoration is fully built up. The lingual supporting matrix and mylar strip are now removed and curing from lingual side is done for better curing of the composite. If any gross excess is present, it is removed with carbide burs.

18. Occlusion is checked in centric and eccentric postions.

**143. HOW IS COMPOSITE RESIN APPLIED TO A FINISHED CLASS II CAVITY?**

**A:** 1. Proximal matricing is important. An ultra thin 0.001 inch metal matrix or thicker polyester matrix can be used in a tofflemire retainer. Polyester light cure matrix is needed for light transmission, if visible light cure composite is used. Custom made compound supported metal matrix can also be used. Matrices should be suitably contoured. A plastic translucent wedge should be used if light activated composite is to be used.

2. Acid etching and conditioning of enamel and dentine done as per manufacturer's directions for 15 seconds. Cavity is washed for 20 seconds and dried.

3. Bonding agent applied in etched area but pooling in one area should be avoided. Light activated.

4. Composite resin, if chemically activated, is mixed from the two pastes supplied to a homogenous colour.

5. The mixed chemically activated composite or the visible light activated composite can be applied to the cavity either with hand instruments made of plastic, anodized aluminium or Teflon coated steel or with special applicator guns. The applicator guns are of two types. In the first type, the composite is loaded on to the applictor tip by the operator. The tip is transparent for chemically activated composite and the applicator tip may be black or orange for light activated composite resins. The second type of guns use the preloaded corpule tips supplied by the manufacturer. If chemically cured composite is applied with, guns starting from deepest portion, it is offloaded in one stretch and as quickly as possible and withdrawing the gun as material is ejected out. If light cure composite is used, the first small layer applied in gingival seat is for 0.5 millimeter thickness and cured through the transparent matrix & wedge of proximal side. Subsequent additions are made in 2 millimeter thickness and cured till cavity is completely filled up.

6. Wedge and matrix removed. If any deficiency is present more composite added and photocured. Any gross excess, if present is removed.

**144. HOW ARE GLASS IONOMER SUPPLIED FOR RESTORATIVE PURPOSE?**

**A:** 1. Powder & liquid

2. Powder only (anhydrous type)

3. Encapsulated form

4. Light activated (powder & liquid)

**145. HOW ARE GLASS IONOMER RESTORED FOR A CLASS V ABRASION DEFECT?**

**A:** As no carries is involved, cavity cutting is not needed.

1. Tooth is isolated (in patient's mouth) matrix selected

2. Pumice prophlaxis done in the affected area with a bristle brush in a slow speed contra angle hand piece.

3. Tooth cleaned with water and dried.

4. 10 percent polyacrylic acid is applied over the surface of the lesion to expose clean tooth surface to the restoration.

5. Tooth is washed and dried

6. Powder liquid ratio is 3:1 by weight. By volume, it will be 2 scoops of powder to 1 drop of liquid dispensed onto a paper pad. If it is anhydrous powder, it is dispensed 3:4:1 by weight. Plastic spatula is used for mixing. Powder divided into two halves. One half of powder is incorporated into the liquid and mixed by collecting the mix and folding back for 15 seconds. The other half is incorporated & mixed for another 15 seconds.

7. The shiny mix of glass ionomer is applied over the clean tooth surface & matrix applied and held in position for 5 minutes. Any excess present is removed with sharp probe.

8. Matrix removed and the new restoration is immediately protected with light cured bonding agent (resin) to prevent drying up of the restoration.

9. If encapsulated glass ionomer is used, mixing is done by capsulator. After mixing, the capsule with nozzle is kept in the application gun and glass ionomer ejected onto the tooth surface and matrix applied. After matrix removal, light enamel cured resin applied on the surface for protection. If light cured glass ionomer is used, the powder and liquid are proportioned as per manufacturer's instruction and mixed over a paper pad. The slow curing provides ample working time & material is manipulated over the lesion and photocured.

**146. HOW IS CAVITY RESTORED WITH SILICATE CEMENT?**

A: Silicate cement is supplied either as powder and liquid or in capsules.

1. Cool dry slab and an agate or plastic spatula is used for mixing.
2. Powder and liquid are dispensed over the slab as per manufactuer's instructions. Liquid is dispensed last to prevent evaporation.
3. Powder is introduced into the liquid in large increments
4. Rapidly spatualated in a small area of the slab (wiping & folding motion).
5. Mixed within one minute into a putty consistency
6. Mix should be used before the shine is lost.
7. Celluloid matrix strips used for confining the restoration. The silicate cement is placed in the cavity with protective base cement and matrix pressed over the restoration. Excess cement removed along the margins with a sharp probe.
8. After material sets, matrix is removed and protective varnish or cocoa butter applied to prevent drying up of restoration.

**147. HOW ARE DIRECT FILLING GOLD APPLIED TO THE CAVITY?**

**A:** 1. Complete isolation of the cavity from moisture and absolute cleanliness are necessities for doing a direct gold restoration.

2. Degassing (desorbing, anealing) by piece method or bulk method.

3. Selection of condenser points depending on the cavity size and condensation method - Hand condensing, mallet and condenser, spring loaded mallet, Hollenback's pneumatic condenser & McShirley's electro mallet.

4. Application of cavity varnish in the dentine walls and floor & application of base, if necessary.

5. An annealed piece of gold foil is placed in a retentive starting pit and condensed with a holding instrument, another annealed piece of gold foil is placed against the first piece and condensed. Further pieces are condensed till the gold is securely locked into the pit without moving. Condensing starts with the least accessible retentive pit.

6. Further pieces of annealed gold are added to the locked mass by overlapping the prevsiously laid piece by one third. Fresh piece of annealed gold is laid into position, straightened, kept overlapping the previous piece continued till the opposite pit. Such condensation of gold foil from one retentive point to another leads to tie formation.

# CHAPTER : 11

# POLISHING OF RESTORATIONS

**1. WHY SHOULD RESTORATIONS BE POLISHED?**

**A:** 1. Deposition of materia alba, salivary cuticle and plaque formation are easy to occur over a rough surface. Smooth surfaces do not have stagnation areas.

2. Smooth polished metals and alloys do not tannish or corrode easily.

3. Polished surface reflect light evenly and are pleasing to look at.

4. Rough surfaces can mechanically irritate soft tissues like gingiva and oral mucosa.

5. Smooth polished surfaces are easy to keep clean.

**2. WHAT IS THE DIFFERENCE BETWEEN FINISHING AND POLISHING?**

**A:** Finishing refers to removal of gross excesses along the margins and alteration of contour, if needed. It is done usually immediately after the placement of restoration. Polishing refers to improving the surface texture of the restoration and is done usually one or more days after placement of restoration, to ensure completion of chemical reactions & hardening.

**3. HOW ARE THE POLISHING MATERIALS USED?**

**A:** The polishing materials could be in the form of powders, incorporated in pastes, glued to paper, resin or cloth, impregnated into rubber and supplied as wheels or points or bonded with ceramics and supplied as wheels, cylinders or points. They are supplied in different grades of abrasiveness. For any polishing procedure, coarser abrasives are used initially and finer abrasives later. Sequential use of descending grades of abrasiveness results in smoother surface.

**4. WHY SHOULD POLISHING BE DONE AT SLOWER SPEEDS?**

**A:** Higher rotational speeds increase the friction and the resultant heat. Higher heat generation during polishing is harmful to the pulp. Slower speed produces lesser frictional heat which can be dissipated easily with efficient coolants.

**5. WHY DRY POLISHING IS NOT ADVICED?**

**A:** Coolants not only dissipate frictional heat generated, but also tend to wash away the abrasive particles quicker. Dry polishing can elevate the temperature of the restoration and tend to spray the abrasive particles into air which might be inhaled by the dental staff as well as the patients. Some rubber polishing points will also disintegrate at higher roational speed.

**6. HOW IS SILVER AMALGAM POLISHED?**

**A:** Polishing of silver amalgam is done usually after 24 hours. If more restorations are planned over a period of days, it is preferable to complete all the restorations and do the polishing later simultaneously.

1. Removal of roughness of the restoration either with green carborundum stone or white fused alumina stone with the stone's long axis held at right angle to the margins. Centric holding areas should not be reduced. The unprepared tooth surface can guide the point to have continuity between tooth and restoration.
2. Coarse rubber impregnated abrasive points can be used for polishing at low speed to get a smoother, shiny appearance. Overheating is to be avoided as it can bring mercury to the surface to appear polished but cloudy. This mercury rich surface will be weak & prone for corrosion.
3. After washing the area to remove the abrasive particles, fine abrasive points are used at low speed and within a few seconds high Lustre should appear.
4. Instead of using abrasive impregnated rubber points, rubber cups & pumice slurry to be folowed by rubber cups and precipitated chalk can also be used to get high degree of polish.

**7. HOW IS AN ALLOY CASTING FINISHED & POLISHED?**

**A:**

1. The recovered casting is checked for contaminating investment materials and nodules on the fitting surface of the casting are removed with a proper sized round bur in an airotor handpiece.
2. Casting should be carefully seated on the die & if any other irregularity prevents complete seating of the casting, it is judiciously removed without damaging the die. External surface is also smoothened.
3. Once the casting is seated properly in the die, sprue former attached to the casting can be removed carefully as close to the casting as possible. Instead of passing the carborundum separating disc through and through, which may result in the casting accidentally flying off, the spure - casting junction can be sufficiently thinned out so as to bend and separate the sprue former easily.
4. Remnants at sprue casting junction is smoothed away with a heatless store or a corborandum disc.
5. Grooves may be accentuated by applying a dull Number 1 round bur, lightly over the grooves.
6. Knife edge rubber polishing wheels are used on accessible areas to polish them.
7. Smaller rubber knife edged wheels are applied for deeper inaccessible areas.
8. Grooves and pits are smoothened with rubber abrasive points.
9. A bristle wheel brush and tripoli or pumice can be used for further smoothening of the surface. A small felt wheel can also be used.
10. A felt or chamois wheel and rouge are applied for a few seconds to incorporate the final lustre.

If the casting is not held in the die while polishing, it should be held in an inlay holder (vice like device) to present slippage and loss.

After polishing, the casting is washed clean to remove the polishing materials, with soap and water.

**8. HOW IS A COMPOSITE RESIN RESTORATION POLISHED?**

**A:** A resin rich surface left by a matrix is probably the best finish that is possible for a composite resin. For light activated composite resins also, manufacturers suggest final application of bonding agent over the surface to create a glazed surface. But with the low abrasive resistance of resins, for how long the polish could be retained will remain a question mark.

1. Flame shaped carbide finishing bur or a fine diamond point could be used to remove excess composite and medium speed with light, intermittant brush strokes could be used.
2. A rubber polishing point and an aluminium oxide polishing paste can be used for final polishing.
3. Sof-lex and Pop-on discs are also available for contouring and polishing. They are flexible abrasive coated resin discs supplied by manufacturer in different colours with abrasives of coarse, medium, fine and extra fine particles. They are to be used in the suggested sequence.
4. In embrassure areas, to remove excess, gold foil knife could be used. Proximal abrasive strips could also be used, by folding over the restored tooth and using the strip in shoe shining action.

**9. HOW IS GLASS IONOMER RESTORATIONS POLISHED?**

**A:** A matrix is usually used for glass ionomer restoration & a smooth finish is obtained. Excess around the margins are removed with a sharp knife. If rotary instrumentations is to be used Micron finishing diamonds can be used with a petroleum Lubricant to prevent drying up. Flexible abrasive discs like sof-lex discs can also be used with a lubricant. Aluminium oxide polishing paste can also be used with a rubber cup.

**10. HOW IS A GOLD FOIL RESTORATION POLISHED?**

**A:** Gold restoration done directly in the mouth can be finished immediately as no setting is involved. If gross excess is present, it can be removed with a fine cuttle disc. If marginal excess is present, it can be removed with a gold foil knife from the gold to the tooth or with discoids and cleoids from the tooth to the gold. Cuttle discs can be used sequentially (as coarse, medium and fine) to get smoothness. Light brush strokes are used, maintaining the contour of the restoration, polishing done with pumice, tin oxide or white rouge applied with a soft webless rubber cup.

**11. HOW IS PORCELAIN POLISHED?**

**A:** During fabrication of porecelain itself, after patient trial and all occlusal adjustment are over, the restoration, on its external surface is covered with low fusing glasses (this is also porcelain, but with more glass modifiers) and fired in the furnace. Such glazing of porcelain results in a highly smooth scratch resistant polished surface. Some of the newer precelains are self glazing in nature.

If a highly glazed porcelain surface is highly reflective and too artifical to look at, the surface glaze can be removed by grinding and surface polished with a series is of abrasive impregnated rubber points followed by a creamy mix of Levigated (powdered when wet) alumina and water. Special porcelain polishing pastes are also available.

# CHAPTER : 12

# ALLOY CASTING PROCEDURE

**1. WHAT METERIALS ARE USED FOR PREPARING A CAST RESTORATION?**

**A:** Noble metal alloys, base metal alloys and castable ceramics are materials used for preparing a cast restoration.

**2. IS THE CASTING PROCEDURE SAME FOR THE ABOVE MATERIALS?**

**A:** The procedure is similar, but for castable ceramics special equipment are needed.

**3. WHAT IS LOST WAX PROCESS ?**

**A:** It is a restoration fabrication procedure wherein the restoration is initially made in wax, a mould created around it, wax is elimiated from the mould to create an empty space within the mould and the final restorative material in a liquid or plastic stage is packed into the mould.

**4. DO THE PHRASES 'CASTING PROCEDURE' & 'LOST WAX PROCESS' DENOTE THE SAME MEANING?**

**A:** No. Lost wax process is also used in acrylic denture fabrication which is not a casting procedure. The denture base is initially made in wax, flasked to create a mould, wax elimiated to create mould space, acrylic resin packed in a plastic stage into the mould and curing done.

Though casting procedure generally denotes fabrication of restoration by lost wax technique sometimes, instead of wax, resins and plastics may also be used for fabricating the initial restoration which is burnt out later to create the mould space.

**5. WHAT WAXES ARE USED FOR PREPARING THE WAX PATTERN?**

**A:** Inlay waxes type I and Type II are used for preparing the wax pattern.

**6. WHY THERE ARE TWO TYPES OF INLAY WAXES?**

**A:** Type I inlay wax is used for taking direct wax pattern and has hardening temperature of around 37 degrees centigrade. Type II inlay wax is used for taking indirect wax pattern and has a hardening temperature of 30 degrees centigrade. (room temperature)

**7. WHAT IS MEANT BY DIRECT AND INDIRECT WAX PATTERNS?**

**A:** After cavity preparation, if the wax pattern is made directly in the patient's mouth, it is a direct wax pattern. If an impression is taken of the prepared tooth and a removable die prepared and a wax pattern is made from that die, it is an indirect wax pattern.

**8. WHAT ARE THE ADVANTAGES OF A DIRECT PATTERN?**

**A:**
1. Elimination of impression taking and die making thereby avoiding possible dimensional changes due to impression materials and die materials.
2. Occlusal relationship of the pattern directly checked in the patient's mouth.
3. Time saving procedure (not chairside time) as impression taking and die making are avoided.

**9. WHAT ARE THE DISADVANTAGES OF DIRECT PATTERN?**

**A:**
1. More chairside time & possible inconvenience for the patient.
2. Possible thermal contraction (though minimal) due to difference in hardening, temperature of inlay wax Type I (37°C) and investing temperature (room temperature).
3. Difficult access to proximal & lingual area.

4. Possibility of distorsion of wax pattern unless immediately invested & confined.

**10. WHAT ARE THE ADVANTAGES OF INDIRECT PATTERN TAKING?**

**A:** 1. Saving of chair side time for dental surgeon and the patient, as die making and pattern forming are done in the dental laboratory.

2. Thermal contraction of inlay wax is not present as hardening temperature of wax and mold formation temperature are the same.

3. Better access to all the prepared surfaces of the cavity

4. Possibility of distortion is less as the pattern need not be removed from the die till just before investing.

**11. WHAT ARE THE POSSIBLE DISADVANTAGES OF AN INDIRECT PATTERN?**

**A:** 1. Possibility of dimensional changes due to expansion or contraction of impression & die materials

2. Occlusion of the pattern is not directly checked in patient's mouth.

**12. WHAT IS AN INDIRECT - DIRECT METHOD?**

A: When the wax pattern is made originally in a die, replaced in the mouth to assess the fit and occlusion, is later processed in the laboratory, it is an indirect - direct method.

**13. WHAT IS A DIE?**

A: Die is a positive replica of a single prepared tooth.

**14. WHAT IS A REMOVABLE DIE?**

A: A die that can be removed from the working cast is a removable die.

**15. WHAT MATERIALS ARE USED TO FORM DIES?**

**A:** 1. Commonly used materials are Type IV & Type V improved stone.

2. Divestment

3. Amalgam (Silver analgam)

4. Acrylic resin

5. Silico phosphate cement

6. Epoxy resin dies

7. Electro formed metals.

**16. DESCRIBE A METHOD OF PREPARING A REMOVABLE DIE?**

**A:** There are many ways of preparing dies. One way of preparing a removable stone die will be described.

1. An alginate impression is taken

2. Stainless steel strips are cut from ribbon of matrix or matrix or orthodontic bands of size 8 millimeters height and 0.002" thick. The width of the material should be trimmed to a size when it is just short of touching the impression. Two strips are needed for each die preparation. Every strip is customized for its position, where the edges will be just short of touching the impression.

3. Utility wax is flowed onto the buccal and lingual flange regions of the impression to a thickness of 1 or 2 millimeters. Care is taken that wax doesn't flow into the impression areas.

4. Cut strips for each place is warmed and carefully positioned into the utility wax so that the pair of strips for each die converge towards the base of the cast (to facilitate removal of die)

5. Die stone is mixed and first pour is made upto 1 millimeter short of the strips

6. As the stone sets, die pin is inserted into the first pour till the head of the pin is within the setting stone. Die pin is centrally postioned with reference to the strips. If the die pin is unstable, a paper pin could be inserted through

the buccal & lingual flanges & die pin attached to it with sticky wax.

7. Once the first pour has hardened, any paper pin & sticky wax, if used to hold the die pin in postion when the first pour sets, are removed and vaseline (as a separating media) applied over the first pour & die pin except in areas where removable die is not needed.

8. Impression is boxed up & second pour of die stone is mixed and poured upto 2 millimeter short of the die pin tip. The second pour unites with the first pour only in areas where no separating media is applied.

9. Once the stone cast hardens, gentle tapping of the die pin with an instrument pushes the die with strips out. Strips are removed.

**17. HOW CAN INLAY WAX BE SOFTENED TO TAKE A WAX PATTERN?**

**A:** The best way of softening an inlay wax is to use a controlled temperature oven. Inlay wax is a poor thermal conductor. So a controlled heating device for a sufficiently prolonged period ensures uniform softening.

**18. WHAT OTHER METHODS OF SOFTENING INLAY WAX ARE AVAILABLE?**

**A:** Heating over a flame is an accepted method. But the quicker heating tends to melt the superficial layer while the inner core might remain hard. So the wax stick is contantly kept rotating along its long axis and periodically kneaded with fingers to bring the inner side out and outer side in. This is repeated till the wax is uniformly soft.

Some dental surgeons tend to soften the inlay in hot water. The might not be deleterious if done for a short period but prolongd heating in hot water might make some of the ingredients of the inlay wax leach out.

For indirect pattern, liquid paraffin is used as a separating media on the die and molten wax could be added in layers, to overfill the cavity & pattern carved after wax hardens.

Another way of preparing a wax pattern in the indirect method is by water swaging. In this technique, the die and the softened wax kept in the die are mounted into a closed vessel containing water and a piston. When piston is pressed, hydrostatic pressure is evenly applied over the wax pattern to closely adapt it to the cavity.

**19. HOW IS THE SOFTENED INLAY WAX SHAPED?**

**A:** For class I or V wax patterns, the softened inlay wax is shaped to a cone. For class II or M.O.D. cavities it is bifid shaped. The shaping of the softened wax is to ensure easier & complete flow into all the cavity details.

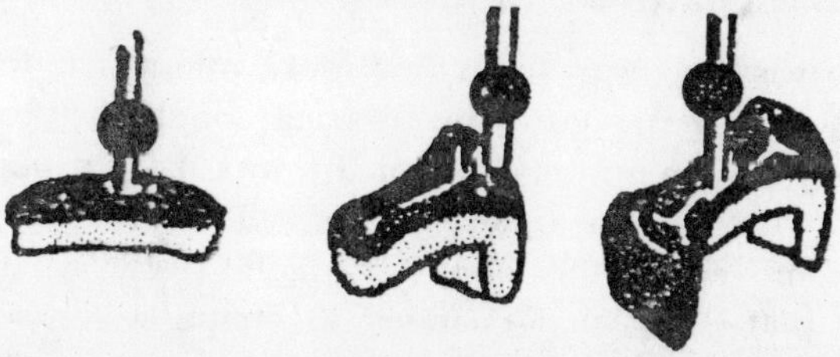

*Fig. 12.1. Softened wax shape for Class I & Class II cavities*

**20. IN WHAT WAY LIQUID PARAFFIN IS SUPERIOR TO OIL OR GLYCERINE AS A SEPARATING MEDIUM?**

**A:** If oil is used as separating medium between cavity walls and inlay wax, some of the oil might stick to the wax pattern and later preventing close adaptation of the investment to the pattern. If glycerine is used as a separting media, because of its thickness, it will prevent closer adaption of the wax pattern to the die.

**21. HOW IS THE WAX PATTERN MADE?**

**A:** The correctly, softened and shaped inlay wax is pressed into the cavity and if it is a direct pattern, patient may be asked to bite over the pattern. If it is an indirect pattern, firm finger pressure is kept over the pattern for a few minutes.

**22. WHY SHOULD PRESSURE BE APPLIED WHEN THE SOFTENED INLAY WAX HARDENS?**

**A:** 1. Pressure applied over the softened inlay wax ensures good flow of the inlay wax into all the portions of the cavity.

2. As wax hardens, it shrinks & because the coefficient of thermal expansion of inlay wax is very high the shrinkage might affect the fit of the restoration. Pressure appliction might partially offset the disadvantage of shrinkage.

**23. CAN THE WAX PATTERN BE REMOVED AS SOON AS THE OUTER SURFACE HARDENS?**

**A:** It is wiser to wait for a few more minutes before the wax pattern is removed. The thermal conductivity of inlay wax being low, the outer layer of the wax pattern might become hard, though the inner core is still warm. If the pattern is removed at this stage, it might result in distortion of the pattern. Such changes in shape will result in an ill fitting casting.

**24. WITH WHAT INSTRUMENT IS THE WAX PATTERN CARVED?**

**A:** 1. Sharp instruments are used for carving

2. It is also desirable to use warm instruments for carving.

**25. WHAT CAN HAPPEN IF DULL COLD INSTRUMENTS ARE USED FOR CARVING ?**

**A:** Dull, cold instruments tend to drag the wax, incorporating lot of stresses in the pattern.

**26. WHY THE INLAY WAXES ARE COLOURED DEEP RED OR DARK BLUE?**

**A:** Such dark colours are given for contrast. These colours stand out against the white tooth or the common die materials and help in delineating the margins.

**27. HOW IS THE WAX PATTERN CARVED?**

**A:** If sufficient tooth structure is present, the carving instrument is held partly over the remaining tooth substance to guide the instrument for carving the morphology correctly. When gross tooth structure loss in present, the shape of neighbouring teeth, the location of marginal ridge on the neighbouring teeth, the occlusal morphology of the antagonist tooth are all taken as the guiding factors for carving.

**28. HOW IS THE WAX PATTERN FINISHED?**

**A:** In accessible aras, careful smoothening with a silk cloth is permitted. In inaccessible areas like a deep groove, cotton fibres wrapped around a toothpick may be used to smoothen them.

**29. WHAT IS SPRUE?**

**A:** Sprue is a pathway for wax elimination and molten alloy to enter the mould.

**30. WHAT IS A SPRUE FORMER?**

**A:** Sprue former is a device made of metal, plastic or wax to create a sprue.

**31. WHERE ARE METAL OR PLASTIC SPRUE FORMERS USED?**

**A:** For smaller restorations, a metal or plastic sprue former is used. For larger restorations, wax sprue formers are utilized.

**32. HOW IS A SPRUE FORMER SELECTED?**

**A:** The selection of sprue former depends on size of the pattern, length of the casting ring and type of casting machine used.

**33. HOW DOES THE SIZE OF THE RESTORATION DECIDE SPRUE FORMER SELECTION?**

**A:**
1. A smaller pattern needs a metal or plastic sprue former. Wax sprue former is used for larger pattern.
2. A larger diameter sprue former can distort a smaller pattern.

**33. HOW DOES THE TYPE OF CASTING MACHINE AFFECT THE DIAMETER OF THE SPRUE FORMER SELECTION?**

**A:** When pressure casting (steam pressure or air pressure casting) is done, the alloy is melted on the crucible of the mould. If the sprue former used is thick, the resultant larger pathway might permit flow of some molten metal into the mould even before steam or air pressure is applied. Such premature entry and solidification of molten alloy can result in blockage of the pathway and even casting failure. So thinner sprue formers are used for Solbrig (steam pressure) casting machine and air pressure casting machines. If centrifugal casting machine is used, a larger sprue former is used as the melting of alloy is not done on the crucible of the mould but on a separate crucible.

**35. HOW DOES THE LENGTH OF THE CASTING RING AFFECT THE SELECTION OF SPRUE FORMER?**

**A:** To avoid back pressure porosity, the bottom of the pattern should be just 1/4" (6 millimeter) from the base of the ring for gypsum bonded investments. For phosphate bonded investments, which are dense, the back up investment could be 1/8" (3 millimeter). Accordingly, the sprue former is selected to match the length of the casting ring, to position the pattern suitably.

**36. WHERE IS THE SPRUE FORMER ATTACHED?**

**A :** The sprue former is attached to the bulkiest portion of the wax pattern.

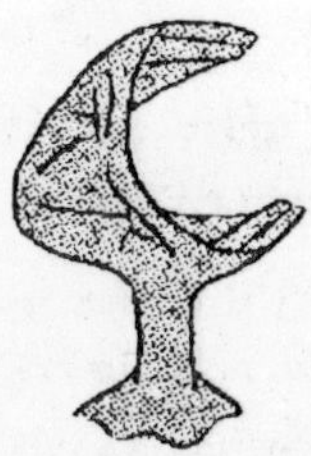

*Fig. 12.2. Sprue Former attachment*

**37. WHY IS THE SPRUE FORMER ATTACHED TO THE BULKIEST PORTION OF THE WAX PATTERN?**

**A:** If a heated metal sprue former is attracted to the bulkiest portion of the wax pattern, the extent of stress incorporation and resultant distorion could be minimal. If it is attached to a thinner area, possibility of distortion is higher. Moreover, thickest portion of the pattern will be the last to solidfy in the casting as more heat has to be lost from that area. The solidification shinkage of the molten alloy might be seen in the thickest portion and if further molten alloy is to flow from the reservoir to compensate for the shrinkage, the sprue former shoud be attached to the thickest portion of the pattern. If the sprue former is attached to a thinner portion of the pattern, that portion might solidify earlier and block compensatory flow of molten alloy from the reservoir through the sprue.

**38. WHY SHOULD THE SPRUE FORMER ATTACHMENT BE FLARED?**

**A:** The flaring of sprue former atachment area enhances the flow of high density alloys.

**39. WHAT SHOULD BE THE DIRECTION OF ATTACHMENT OF THE SPRUE FORMER?**

**A:** 1. The sprue former should not be attached perpendicular to any wall or floor to avoid creating a hot spot with resultant suckback porosity.

2. The sprue former should also not be directed towards any thin, delicate portion of the mould, lest it break at the impact of the molten alloy.

**40. WHAT SHOULD BE THE RELATIONSHIP OF THE SPRUE FORMER TO THE RING?**

**A:** If only a single sprue former is used, it should be placed in the centre of the ring, to permit even expansion of the investment mould.

**41. HOW MANY SPRUE FORMERS SHOULD BE USED?**

**A:** If it is a single inlay, a single sprue former is adequate. For a large M.O.D. inlay or a full crown, two sprue formers might be needed. If it is a multi unit bridge, more sprue formers might be needed.

**42. WHAT IS THE THICKNESS OF SPRUE FORMER FOR A CENTRIFUGAL CASTING TECHNIQUE?**

**A:** A 14 gauge wire can be used as a sprue former for a centrifugal casting technique. For pressure casting, a 19 gauge wire can be used.

**43. HOW IS THE METAL SPRUE FORMER ATTACHED TO THE WAX PATTERN?**

**A:** That end of the metal sprue former which will enter the wax pattern, is roughened to get a grip on the pattern. It is slightly warmed (but not heated too much) to penetrate the pattern by 1 to 2 millimeters. Inlay wax is added to the attachment area for flaring the area. The sprue former is attached at an angle to the pulpal floor. If it is a class II restoration, sprue former is attached at the isthumus, area of greatest bulk.

**44. WHAT IS A RESERVOIR?**

**A:** Reservoir is a storage area for molten alloy to permit flow of the liquid alloy into the mould through the sprue to compensate solidification shrinkage and prevent localised shrinkage porosity.

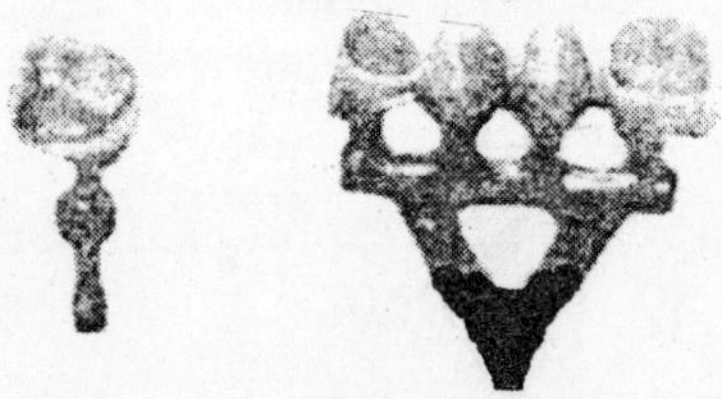

*Fig. 12.3. Reservoir*

**45. WHAT SHOULD BE THE SIZE OF THE RESERVOIR AND WHY?**

**A:** The reservoir should be thicker than the bulkiest portion of the pattern to permit the molten alloy in the reservoir to remain molten after the bulkiest portion of the pattern solidfies. If the reservoir is thinner, it may solidify earlier & no molten alloy will be available to enter the mould to compensate the solidification shrinkage.

**46. HOW IS A RESERVOIR CREATED IN THE MOULD?**

**A:** A piece of wax, thicker than the thickest portion of the pattern is attached to sprue former and this creates the reservoir in the mould.

**47. CAN THE RESERVOIR BE ATTACHED 3 OR 4 MILLIMETERS ABOVE THE PATTERN?**

**A:** If the reservoir is attached more than 1 or 2 millimeter the alloy in the intervening sprue between the reservoir and pattern may solidify earlier (because of the thin size) preventing flow from reservoir to the mould space.

**48. IS A RESERVOIR ALWAYS NECESSARY?**

**A:** A reservoir is superfluous if a thick sprue is used. Thicker wax sprues themselves will act as reservoirs.

**49. IF A THIN METAL SPRUE FORMER IS AVAILABLE, AND A THICKER SPRUE FORMER IS NEEDED, WHAT CAN BE DONE?**

**A:** After attaching the thin sprue former onto the pattern, wax can be coated around the metal sprue former to make it thicker.

**50. IN WHAT SIZES ARE CASTING RINGS AVAILABLE?**

**A:** Casting rings are available in different sizes to accomodate single inlay or crown, multiunit bridges or denture bases. Different cradles with varying concavities are available and appropriate cradle should be chosen for the selected ring to align the sprue hole with the flow hole in the crucible.

**51. WHAT SHOULD BE THE SIZE OF THE CASTING RING FOR A SMALL CASTING?**

**A:** It could be approximately 1½" long 1¼" diameter hollow cylinder.

**52. WHAT ARE THE TYPE OF 52 S CASTING RING?**

**A:** Casting rings could be made from metal or rubber. Rubber rings are intended to be used for investments that are used for getting maximum hygroscopic expansion. Metal casting rings are rigid and might not expand sufficiently to accomodate the expansion of investment. Split metal rings, however could move sufficiently to provide the required space for expansion.

**53. WHAT ARE CASTING RING LINERS?**

**A:** When a rigid metallic casting ring is selected for the casting procedure, expansion of the investment mould is difficult. To provide the required space for expansion, resilient casting ring liners are kept on the inner side of the ring. Asbestos liners were used earlier. As asbestos are considered to be carcinogenic, it is no longer used. Non asbestos materials like aluminium silicate ceramic material, cellulose paper or ceramic cellulose combination are used.

**54. HOW IS THE CASTING RING LINER ADAPTED ON THE RING?**

**A:** The width of the liner strip is cut so that it is 3.5 millimeter less on both ends of the casting ring. It is wetted with water and adapted on the inner aspect of the casting ring with no overlap and fixed with sticky wax.

**55. WHY IS THE CASTING RING LINER ADAPTED ON THE INSIDE OF THE CASTING RING 3.5 MILLIMETER SHORT ON BOTH ENDS OF THE RING?**

**A:** The provision of 3.5 millimeter space on both ends of the casting ring is to permit the investment to lock with ring and prevent slippage of the investment mould from the ring.

**56. WHAT ARE THE FUNCTIONS OF A CASTING RING LINER?**

A: 1. Ring liners provide space for the expansion of the mould

2. Liners provide water for hygroscopic expansion.

3. Casting ring liners retain the heat while the ring is transferred from the furnace to the casting machine and casting is done.

**57. IF MORE SPACE FOR EXPANSION IS NEEDED, WHAT CAN BE DONE?**

A: By increasing the number of liners, the extent can be increased.

**58. WHAT IS CRUCIBLE?**

A: In casting procedure, crucible is the portion where alloy is melted. It could be the top portion of the investment mould, if Solbrig steam pressure casting machine or air pressure casting machine is to be used. If centrifugal casting machine is used, separate melting crucibles are made use of.

**59. WHAT IS A CRUCIBLE FORMER?**

A: Crucible former is a device used to produce a funnel shaped depression (crucible) on the top of the investment mould.

**60. FROM WHAT MATERIALS IS A CRUCIBLE FORMER MADE?**

A: Crucible former can be made of metal, rubber (commercially available) or from wax (custom made).

**61. HOW IS A WAX CRUCIBLE FORMER MADE?**

A: A square piece of wax sheet is taken. About 1/8 of the sheet is cut off. The cut ends are brought together and luted to form a cone with an internal angle of $120^0$. The ring is postioned over the cone so that the tip of the cone is in the central axis of the ring. The excess wax is cut off, so that a cone of wax crucible former remains. This is how a wax crucible former is made.

## 62. WHAT IS A DEBUBBLISER?

**A:** To get an accurate metallic reproduction of the wax pattern, the mould created around the pattern should closely adapt to it. Investment is mixed with water or water based special liquids. Wax is water repellant. To ensure closer adaptation of the investment around the pattern, a debubbliser is applied to the wax pattern as a thin coating. As the debubbliser acts by lowering the surface tension of the wax, it is also called a surfactant or wetting agent. Commercial wax pattern cleaners are also available. Dilute synthetic detergent soap solution can also be applied.

## 63. HOW IS THE WETTING AGENT APPLIED?

**A:** Holding the sprued wax pattern on the left hand, the soap solution or the commercially available surfactant solution is applied with a camel hair brush as a thin layer around the pattern and the reservoir. Excess debubbliser solution is shaken off. The pattern is not washed in water before investing lest the surfactant effect is lost.

## 64. HOW IS THE CASTING RING ASSEMBLED?

**A:** The selected casting ring with the liner adapted on the inner surface, 3.5 millimeter short of the ends of the ring is kept

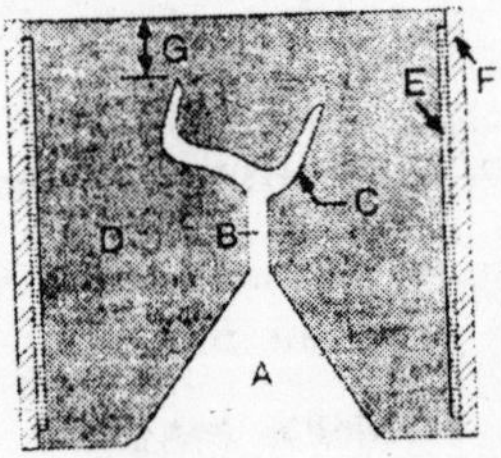


*A*, crucible former; *B*, sprue; *C*, cavity formed by wax pattern after burnout; *D*, investment; *E*, liner; *F*, casting ring; *G*, recommended maximum investment thickness of approximately 6 mm between the end of the mold cavity and the end of the invested ring, to provide pathways for sufficient gas escape during casting.

*Fig. 12.4. Assembled casting ring*

aside. The surfactant applied pattern with the sprue former and reservoir is attached to the tip of the crucible former with a piece of utility wax. The sprue former is so adjusted that when the casting ring is placed over the crucible former, the bottom of the pattern is 3 to 6 millimeters from the base of the ring, depending on the type of investment to be used. When placed inside the casting ring, the sprue former and pattern should be in the central axis. With the sprue former firmly attached to the crucible former, the casting ring is united with the crucible former by using wax along the edges of the ring. This assembly is for single investment technique.

**65. WHAT IS MEANT BY SINGLE INVESTMENT TECHNIQUE?**

**A :** During investing the pattern, the mixed investment could be poured into the assembled casting ring as a single pour with the ring kept over a vibrator. If vaccum investing is done the chances of air bubble incorporation is nil. When vaccum investing facility is not available, double investing technique should be done.

**66. WHAT IS MEANT BY DOUBLE INVESTING TECHNIQUE?**

**A:** In this technique, investing is done in two stages. After attaching the sprue former with reservoir and pattern to the crucible former and before luting the crucible former to the casting ring, wetting agent is applied over the pattern with a camel brush, excess is shaken dry. Investment is mixed to a creamy consistency and is applied over the pattern with a camel hair brush. Dry powder is sprinkled over the creamy investment to make it thick. The layers of investment around the pattern are built up by alternatingly applying creamy mix of investment and sprinkling dry powder. Such careful addition ensures avoiding air bubble entrapment around the pattern once a blob of investment completely covers the pattern and reservoir, the crucible former with the sprue former and the pattern are luted to the casting ring and the second pour of investment is made to fill the ring flush upto the base.

**67. HOW IS THE INVESTMENT MIXED?**

**A:** The manufacturer's instructions should be followed. About 50 grams of investment powder and 11 millilitre of water (or special liquid) is taken, in a clean bowl & mixed with a stiff plaster spatula manually or a mechanical spatulator is used for mixing.

**68. AFTER INVESTING, ATLEAST HOW MUCH TIME SHOULD LAPSE BEFORE HEATING THE RING FOR WAX ELIMINATION?**

A: After investing atleast 1 hour should lapse before the casting ring is kept in the furnace for wax elimination.

**69. WHAT SHOULD BE DONE BEFORE KEEPING THE CASTING RING IN THE FURNACE?**

A: 1. If a rubber ring was used for investing, it should be removed.

2. The crucible former should be removed.

3. If a metal sprue former was used, it should be removed.

**70. HOW SHOULD THE METAL SPRUE FORMER BE REMOVED FROM THE INVESTMENT MOULD?**

A: The investment mould is held upside down with the crucible surface facing down and the exposed metal sprue former tip is gently heated to soften the wax attached to it. Once the sprue former is warm, the tip is held with a nose plier and with the mould held upside down, the sprue former is gently teased out. The purpose of holding the investment mould upside down during sprue former removal is to prevent any small piece of broken investment, accidentally falling into the mould space to contaminate the casting, or block the sprue.

**71. HOW IS THE CASTING RING KEPT IN THE FURNACE?**

A: Initially the casting ring is kept in an upside down (crucible side down) position. This facilitates the gravitational flow of the molten wax to the floor of the furnace. If the casting ring is kept with crucible side up, the liquid wax might be absorbed into the mould walls and there might not be complete wax burn out and some carbon residue might block the pores in the investment. So, initially the investment mould is to be kept upside down. (Crucible side down) and after 200$^0$ C when all the molten wax has fallen out, the investment ring should be turned so that the crucible side is facing up. This is needed for good air circulation and burnout of wax in an oxidizing atmosphere.

**72. HOW SHOULD THE INVESTMENT MOULD BE HEATED?**

**A:** The investment mould kept in the furnace should be gradually heated to avoid crack formation in investment due to too rapid heating. Gradual heating is continued upto the casting temparature. The mould is kept inside the furnace till just before the casting is done.

**73. WHAT METHODS ARE AVAILABLE FOR MELTING ALLOYS?**

**A:** 1. Commercial gas and compressed air blow torch.

2. Commercial gas and oxygen blow torch
3. Oxygen acetylene blow torch
4. Electric resistance melting
5. Carbon arc melting
6. Induction melting

The first three types produce a flame which has to be shown over the alloy to be melted to liquify them. The last three types do not involve any flame.

**74. HOW SHOULD CONVENTIONAL GOLD ALLOYS BE MELTED?**

**A:** Conventional gold alloys could be melted by gas-air flame or electrical resistance melting.

**75. HOW SHOULD LOW GOLD OR NO GOLD ALLOYS BE MELTED?**

**A:** Low gold or no gold alloys, having a melting temperature around 1037°C need gas-oxygen flame or electrical resistance melting.

**76. HOW ARE NICKEL CHROMIUM ALLOYS AND CHROME COBALT ALLOYS MELTED?**

**A:** For high fusing base metal alloys, oxy-acetylene flame, carbon are melting or induction melting are used.

**77. WHAT ARE THE ADVANTAGES OF ELECTRICAL RESISTANCE MELTING?**

A: 1. Chances of contamination is less for low fusing alloys if electrical resistance melting is used

2. In electrical resistance melting, the temperature can be controlled and the alloy is not subjected to super heating

**78. WHAT ARE THE ADVANTAGES AND DISADVANTAGES OF INDUCTION MELTING METHOD?**

A: 1. Chances of contamination are less, if induction melting is done.

2. Induction melting is very fast and alloy is ready for casting in 40 seconds.

3. The melting environment can be protected by an inert gas like argon or vacuum so that contamination of gases at high temperature doesn't occur.

One disadvantage of induction casting is, it is unsuitable for low fusing alloys & other disadvantage is its cost.

**79. WHAT CAN HAPPEN IF AN ALLOY IS HEATED AT A MUCH HIGHER TEMPERATURE THAN ITS MELTING POINT?**

A: Excess heating might not affect noble metals like gold, precious metal like silver or base metal like copper. But metals like iron, zinc or indium might be lost during superheating.

**80. WHAT ARE THE CRUCIBLES AVAILABLE FOR CENTRIFUGAL CASTING MACHINES?**

A: 1. Clay crucibles are used for gold based and silver palladium alloys for crown and bridges.

2. Carbon crucibles are used for gold based crown & bridge alloys and gold based metal ceramic alloys

3. Quartz crucibles are used for any high fusing alloy.

**81. HOW IS A CENTRIFUGAL CASTING MACHINE DRIVEN?**

**A:** Centrifugal casting machine is driven by either a mechanical spring or an electrical motor. An electrical motor driven casting machine has quicker acceleration.

**81. HOW IS THE CENTRIFUGAL CASTING MACHINE PREPARED FOR THE CASTING?**

**A:** With the casting ring on the cradle and the melting crucible kept in portion, the counter weight on the balancing arm is adjusted and locked to ensure equal weight on both balancing arm and crucible arm. Such balancing enhances prolonged and even rotation of the arms without drag. The flow hole in the crucible and the sprue of the investment mould should be aligned. If the alignment is not proper, the cradle should be changed to get proper alignment. If the casting machine is spring activated, the balancing arm is given 2 to 5 turns in the clockwise direction and the locking pin applied. The hinged end of the crucible arm is conveniently turned for better access for the flame.

**83. WHY DOES THE CRUCIBLE ARM OF THE CASTING MACHINE HAS A HINGE TO PERMIT A QUARTER TURN OF THE PORTION HOLDING THE CRUCIBLE AND THE CASTING RING?**

**A:** 1. To provide better access for the blow torch flame

2. To provide greater initial acceleration.

**84. DESCRIBE THE BLOW TORCH FLAME?**

**A:** The gas-air or gas-oxygen should be properly proportioned.

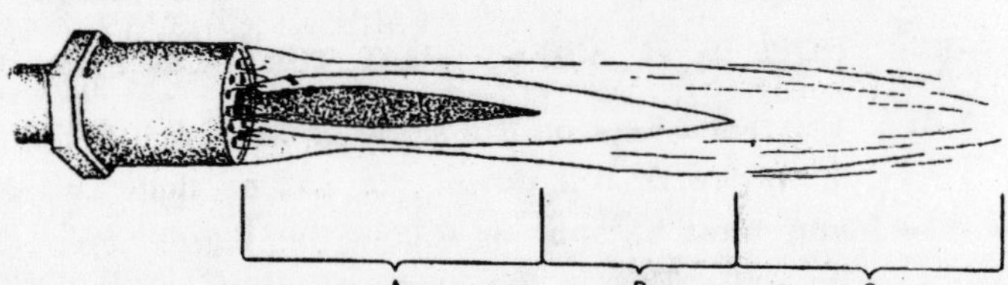


*A*, Air and gas combine in this zone. The junction of A and B is the combustion zone. *B*, This area represents the reducing zone and is most effective as it moves toward junction with C. C,Oxidizing zone.

*Fig. 12.5. Blow torch flame*

First the gas is lit at the torch tip and then air or oxygen is added to get a nonluminous brush flame wherein different combustion zones are seen. The innermost zone is dark and it is the mixing zone for gas and air. The next zone is green in colour where partial combustion has started and it is an oxidizing zone. The next zone is dim blue in colour and is the reducing zone. The outermost zone is the oxidising zone. The blue reducing zone which is just next to the green zone is the hottest, and that is the zone to be shown to the alloy to be melted.

**85. CLINICALLY, IS IT POSSIBLE TO KNOW WHETHER A REDUCING OR OXIDIZING ZONE IS IN CONTACT WITH THE ALLOY?**

**A:** The melting alloy surface is bright and mirror like if the reducing flame is in contact. The surface of the alloy is dull if the oxidizing zone is in contact.

**86. WHERE IS THE ALLOY KEPT IN THE CRUCIBLE?**

**A:** The alloy pellets are kept in the slope of the crucible and the reducing zone of the flame is shown on it.

**87. HOW IS OXIDATION OF MOLTEAN ALLOY PREVENTED?**

**A:**
1. By showing the reducing zone of a properly adjusted flame or using electrical resistance melting.
2. By using a carbon crucible
3. By adding a flux (usually fused borax powder and boric acid powder are added in equal parts).

**88. HOW IS IT KNOWN THAT THE ALLOY IS MELTED?**

**A:** The pellet kept on the slope of the crucible tend to become a sphere & roll down. It will be light orange in colour and tend to spin or follow the flame when the flame is moved. This is the stage of casting. Holding the flame over the molten alloy, the other hand of the operator gently turns the balancing arm in a clock-wise direction to let the locking pin drop down. Then simultaneously the balancing arm is left off and torch removed. The gas is first turned off and then air (or oxygen) closed. The rotating arms of the casting machine are permitted to come to rest of its own accord.

**89. WHAT IS DONE AFTER THE ARMS OF THE CASTING MACHINE STOP?**

**A:** The casting ring containing the investment mould is carefully removed with a locking tongs and when the button of alloy on the crucible becomes dull in colour, the investment is quenched in cold water.

**90. AFTER CASTING WHY IS THE INVSTMENT QUENCHED IN COLD WATER?**

**A:** 1. The sudden quenching of heated invstment violently disintegrate the mould making recovery of casting easy.

2. Quenching leaves the casting in an annealed condition, permitting further cold working.

**91. WHAT CARE SHOULD BE TAKEN WHILE RECOVRING THE CASTING?**

**A:** It is preferable to do the quenching in cold water kept in a vessel. If the quenching is done in a sink under tap water, there is a possibility of the casting falling into the drain. If quenching is done in a sink, it is advisable to cover the drain hole with a piece of cotton guaze.

**92. DESCRIBE THE SOLBRIG CASTING MACHINE?**

**A:** Solbrig casting machine consists of a flat rectangular metal base with a movable arm attached to one end. Suspended on the movable arm in the middle, is a lid like structure, approximately 4 inches in diameter. A mark is present in the base for positioning the casting ring.

93. **DESCRIBE STEAM PRESSURE CASTING PROCEDURE?**

**A:** The solbrig casting machine is kept on a flat work table. The movable arm is extended to the full extent to lie on the table top, with the hanging lid facing upwards. Into the hollow of the lid is fitted 4" circular asbestos sheet soaked in water. The casting ring, which is heated to the casting temperature, is removed from the furnace and positioned in the marked place on the base, with the crucible of the ring facing up. The alloy pellet is kept on the slope of the crucible and gas-air open flame (its reducing zone) is used to melt it. When the alloy is melt, the movable arm is brought up so that the lid lies over the ring and hand pressure applied. The wet asbestos seals the top of the ring. The heat from the ring converts the water in the asbestos into steam. Having no means of escape, the steam builds up pressure on the crucible, forcing the molten alloy into the mould. After two or three minutes, the movable arm is opened. When the button of excess alloy on the crucible becomes dull, the investment is quenched in cold water to recover the casting.

94. **WHEN THE ALLOY IS KEPT AND MELTED ON THE CRUCIBLE OF THE CASTING RING, WHY GRAVITATIONAL FLOW INTO THE SPRUE AND MOULD DOES NOT OCCUR?**

**A:** The thinner sprue and the higher viscosity of the molten alloy do not permit gravitational flow into the mould. Only when steam pressure builds up between the ring and the lid, does it force the molten alloy into the mould.

95. **HOW IS AIR PRESSURE CASTING DONE?**

**A:** Air pressure casting machine has a ring table on which the ring is positioned and a flexible piston through which air pressure could be applied. The ring table could be connected to a vacuum pump. The ring is kept on the table. The alloy pellet is melted on the crucible with the reducing zone of the an open flame. Once the alloy is melted the piston is brought down to snugly cover the ring, 10 to 15 PSI air pressure applied and vaccum started. After a minute the vaccum is released and air pressure shut off and piston removed. The ring is quenched and the casting recovered.

**96. WHAT IS PICKLING?**

**A:** Pickling is a prcedure done to remove the surface oxidation or other contamination form the casting. 50% hydrochloric acid or 50% sulfuric acid is taken into a porcelain or glass beaker, the casting dropped into it and warmed. Sufficient ventillation should be there. It is advisable not to inhale the acid fumes. Ultrasonic cleaners are also available for removing the clinging investment.

# CHAPTER - 13

# INTRODUCTION TO ENDODONTICS

**1. WHAT IS ENDODONTICS?**

**A :** Endodontics is that branch of dentistry that deals with diagonosis, treatment and prevention of pulpal and periapical diseases.

**2. WHAT ARE THE TREATMENTS RENDERED IN ENDODONTICS?**

**A:**
1. indirect pulp capping.
2. Direct pulp capping.
3. Pulpotomy and apexigenesis.
4. Pulpectomy or root canal treatment.
5. Periapical curettage.
6. Apicectomy and retrograde filling.
7. Replantation.
8. Transplanatation.
9. Radisection and hemisection.
10. Endodontic endosseous implants
11. Bleaching.
12. Perforation / resorption repair..
13. Apexification.
14. Management of traumatic injuries.
15. Post endodontic restorations.

**3. WHAT ARE THE AIMS OF ENDODONTICS?**

**A:**
1. Preservation of healthy pulp.
2. Curing a diseased pulp, if possible.

3. Removing the dead pulp, cleaning and shaping the canal space and filling it with inert materials.

4. To restore and maintain the function and appearance of a non vital tooth.

5. To cure a periapical disease, if present.

**4. WHY DOES A TOOTH BECOME NON-VITAL?**

**A:** Trauma & caries are the commonest causes for non vitality of a tooth. Attrition, abrasion, & iatrogenic causes can also make a tooth non vital. Erosion and resorption can also cause non vitality, though, rarely.

**5. WHAT ARE THE EFFECTS OF NON VITALITY?**

**A:** 1. A non vital tooth is discoloured. From a slight loss of the translucency, the tooth may appear from light brown to dark brown or down right black.

2. The non vital tooth is weaker than the natural tooth. This is mainly because of the loss of water content of the enamel & dentine.

3. The non vital tooth is a potential source of infection. The remnants of pulp tissue and the accumulation of tissue fluid can act as nutrients for bacterial growth. The infection may be confined to pulpal area or may spillover to the periapex. The infection may be dormant or active depending on the general health of the individual.

4. The infection if confined to the tooth, may cause systemic changes and spread to other areas of the body during periods of acute exacerbations (flare ups).

**6. WHAT ARE THE AIMS OF ROOT CANAL TREATMENT?**

**A:** The aims of root canal treatment are

1. Complete removal of damaged tissues within the root canal system

2. Properly cleaning and shaping the root canal system and

3. Filling the root canal system completely without any gap to prevent future stagnation of tissue fluid.

**7. HOW ARE THE CONTENTS OF ROOT CANAL REMOVED?**

**A:** If a fracture of the tooth has already exposed the pulp chamber, it is suitably enlarged to gain access into the root canal. If the non vital tooth is intact, an opening is made in the crown to reach into the pulp chamber.

**8. IN WHICH PART OF THE CROWN AN ACCESS CAVITY IS PREPARED?**

**A:** It can vary from tooth to tooth. Usually on the occlusal surface of a posterior tooth and lingual surface of an anterior tooth the access opening is made.

**9. WHY IS THE ACCESS OPENING MADE ON THE LINGUAL SURFACE OF AN ANTERIOR TOOTH?**

**A:**

1. For aesthetics the hole prepared is not visible from the front.
2. The lingual concavity of an anterior tooth permits easier reach into the pulp chamber.

**10. IS ANY OTHER SURFACE OF THE TOOTH USED FOR GAINING ACCESS?**

**A:** In an anterior tooth, if the labial surface is severely abraded and lingual surface is intact, the labial surface approach is easier and more sensible. In severely attrided tooth or teeth with half its crown structure lost to caries, an incisal approach may also be used.

**11. IS A PROXIMAL ACCESS CAVITY PREPARED IN ANY TOOTH IF PROXIMAL CARIES HAS INVOLVED THE PULP?**

**A:** Proximal access cavity is never prepared as it will not be possible to have straight line access to the root canal system.

**12. WHAT SHOULD BE THE APPEARANCE OF AN ACCESS CAVITY?**

**A:** The access cavity should be an occlusal continuation of the pulp chamber.

**13. WHAT FACTORS DECIDE THE SIZE, SHAPE & LOCATION OF THE ACCESS CAVITY?**

**A:** 1. The size and shape of the pulp chamber.

2. Curvature of the root canal.

3. The existing damage on the surface of the tooth (extent of caries, fracture, attrition or abrasion).

**14. WHAT ARE THE PRINCIPLES INVOLVED IN ACCESS CAVITY OPENING?**

**A:** 1. Direct line access.

2. Removal of the entire roof of pulp chamber.

3. Flaring the access opening.

4. Preservation of remaining tooth structure.

**15. WHAT IS MEANT BY DIRECT LINE ACCESS?**

**A:** It means instruments must reach the apex directly, without being deflected by coronal tooth structure. Sometimes, to get direct line access even half the cusp must be sacrified. Care should be taken in tilted teeth and teeth with severe root curvature to get good access.

**16. WHAT IS MEANT BY REMOVAL OF THE ENTIRE ROOF OF THE PULP CHAMBER?**

**A:** To reach into a large pulp chamber even a small hole in the pulp chamber roof may be adequate and it may be possible to reach even upto the apex. But during cleaning and shaping the canal, the remaining roof of the pulp chamber will prevent instrumentation and removal of tissues just below it. With limited removal of only a portion of the pulp chamber roof, thorough cleaning will not be possible. The entire roof of the pulp chamber should be removed so that the access cavity will truly be a coronal extension of the pulp chamber to facilitate easy cleaning. This prevents portions of debris remaining in pulp horn areas.

17. **WHAT IS MEANT BY FLARING THE ACCESS OPENING?**

**A:** Flaring of access opening is done to gain good access. In an anterior tooth, there might be a thickening of dentine called lingula which has to be removed to gain better access. The occlusal flaring of the access cavity also offers good resistance to the seating of the temparary filling given in the access cavity. It prevents sinking of the temporary restoration into the pulp chamber.

18. **WHAT IS MEANT BY PRESERVATION OF REMAINING TOOTH STRUCTURE?**

**A:** For gaining access into the pulp chamber, some destruction of healthy tooth structure is permitted. However, only the absolutely necessary removal of tooth tissue is permitted. Unnecessary weakening of the crown is to be avoided so that sufficient core of remaining tooth structure is available for post endodontic restoration.

19. **WHY IS THE INTERNAL ANATOMY OF A TOOTH TAUGHT IN TOOTH MORPHOLOGY?**

**A:** Knowledge of internal anatomy of teeth is absolutely essential for endodontic work. Though each root canal system can vary from one another, the common incidence in number and shape of root canals, the location of pulp chamber, the curvatures should be known for anticipating and identifying them.

10. **WILL THE PULP SIZE REMAIN THE SAME FOR A TOOTH THROUGHOUT THE LIFE OF A PERSON?**

**A:** Production of repairative dentine, calcifications in the pulp can alter the dimension of pulp and these changes are due to diseases of dentine and pulp. Even in normal healthy teeth, in aged individuals, the continuous deposition of physiological secondary dentine would have reduced the size and location of the pulp chamber.

21. **IF THE LOCATION OF THE PULP CHAMBER IS GOING TO VARY, HOW WILL THE DENTAL STUDENT KNOW WHERE TO MAKE THE ACCESS CAVITY?**

A: An undistorted pre operative radiograph will be of great use. It reveals the size and location of the pulpchamber. Radiographs can also give the curvature of roots, number, size and branching of root canals etc. The radiograph also gives an idea about the thickness of tooth structure to be removed before reaching the pulp. The bur in the hand piece is held over the radiograph to know approximately to what level the bur should penetrate for entering the pulp chamber.

**22. WHAT INSTRUMENTS ARE USED FOR MAKING THE ACCESS CAVITY?**

A: A high speed handpiece is used. A tapering fissure diamond can be used for entering through enamel and dentine into the pulp chamber. Once the point has dropped into the pulp chamber, a round bur could be used to define the cavity by drawing the bur from inside out.

If a slow speed instrument is used, a round bur is used initially and once the pulp chamber is reached, a fissure bur is used to define the access cavity.

**23. ON THE LINGUAL/PALATAL SURFACE OF THE ANTERIOR TOOTH, WHERE EXACTLY IS THE ACCESS CAVITY MADE?**

A: The access cavity is made on the lingual / palatal surface of an anterior tooth just coronal to the cingulam. The bur should be kept at an angle so as to reach the pulp chamber as evidenced in the radiograph. If the pulp chamber is not reached even after penetrating the tooth structure for the previously assessed depth, further cutting should immediately be stopped and a check radiograph be taken to diagnose any wrong angulation of the bur. Correction in angulation of the bur, if necessary is made & pulp entered into. After entering the pulpchamber, further penetration is avoided and in a smaller pulp chamber round bur is used along the walls of the pulp chamber to drag out the bur from inside out. For a larger pulp chamber, the lateral cutting of the fissure bur ensures removal of most of the roof of pulp chamber. Then the walls are smoothened and flared out.

**24. WHAT IS MARTIN'S ENDO BUR?**

**A:** It is a diamond point with a tapering head with a spherical tip. The round tip is used for initial penetration and the tapering portion is used for flaring the sides of the access cavity.

**25. CAN PERFORATION OCCUR WHILE MAKING AN ACCESS CAVITY?**

**A:** Yes. If the pulp chamber has retreated and the bur entering through lingual enamel, through the dentine can penetrate through labial enamel and perforate. Some times, not aware of having entered the thin pulp chamber the penetration might be injudiciously continued through the labial side to perforate.

**26. WHAT IS THE BEST WAY OF AVOIDING A PERFORATION?**

**A:** Assessing the location and size of pulp chamber in the preoperative radiograph correctly and assessing the required depth of penetration and not exceeding that depth. Taking a check radiograph with bur inside the preparation, midway, could also clear the doubt, if any.

**27. WHAT WILL BE THE SHAPE OF THE ACCESS CAVITY FOR AN ANTERIOR TOOTH?**

**A:** Triangular access cavity is made for upper central, lateral and molars. It could be triangular with a smaller base for lower anteriors too. For canines and premolar, it is oval. However it depends on the size and shape of the crown.

**28. HOW IS THE CORRECTNESS OF THE ACCESS CAVITY ASSESSED?**

A: By checking

1. Direct line access.
2. Absence of overcutting.

3. Absence of ledges.

4. Outward flaring of cavity.

5. Removal of entire roof of pulp chamber.

**29. WHAT IS THE NEXT STEP AFTER ACCESS CAVITY OPENING?**

**A :** Determination of working length of the tooth.

**30. WHAT IS MEANT BY WORKING LENGTH?**

**A:** Working length denotes to what extent the instruments are worked in the root canal. Usually the cleaning and shaping of the canals (called biomechanical preparation) is limited upto apical constriction which may be 0.5 to 2.5 millimeter from the apical foramen. This means that the working length will be always shorter than the actual length of the tooth.

**31. HOW IS THE WORKING LENGTH OF THE TOOTH DETERMINED?**

**A:** There are radiographic and non-radiographic methods available. But only one radiographic method will be described. From the pre operative radiograph, the length of the tooth image (distance between the the incisal edge and apical tip) is measured (Say 22m.m.) From this measurement, about 3 millimeter is reduce as a safety measure for possible elongation of image (22-3=19m.m.). The obtained value (19m.m) is transferred to a root canal file or reamer by adjusting the stopper so that the distance between the stopper and instrument tip is 19 millimeter. After access cavity is opened, the file with the stopper adjusted to 19 millimeter, is inserted into the root canal till the stopper is at the level of the incisal edge and a radiograph is taken. In this length determination radiograph, the relationship between the instrument tip and the apical constriction is checked. The instrument tip could be at the level of apical constriction, well short of the apical constriction, or gone beyond it. If the instrument tip is at the level of the apical constriction, then the working length is 19 millimeters since that is the length of the inserted instrument. If there is a deficiency or over extension, it is measured with a scale and added or substrated accordingly to calculate the working length.

**32. WHAT IS DONE AFTER LENGTH DETERMINATION?**

A: Biomechanical preparation is done for the root canal system to clean and shape the canals.

**33. WHAT INSTRUMENTS ARE USED FOR BIOMECHANICAL PREPARATION?**

A: Hand instruments, engine driven instruments or ultrasonic instruments may be used either singly or in conjunction.

**34. HOW IS BIOMECHANICAL PREPARATION DONE?**

A: Only one method of bio-mechanical preparation will be described. During biomechanical preparation, the side walls of the root canal are smoothened to remove the irregularities in dentine that has been penetrated by bacteria (commonly known as infected dentine). During biomechanical preparation, the canal walls are tapered smoothly with creation of an apical stop at the apical constriction. The files are used along the sides of the root canals in an up and down direction to smoothen the walls. Some rules are followed during biomechanical preparation.

**35. WHAT ARE THE RULES FOLLOWED DURING BIOMECHANICAL PREPARATION?**

A:

1. Instrumentation is done only in wet canals. Frequent irrigation with sodium hypochlorite, normal saline, EDTA, hydrogen peroxide or RC prep is necessary during instrumentation to remove the debris and for lubrication.
2. Standardized instruments are used sequentially. No skipping of instruments is permitted. Smaller canals are enlarged atleast upto size 40 and, larger canals atleast three sizes larger than the first instrument used.
3. A file is used only in an up and down stroke with an

amplitude of 0.5 to 1 millimeter and the emphasis is on the down stroke.

4. All instruments are fitted with a stopper to limit the instrumentation only upto the working length determined.

**36. HOW IS THE FIRST INSTRUMENT SELECTED FOR THE PARTICULAR ROOT CANAL?**

**A:** By looking at the width of the root canal an approximate size of file is chosen and tried in the canal. If the instrument goes beyond the calculated working length of the tooth, it is too small. If the instrument goes upto the working length, it is also small. If the instrument goes 1 or 2 millimeter short of the calculated working length, it will be the first instrument to be used in the root canal. Next three sizes of the instrument also should be used for enlarging the canal.

**37. HOW EXACTLY IS THE FILE USED IN THE CANAL?**

**A:** In a wet canal the file is inserted into the canal and when it is short of the working length by 0.5 or 1 millimeter, it is forced apically. The file manages to go because of the elasticity of dentine. The subsequent forcible removal of the file, manages to remove the dentine because of the cutting edges of the file. The procedure is repeated till the instrument is able to go to the determined working length. Then the next larger instrument is able to go to the determined working length. Then the next larger instrument is used with copious irrigation till the instrument is able to go to the determined working length.

**38. AFTER BIOMECHANICAL PREPARATION, WHAT IS DONE?**

**A:** After the root canal is thoroughly prepared, the canal is ready for filling (obturation).

**39. WHEN IS A ROOT CANAL READY FOR OBTURATION?**

**A:** 1. When biomecnanical preparation is complete.

2. When the canal is dry & free from discharge (in a clinical patient)

3. When there is no pain (in a clinical patient)
4. When the sinus (if present) has healed (in a clinical patient)
5. When the temporary access filling given in the previous appointment is intact (in a patient)
6. When there is no foul odour in the root canal (in a clinical patient)

**40. WHAT MATERIALS ARE USED FOR FILLING THE ROOT CANALS?**

**A:** Gutta percha with or without root canal sealant is the commonest root canal filling material. Other materials are silver points, paste materials of zinc oxide eugenol, Cavit, AH26, Diaket, silicone rubber etc.

**41. HOW ARE ROOT CANALS FILLED?**

**A:** There are plenty of obturation techniques like lateral condensation technique, vertical condensation technique chloropercha & Eucapercha techniques Endotec system Thermopact technique, single cone technique, reversed cone technique, rolled cone technique, obtura, ultrafil Thermofil technique, Successfil & Trifecta technique. Only one technique of obtuation will be described now.

**42. WHAT IS LATERAL CONDENSATION METHOD OF OBTUARATION?**

**A:** After biomechanical preparation is complete and the tooth is asymptomatic, the tooth is isolated. A master cone of standarized gutta percha point is chosen which has the same number as the last reamer/file used in the root canal. The master cone is inserted into the root canal to the full working length, and the good fit in the apical region checked. Instruments called spreaders are chosen that can reach upto 1 millimeter short of the apical stop. Root canal sealant pastes like zinc oxide eugenol is mixed to a creamy consistency and applied either with a lentulo spiral rotated clockwise or a reamer in anticlockwise direction upto the working length. Master cone is seated into position. The selected spreading instrument is inserted into the canal as for as possible by the side of the master cone and kept in position for atleast one minute. Then the spreader is withdrawn and a gutta percha cone of similar size is inserted to the canal as for as the spreader went. Then the spreader is firmly reinserted as far as it could go & the procedure repeated till the canal can take no further points. The ends of the points projecting out of the access cavity are cut off and a heated plastic instrument is used to soften the gutta percha & condensed with a cold condenser. Excess gutta percha is removed from the pulp chamber and an entrance filling is given.

**43. IS ENDODONITA THIS SIMPLE?**

**A:** Root canal treatment is not the only treatment given in endodontics though it forms a major part. It is erroneous to assume that endodontic treatment is so simple merely because root canal treatment procedure is explained in very few pages. Only a very brief description is given about the basic outline of treatment so that a II B.D.S. student can easily understand. In many preclinical training programmes, endodontic access cavity preparation in an upper incisor forms the last exercise and hence an introduction to endodontics form the last chapter of this book.

**"GOOD LUCK!"**